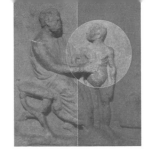

Pediatric Gastroenterology and Clinical Nutrition

Authors

Donald Bentley, MB, MSc, FRCP, FRCPCH
Hon. Clinical Senior Lecturer
Imperial College of Science Technology & Medicine
London
UK

Carlos Lifschitz, MD
Associate Professor
Baylor College of Medicine
Houston TX
USA

Margaret Lawson, MSc, Cert Ed, PhD, FBDA, SRD
Nestlé Senior Research Fellow
Childhood Nutrition Research Centre
Institute of Child Health
Honorary Research Dietitian
Great Ormond Street Children's Hospital
London
UK

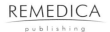

REMEDICA
p u b l i s h i n g

LONDON • CHICAGO

Acknowledgements

To my beloved wife Elaine and our children Russell Daniel, Melissa Sarah, Elliott Saul and Davina Shula for allowing me to irretrievably erode precious family time. To my mother Marie and father the late Reuben for faith and forebearance. Without the tireless support and IT skills of Elliott Bentley this book would not have been completed.

We have had much encouragement and advice throughout this book's protracted gestation. We wish to thank Alex Ashmore, pharmacist, Bridget Wardley and Rosemarie Jundt, dietitians, our colleagues Drs Alastair Baker, Martin Brueton, Anil Dhawan, Sonny Chong, Muftah Eltumi, John ME Fell, Nathan Hasson, Warren Hyer, Colin Michie, Nigel J Meadows, Ragai P Mitry, Michael A Thomson, Sue Packer and the librarians at The Royal Society of Medicine and The Royal Pharmaceutical Society, London. Also we would like to express our gratitude to our committed editors Alyson Colley, Charissa Deane and Helen James for their tireless endeavors. Finally we wish to acknowledge the act of faith and support received from Dr Andrew Ward and Arlene Seaton of Remedica Publishing.

Donald Bentley

I wish to dedicate this book to Leigh Emerson for her love, Robert Shulman, MD, and his family for their friendship and to Barbara Stoll, PhD, for teaching me to "enjoy what you get".

This work is a publication of the US Department of Agriculture, Agricultural Research Service (USDA/ARS) and the Children's Nutrition Research Center (Department of Pediatrics, Baylor College of Medicine, Houston, TX); it has been funded by the USDA/ARS under Cooperative Agreement No. 6250-51000. The contents of this publication do not necessarily reflect the views or policies of the US Department of Agriculture, nor does mention of trade names, commercial products, or organizations imply endorsement by the US Government.

Carlos Lifschitz

A knowledge of dietetics is practically one of the most helpful things in the field of medicine, because of the constant need for food, which is never ending, during health as well as during illness.

De Alimentorum Virtutibus
Maimonides (Rabbi Moses ben Maimon) 1135–1204

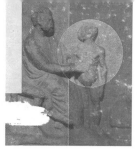

Pediatric Gastroenterology and Clinical Nutrition

Published by the REMEDICA Group

REMEDICA Publishing Ltd, 32–38 Osnaburgh Street, London, NW1 3ND, UK
REMEDICA Inc, Tri-State International Center, Building 25, Suite 150, Lincolnshire, IL 60069, USA

E-mail: books@remedica.com
www.remedica.com

Publisher: Andrew Ward
In-house editors: Alyson Colley, Charissa Deane, Helen James
Design: REGRAPHICA, London, UK

© 2002 REMEDICA Publishing Limited

ISBN 1 901346 43 9
British Library Cataloguing-in Publication Data
A catalogue record for this book is available from the British Library

Printed at Ajanta Offset & Packagings Limited, India.

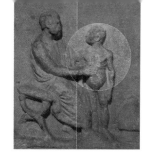

Contents

NON-ENTERIC DISORDERS

APPENDICES

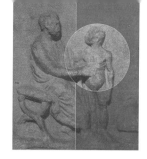

Foreword

This book provides in-depth coverage of major clinical nutrition problems in pediatrics, and underscores the importance of nutrition in the care of complex gastrointestinal problems. As such, it will be a valuable reference source for pediatricians, family practice physicians, nutritionists caring for children and pediatricians-in-training or students with a pediatric interest.

Unlike many textbooks of this magnitude dealing with clinical nutrition, this book is written entirely by three authors: Drs Donald Bentley and Carlos Lifschitz, seasoned Clinical Academicians with enormous personal experience in nutrition and gastroenterology, and Dr Margaret Lawson, a Nutritionist with both practical and theoretical experience in pediatric nutrition. In fact, it was my privilege to have contributed to Dr Bentley's formal training in pediatric gastroenterology and nutrition during his stay in Boston in the early seventies. This collaboration has meant that, instead of a collection of chapters written by multiple authors about their personal research interests, this book involves an important theme and has a continuity of approach that allows for ease of reading and access as a reference source.

The text itself comprises seventeen chapters and seven appendices. The first two chapters deal with nutrient requirements and delivery of parenteral and enteral nutrition; the remaining fifteen cover common clinical problems occurring during infancy and childhood. These include chapters on topics such as malnutrition, malabsorption, inflammatory bowel disease and hepatobiliary disease. Each is a practical approach to diagnosis and management of these conditions. Of particular importance are the appendices which provide an invaluable reference for normal growth and development and nutritional data for unique problems in pediatrics such as prematurity, as well as approaches to diseases, use of intravenous nutrients and further reference to manufacturers and their products.

All in all this textbook should be strongly considered by any physician or student physician dealing with infants and children for whom nutrition is considered to be an important part of their approach to practice. My congratulations to Drs Bentley, Lifschitz and Lawson on their enormous efforts to provide a practical textbook dealing with gastroenterology and nutrition in pediatrics.

Professor W Allan Walker
Conrad Taff Professor of Nutrition
Director, Division of Nutrition
Professor of Pediatrics
Harvard Medical School
Director, Mucosal Immunology Laboratory
Massachusetts General Hospital
Boston, MA
USA

chapter 1

Nutrients and Dietary Recommendations

Many international bodies publish recommendations for all or some essential nutrients. Variations between the recommended dietary allowances (RDAs) set by different countries or organizations can be attributed to several factors, but comparison between the assorted sets of recommendations is difficult because the age groupings used are not standardized. Reasons for the disparity in recommended intakes include the quality of the customary diet in a particular region and the bioavailability of nutrients therein, both of which will affect requirements. Protein quality is important. Breast milk and egg protein contain a balance of amino acids that closely approximates to human requirements. These proteins are efficiently utilized by the body and requirements are correspondingly low. Most recommendations assume a lower efficiency of use for a mixed diet. However, if the only proteins available are of a poor nutritional quality, requirements will be higher. The form in which folate and iron are present in the diet, and the proportions of trace elements such as zinc and copper, will affect the bioavailability, and therefore requirements, of proteins.

Environmental factors may need to be considered: the ambient temperature will marginally affect energy needs, and exposure to sunlight will alter vitamin D requirements.

Physical and social aspects of a community may also have an influence: the age at which children undergo the adolescent growth spurt, menarche commences or childbearing begins will each affect the requirements for all nutrients.

Levels of requirement can be set at the lowest intake that will prevent clinical signs of deficiency, the physiologic minimum, which will maintain normal metabolism and growth, or at an intake that will give maximum values in function tests and/or tissue saturation. The USA recommendations for vitamin C are appreciably higher than those set by most other regions, as tissue saturation was felt to be desirable.

Recommendations usually ensure that the requirements of the majority of the population are met. Countries such as the USA and UK include a large safety margin; other bodies, for example the FAO/WHO, have a smaller one, hence the requirements of some people may be above the recommendations. The FAO/WHO values can therefore be considered as minimum intakes for normal growth and development, while those of the UK and USA represent desirable intakes for the pediatric population.

It is important to remember that the recommendations are designed for groups, not individuals. A normal child may have a requirement that is considerably above or below the recommendations for his or her age or size.

Appendices I.1–I.7 give the recommendations for most of the known essential nutrients for the UK (DHSS, 1991) and the USA (National Academy of Sciences, 1989 and 1998). UK recommendations suggest a range of intakes or dietary reference values (DRVs) based on the distribution of requirements for each nutrient. The estimated average requirement (EAR) is the notional mean requirement of the age group. The reference nutrient intake (RNI) is set at two standard deviations above the EAR, and intakes at or above the RNI should be adequate for all but a small proportion (2.5%) of the age group. The lower reference nutrient intake (LRNI) is set at two standard deviations below the EAR. Intakes close to this level will meet the needs of a small proportion (2.5%) but will be inadequate for the majority of individuals within the age group. Data on the requirements for some nutrients are insufficiently precise as a basis on which to make recommendations: an 'estimated safe and adequate daily intake' has been issued in the USA – and 'safe intakes' in the UK – for the nutrients. In addition, an upper limit has been suggested for some nutrients because adverse effects can occur at levels not greatly in excess of the estimated requirements.

RECOMMENDATIONS FOR INFANT MILKS

Because the whole of an infant's nutritional requirements must be met by one food, standards for the composition of infant formulas have been suggested by several bodies. The recommendations of the American Academy of Pediatrics (1985) and the UK (EEC 1991/1996) are given in Appendices II.1–II.5. Recommendations refer to formulas used for healthy full-term infants. Recommendations for the composition of formulas used for preterm and low-birth-weight infants (ESPGAN 1991, Tsang 1993) are included in Appendix III.4. The sick infant may well have an amended requirement for some nutrients, and these variations are covered in the sections dealing with the specific disorder. The requirement for most nutrients will remain unaltered, and any special formulas must meet the total needs of the infant. The standards for normal formulas given here should provide a reference base for all feeds designed to be the sole source of nutrients.

MICRONUTRIENTS

VITAMINS

Vitamins are chemical compounds present in various animal and plant sources in minute quantities. Although vitamins are required in very small quantities, they cannot be synthesized *in vivo*; however, they play an essential role in metabolic processes and the overall maintenance of good nutrition (Table 1.1). Disorders of vitamins include deficiency, toxicity and biochemical dependency states.

Vitamin A

Substances with vitamin A activity comprise retinol (or a group of substances with similar biological activity) and provitamin A carotenoids derived from plant sources, which can be converted to retinol. The activity of the different types of carotenoids varies, but, in general, $6\,\mu g$ of carotene has the biological activity of $1\,\mu g$ of retinol (3.3 IU).

Name	Functions	Dietary sources
Vitamin A	Growth, development and normal differentiation of tissue; β-carotene is an antioxidant Deficiency causes xerophthalmia	Dark-green vegetables, yellow fruit Retinol – liver, fish oils, milk, eggs
Vitamin D	Calcium absorption – bone health Deficiency causes rickets	Oily fish and eggs; added to margarine in some countries
Vitamin E	Protects lipid membranes from oxidation; antioxidant	Vegetable oils, eggs, butter, wholegrain cereals
Vitamin K	Normal blood clotting	Dark-green vegetables, liver
Thiamin (vitamin B_1)	Carbohydrate metabolism Deficiency causes beriberi	Wholegrain cereals, yeast, liver, pulses, nuts, meat
Riboflavin (vitamin B_2)	Oxidation–reduction reactions	Milk, liver, yeast, eggs
Niacin	Part of coenzymes NAD and NADP Deficiency causes pellagra	Liver, meat, fish, yeast, peanuts, wholegrain cereals
Biotin	Involved in metabolism of fats, proteins and carbohydrates	Meat, fish, milk, eggs, wholegrain cereals
Pyridoxine (vitamin B_6)	Cofactor for enzymes involved in protein metabolism	Liver, wholegrain cereals, meat, fish, eggs, peanuts, bananas
Cobalamin (vitamin B_{12})	Works with folic acid in DNA synthesis and myelin formation Deficiency causes megaloblastic anemia	Liver, meat, fish, eggs, milk, milk products
Pantothenic acid	Part of coenzyme A, involved in energy release	Meat, fish, milk, eggs, wholegrain cereals, vegetables
Ascorbic acid (vitamin C)	Integrity of connective tissue; antioxidant Deficiency causes scurvy	Citrus fruit, berry fruits, green vegetables, potatoes
Folic acid (pteroylglutamic acid)	Synthesis of purines, pyrimidines and some amino acids Deficiency causes megaloblastic anemia	Liver, green vegetables, fruit, nuts, pulses, eggs

Table 1.1 Vitamins – sources and functions.

Clinical aspects

There has been renewed interest recently in both vitamin A and carotenoid activity, owing to the antioxidant properties of these substances. Low plasma levels of retinol (<0.7 mmol/l) have been associated with increased rates of infection, as well as raised morbidity and mortality from infectious diseases, in areas where vitamin A deficiency is common. There is evidence that improving vitamin A status in young children living in regions where deficiency is endemic reduces mortality by up to 23% [1,2]. The prevalence of low plasma retinol levels may be in excess of 30% in many developing countries; in the pediatric population in the USA and UK it is 4.5% and 12%, respectively [3].

In developed countries, low levels of vitamin A have been described in conditions where fat malabsorption is a feature, particularly cystic fibrosis [4]. Vitamin A deficiency has also been implicated in the pathogenesis of bronchopulmonary dysplasia [5].

As vitamin A is a fat-soluble vitamin that is poorly excreted and is stored in the liver, toxicity can occur if an excess is consumed or where excretion is compromised – for example, in chronic renal failure [6]. High plasma levels of vitamin A may be teratogenic: in the UK, frequent intake of high-retinol foods, such as liver, is contraindicated throughout pregnancy [7], although consumption of carotenoids appears to be quite safe.

Vitamin D

Vitamin D_3 (cholecalciferol) can be derived from the diet or formed by the irradiation of 7-dehydrocholesterol in the skin as a result of the action of ultraviolet light. Cholecalciferol acts as a hormone precursor and requires two hydroxylation stages – firstly in the liver and then in the kidney – before the active hormone 1,25-dihydroxycholecalciferol is formed (Fig. 1.1). Vitamin D mediates intestinal calcium absorption, bone calcium metabolism and muscle activity. It also has a fundamental and diverse role in controlling cellular proliferation and differentiation. Dietary intake is expressed in International Units or micrograms, and 1 μg of vitamin D equals 40 IU.

Clinical aspects

Deficiency of vitamin D in the growing child leads to rickets. Radiologic diagnosis of rickets is by identification of cupping and fraying of the distal ends of the radius and ulna, and an increased distance between the distal ends of the forearm bones and metacarpals (Fig. 1.2); in addition, the table and base of the skull show demineralization. Biochemical findings include an increased level of plasma alkaline phosphatase (from bone), a normal or reduced level of calcium and phosphate and a normal or increased serum parathyroid hormone level. Reactive secondary hyperparathyroidism can complicate interpretation of biochemical diagnostic data.

The etiology of vitamin D deficiency is multifactorial and may include poor exposure to ultraviolet light, an inadequate dietary intake of vitamin D or calcium or the presence in the diet of chelating agents for either vitamin D or calcium. Low plasma vitamin D levels caused by impaired intestinal absorption of vitamin D have been described in cystic fibrosis [8], celiac disease [9] and other conditions where fat malabsorption is a feature. Particular drugs, such as certain anticonvulsants, will increase the degradation of 25-hydroxycholecalciferol by inducing hepatic microsomal enzymes, and low plasma vitamin D levels have been described in epileptic children receiving such therapy [10]. Decreased activity of hydroxylating enzymes in the liver or kidney (e.g. in renal failure) and Fanconi's syndrome will also give rise to rickets.

Inadequate sunlight may [11] or may not be the entire explanation for vitamin D deficiency rickets in the general population: rickets was common in the 1940s in southern California [12] and more recently in India [13], and has also been described in Africa [14]. Rickets used to be seen commonly in infants consuming unmodified cow milk during the first year of life; most infant formulas are now fortified with vitamin D, and rickets has decreased in incidence.

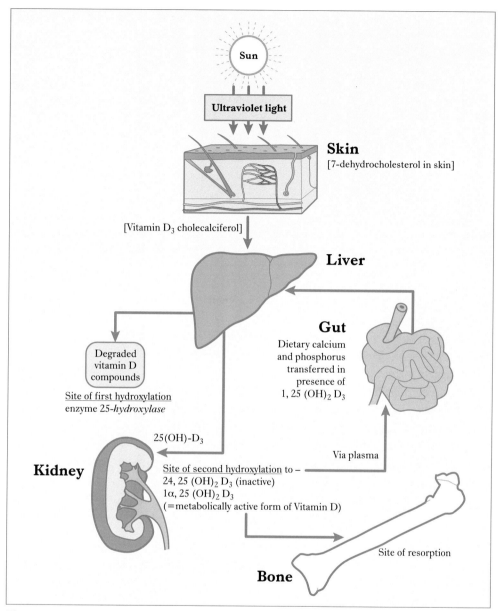

Figure 1.1 Vitamin D is derived from the diet and from the effect of ultraviolet light on the skin. It is hydroxylated in the liver to yield $25(OH)D_3$ and undergoes a second hydroxylation in the kidney to produce the biologically active form, $1\alpha,25(OH)_2D_3$ (1,25-dihydroxycholecalciferol). $1\alpha,25(OH)_2D_3$ acts on the gut and bone to increase gut absorption and bone resorption. $24,25(OH)_2D_3$ = 24,25-dihydroxycholecalciferol. (Courtesy of Professor P Byrne.)

Asian populations appear to have a greater tendency toward vitamin D deficiency than other ethnic groups. Rickets and low plasma vitamin levels have been described in Asian immigrants in the UK [15], other north European countries [16], the USA [17] and Australia [18]. Low plasma levels of 25-hydroxyvitamin D were found in a large survey of Asian 2-year-olds living in the UK [19]. Other dark-skinned immigrant groups (e.g. African

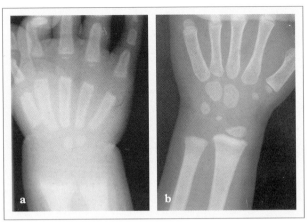

Figure 1.2 (a) Radiograph showing rickets. The lower ends of the radius and ulna are widened, cupped and indistinct – the 'frothing champagne glass' appearance. **(b)** Radiograph of a normal child aged 18 months for comparison. (Courtesy of Dr AMK Thomas.)

and Caribbean) in northern latitudes do not have such a risk of vitamin D deficiency, thus lack of skin exposure to ultraviolet light is clearly not the main issue. Genetic factors, lifestyle (such as less outdoor activity and covering the skin with clothing when outside) and dietary issues are all likely to be involved. It is important that all Asian children receive a daily supplement of 10 μg of vitamin D from the age of 6 months if they are breastfed, or from the time of ceasing fortified infant formula, up to the age of 5 years. Rickets and vitamin D deficiency have been described in adolescents of Asian extraction, particularly girls, and they should receive a vitamin D supplement if they cover their legs, head and arms while out of doors. Pregnant Asian women in the UK have low vitamin D levels [20]. Females with osteomalacia risk having infants with neonatal convulsions and rickets, and need adequate supplements of vitamin D throughout pregnancy and lactation. Typically, rickets is seen in breastfed premature babies and, in the UK, is especially prevalent in those born to Asian mothers. Rickets has also been described in the fetus [21].

Diagnosis
A plasma 25-hydroxycholecalciferol concentration of less than 25 nmol/l is indicative of deficiency.

Treatment
Adequate amounts of dietary calcium and phosphate should be ensured. Vitamin D therapy should be instituted at a level of 40 μg/day (1,600 IU) for mild rickets or 125 μg/day (5,000 IU) for advanced rickets. Once rickets is treated patients should receive 15 mg in a single dose or over 24 h, or, alternatively, 125–250 μg/day (5,000–10,000 IU) for 6–8 weeks.

Prophylaxis
A daily intake of 10 μg (400 IU) of vitamin D is sufficient in most cases. However, patients with cystic fibrosis should receive 10–20 μg/day (400–800 IU), and those with impaired renal function, liver failure or bowel malabsorption should receive 50–125 μg/day (2,000–5,000 IU).

Vitamin E (tocopherols)

Vitamin E is the name given to a group of structurally related tocopherols; α-tocopherol has the highest biological activity. One milligram of vitamin E is equal to 1.5 IU. Vitamin E is absorbed with lipids via the lymphatic system. The vitamin is not associated with a specific enzyme but has a major role as an intracellular antioxidant, maintaining the stability of membranes; it is a free-radical scavenger and also an intermediary in the metabolism of arachidonic acid, prostaglandins, nucleic acids, proteins and lipids. Vitamin E is found in high concentrations in the membranes of immune cells and deficiency may affect immune function. An adequate vitamin E status is thought to be protective against atherosclerosis, the effects of aging and some forms of cancers.

Clinical aspects

Low-birth-weight babies and those of less than 36 weeks gestation are particularly susceptible to vitamin E deficiency. Placental transfer of tocopherol is low, and preterm infants are born with reduced stores. In addition, such infants are more likely to be subject to oxidative stress, with increased lipid peroxidation, through oxygen therapy.

Oxidative stress, and thus vitamin E deficiency, is associated with hemolytic anemia [22], bronchopulmonary dysplasia and other lung diseases [23]. Vitamin E may protect against the development of retinopathy of prematurity [24]; in addition, in one study, the incidence of more severe stage 3 retinopathy was halved by supplementation with vitamin E [25]. The prevalence and severity of intraventricular hemorrhage are decreased in preterm infants who are supplemented with vitamin E [26]. Supplements of vitamin E are recommended for all high-risk infants, particularly those born preterm.

High intakes of polyunsaturated fatty acids (PUFAs) and iron increase vitamin E requirements. The American Academy of Pediatrics recommends that specialized formulas for low-birth-weight babies containing in excess of 1 mg of iron per 100 kcal (418 kJ) should have adequate amounts of both PUFAs and an absorbable form of vitamin E [27]. The addition of long-chain PUFAs to infant formulas is likely to increase requirements for vitamin E. The European Society of Paediatric Gastroenterology, Hepatology and Nutrition recommends that formulas contain 0.9 mg of vitamin E per gram of PUFAs and not less than 0.6 mg of vitamin E per 100 kcal (418 kJ) [28,29].

Secondary vitamin E deficiency may be seen in malabsorption from any cause, especially in steatorrhea due to pancreatic insufficiency [30]. Children with cystic fibrosis are recommended to take a supplement of 50–200 mg/day, as neurological signs associated with vitamin E deficiency have been noted [31]. Children with steatorrhea for other reasons (e.g. biliary atresia and inflammatory bowel disease) fail to absorb vitamin E [32,33] and should also receive a supplement.

Diagnosis

With vitamin E deficiency, erythrocytes are excessively fragile in the presence of hydrogen peroxide, and 30–100% of the red blood cells will hemolyze (normal 5–10%). The tocopherol:cholesterol ratio in blood is low (normal 0.9–5.9), and serum tocopherol – as measured by high-performance liquid chromatography (HPLC) – is less than 5 mg/l.

Treatment
Preterm infants with vitamin E deficiency should receive 75–100 mg daily in divided oral doses. In cases of malabsorption, water-miscible preparations (0.75–1.5 g) can be administered.

Prophylaxis
Preterm babies should receive 5–25 mg/kg daily; for term babies, the vitamin E:PUFA ratio should be 0.4 mg:1 g.

Vitamin K

Vitamin K is a fat-soluble methylnaphthoquinone derivative. The chief source of vitamin K_1 (phylloquinone) is from the diet – mainly green plants – whereas vitamin K_2 (menaquinone) is synthesized by gastrointestinal bacteria. The role of vitamin K_1 is the maintenance of normal levels of prothrombin (factor II) and the normal functioning of the vitamin K-dependent procoagulant proenzyme clotting factors VII, IX, and X. Three other vitamin K-dependent proteins, including osteocalcin, are found in bone, though their function is unclear. Vitamin K requires bile salts and pancreatic juice for its absorption from the small bowel, after which it is stored in the liver. In infants, bacteria are the main source of this vitamin, whereas in older children and adults most vitamin K is obtained from the diet. The estimated requirement for neonates is 0.5–1.0 µg/kg/day.

Clinical aspects
The fetus lacks the prothrombin precursor prothrombinogen. Furthermore, in the newborn infant, fat absorption is impaired, particularly if the baby is immature, and sterility of the intestinal tract prevents vitamin K synthesis (a theory disputed by Keenan et al. [34]).

Hemorrhagic disease of the neonate, a self-limiting disorder caused by deficiency of vitamin K-dependent coagulation, has a prevalence of 1 in 200–400 births [35]. It presents from days 1 to 5, but not within the first 24 h or beyond day 5 in a term baby. It is much more common in breastfed neonates than in those on formula, suggesting that breastfeeding is a predisposing factor. Late hemorrhagic disease occurs between 2 and 6 weeks after birth and is often due to malabsorption of vitamin K caused by hepatic or gastrointestinal problems. Prolonged administration of broad-spectrum antibiotics may also cause vitamin K deficiency. There is often excessive bleeding from the umbilical cord, bruising or increased bleeding after a neonatal screening blood test. Any infant who shows unexplained bleeding or bruising should be fully evaluated for vitamin K status as well as prothrombin and thromboplastin times.

Levels of vitamin K in breast milk are relatively low (15 µg/l); fortified infant formulas contain 25–55 µg/l.

Diagnosis
The prothrombin and partial thromboplastin times are prolonged and levels of factors II, VII, IX and X are low.

Treatment

The initial treatment is vitamin K$_1$ 1 mg intravenously. If the infant has not improved in 6 h, the treatment should be repeated and the prothrombin time checked.

Prophylaxis

A single intravenous or intramuscular dose of 1 mg of vitamin K$_1$ administered on the first day of life is known to be effective in preventing vitamin K deficiency. However, prophylactic injections of vitamin K have been alleged to be associated with a higher incidence of cancers and leukemias during childhood [36]. Other studies have disputed these findings [37], but an increased risk of lymphoblastic leukemia remains a possibility.

High-risk infants should nevertheless receive an intravenous or intramuscular dose soon after birth. Risk factors include a traumatic delivery, cesarean section, maternal drugs that interfere with vitamin K actions (anticonvulsants and antituberculous drugs), preterm delivery, low birth weight and the need for intensive care [38]. Particular attention should be given to infants who cannot absorb fat, as vitamin K will also be inadequately absorbed – in such cases, an intravenous dose should be administered. The American Academy of Pediatrics recommends a single intramuscular dose of 0.5–1.0 mg for all neonates [39].

Oral dosing with vitamin K is common [40,41]. There is no consensus regarding the size or timing of oral doses [42], although an appraisal of effectiveness has shown that three or four divided oral doses are no more effective than a single dose. However, repeated or daily administration does appear to offer an increased level of protection [43]. Regimens commonly in use for breastfed infants include 2 × 1-mg oral dose, 3 × 1-mg oral dose, and 1 mg orally at birth followed by 25 μg daily for 3 weeks [44]. Infants on formula milk should not require repeated oral doses because of the higher vitamin K content of fortified formulas, but should receive one dose soon after birth.

Vitamin B$_1$ (thiamine)

Thiamine pyrophosphate – the phosphorylated, active form of thiamine – plays a major role in the oxidative decarboxylation of α-ketoacids and in the transketolase reactions of the pentose phosphate pathway. Requirements for thiamine are related to the amount of carbohydrate in the diet. Deficiency of thiamine gives rise to two deficiency disorders: beriberi and Wernicke's encephalopathy.

Clinical aspects

Symptoms of thiamine deficiency are due to the essential role of thiamine triphosphate in brain and nerve function, and include peripheral neuropathy leading to infantile beriberi, cardiomegaly with heart failure and Wernicke's encephalopathy. Infantile beriberi has been reported in many developing countries; however, with improved nutritional education, the prevalence is declining. Most infants with beriberi have been breastfed by mothers who were themselves deficient, although low thiamine status has been described in infants fed on canned evaporated milk, as thiamine is destroyed by heat in the canning process [45]. The presence of subclinical thiamine deficiency has been postulated for children who consume large amounts of processed, high-carbohydrate foods that are low in thiamine, but studies have not confirmed this. Parenteral nutrition regimens that contain no fat are likely to precipitate deficiency if thiamine supplements are not used, and associated Wernicke's encephalopathy has been reported [46]. This is characterized by irritability, somnolence, ocular signs and, less frequently, confusion and ataxia.

Children who are malnourished for any reason are likely to become thiamine deficient, and Wernicke's encephalopathy has been described in children treated for malignancies [47,48]. A proportion of children with maple syrup urine disease show a partial response to large doses of thiamine or thiamine pyrophosphate [49].

Diagnosis
Findings include a reduced red cell thiamine pyrophosphate content (<150 nmol/l), as measured by HPLC, and a reduced urinary excretion of thiamine (<15 μg/24 h; normal = 40–100 μg/24 h). An activation coefficient greater than 1.25 for erythrocyte transketolase activity with and without added thiamine pyrophosphate (functional test of tissue saturation) is confirmatory.

Treatment
Beriberi will usually respond rapidly (within 24–72 h) to treatment, but motor weakness may last for 1–3 months. The treatment is oral thiamine (5 mg/day) until all symptoms resolve (up to 6 weeks). Seriously ill children should receive 10 mg of thiamine intravenously twice a day for 2–3 days, followed by oral supplementation as above.

Vitamin B$_2$ (riboflavin)
Riboflavin has an important biochemical role: it is incorporated into flavoproteins and many enzyme systems (e.g. flavin mononucleotide [FMN] and flavin adenine dinucleotide [FAD]) that are involved in oxidation–reduction reactions. Both FMN and FAD function as cofactors for several enzymes. Riboflavin is thought to be necessary for optimal iron absorption from the gut and for the conversion of folic acid to the active form. Anemia is often seen associated with riboflavin deficiency. Vitamin B$_2$ is destroyed by photodegradation; hence, solutions containing riboflavin should not be exposed to light for long periods.

Clinical aspects
Riboflavin deficiency is rarely seen in western countries, although low blood levels have been noted in children on macrobiotic diets [50]. The organic acidemia seen in children undergoing refeeding after severe malnutrition is thought to be due to deficiencies of B vitamins, including riboflavin [51], but has been described in preterm infants fed with expressed breast milk. The latter is probably due to bright-light exposure of the bottles of expressed milk during continuous infusion through an enteral tube, thus causing photodegradation of the riboflavin therein [52]. Preterm formulas are supplemented with riboflavin, but questions have been raised as to whether current supplementation – normally 150–200 μg per 100 kcal (418 kJ) – is excessive [45,53].

Diagnosis
A plasma riboflavin concentration of less than 10 μg/dl, as measured by HPLC, suggests deficiency. An activity coefficient greater than 1.2–1.3 for erythrocyte glutathione reductase activity, with and without added FAD, establishes the diagnosis.

Treatment

Infants aged 0–12 months should receive 0.5 mg of riboflavin twice a day; children aged 1–10 years, 1 mg three times a day. Although response to therapy is usually prompt (within 24 h), treatment should be continued for several weeks.

Niacin

Nicotinic acid and nicotinamide are both referred to as niacin (vitamin B_3). The amino acid tryptophan is a provitamin for nicotinic acid. The quantity of the potential vitamin in food is expressed in niacin equivalents: 60 mg of tryptophan is equivalent to 1 mg of niacin or one niacin equivalent. Conversion of tryptophan to nicotinamide requires vitamin B_6.

Nicotinamide is incorporated into nicotinamide adenine dinucleotide (NAD) and nicotinamide adenine dinucleotide phosphate (NADP), which are important coenzymes needed for oxidation–reduction reactions (including synthesis of high-energy phosphate compounds).

Niacin requirement is closely related to the total energy of the diet: a high energy intake necessitates a correspondingly increased source of niacin.

Clinical aspects

Dietary niacin deficiency gives rise to the disorder pellagra (meaning 'rough skin'), typically seen in communities that consume maize or millet as the staple food. Clinical features of pellagra, known as the three Ds, are: dermatitis, diarrhea and dementia.

Patients receiving isoniazid for tuberculosis therapy can acquire pellagra because the medication competes with pyridoxal phosphate; thus, transformation of tryptophan to niacin is impaired [54].

Subclinical niacin deficiency has been implicated in the etiology of insulin-dependent diabetes [55], and niacin has been used in the treatment of hypercholesterolemia in childhood [56]. In Hartnup's disease, a rare inherited metabolic disorder of the transport of amino acids (including tryptophan), a deficiency state can arise and large amounts of monoamino monocarboxylic acids are recovered in the urine [57].

Diagnosis

Urinary excretion of *N*-methylnicotinamide (NMN) is usually 4–6 mg/day: values less than 3 mg/day suggest niacin deficiency. In pellagra, urinary NMN excretion is 0.5–0.8 mg/day. In single urine samples, an NMN:creatinine ratio below 1.5 mmol:1 mol is indicative of niacin deficiency. The molar ratio of urinary NMN to 2-pyridone is a sensitive test of early deficiency: values below 1 indicate a deficit.

Treatment

This comprises oral nicotinamide, 50–100 mg/day, or parenteral therapy with 5 mg three to five times a day, for 5 days. Within 24 to 72 h, there is marked improvement, including a dramatic resolution of the mental symptoms.

Biotin

Biotin, a coenzyme, is a carrier of activated carbon dioxide and enables pyruvate to be carboxylated. Not only is pyruvate carboxylase important in gluconeogenesis, but it also plays a critical role in maintaining the level of the citrate cycle intermediates. Biotin-dependent enzymes are also important in fatty acid synthesis and branched-chain amino acid metabolism. Gastrointestinal bacteria produce biotin, although the bioavailability of this is not known.

Clinical aspects

Features of deficiency include non-pruritic dermatitis, fatigue, muscle pain, hypoesthesia and, later, nausea, anemia and hypercholesterolemia. The effects of biotin deficiency may be made worse by a coexisting pantothenic acid deficiency. Avidin, a specific protein in raw egg albumin, binds biotin and renders it unavailable. Diets that contain large quantities of raw eggs are likely to give rise to deficiency, although this has only been reported in adults.

There have been several case reports of biotin deficiency associated with total parenteral nutrition, particularly where there is altered bowel flora secondary to the use of antibiotics [58]. A specialized formula feed that was not supplemented caused symptoms of biotin deficiency in one reported infant [59]. Reduced plasma biotin concentrations have been observed in children undergoing long-term anticonvulsant therapy, particularly with carbamazepine and phenytoin [60].

Biotinidase deficiency, an autosomal recessive disorder of biotin metabolism, results in neurological and skin symptoms, and if untreated, will lead to death in severely affected infants. Symptoms are corrected with biotin supplementation [61]. Holocarboxylase synthetase deficiency is similarly an inborn error of biotin metabolism that requires long-term large doses of biotin [62]. Because biotin is involved in the carboxylation of pyruvate, some of the symptoms of pyruvate carboxylase deficiency will also respond to biotin supplements [63].

Diagnosis

The symptoms are relatively non-specific; laboratory investigations include whole blood levels of biotin (normal 0.22–0.75 μg/ml) and urinary biotin excretion (normal 6–50 μg/day).

Treatment

For biotinidase deficiency, the treatment is usually 10–20 mg of biotin daily, although some patients may require up to 100 mg/day for full remission of symptoms.

Vitamin B$_6$ (pyridoxine)

The metabolically active form of the vitamin is pyridoxal phosphate, which is involved in transamination and decarboxylation of amino acids to yield ketoacids and amines, respectively. Two other significant reactions that are pyridoxine dependent are the synthesis of niacin from tryptophan and the initial step of heme synthesis. Recently, there has been renewed interest in pyridoxine metabolism in adults, focusing on its action in lowering plasma homocysteine levels and thus potentially decreasing the risk of coronary heart disease.

Clinical aspects

Breast milk is thought to provide adequate pyridoxine for the growing infant until about 6 months of age, after which an intake from other foods needs to be established [64].

However, the adequacy of pyridoxine in the breast milk of some mothers has been questioned [65]. Breast milk substitutes are supplemented with pyridoxine, but there has been debate about the optimal level of supplementation [66]. Hyperactivity and convulsions have occurred in infants who were inadvertently fed an inaccurately prepared milk formula with a much-reduced pyridoxine content. Symptoms were aggravated by an increased protein intake, but the convulsions responded to 5 or 10 mg of pyridoxine.

A proportion of seizures in infancy and childhood are responsive to pyridoxine supplementation in large doses, and this therapy should be considered in all cases of early-onset intractable seizures [67,68].

Approximately 50% of children with homocystinuria – an inborn error of methionine metabolism due to cystathionine β-synthase deficiency – may respond wholly or partially to pyridoxine supplements [69]. There is a suggestion that pyridoxine therapy should be continued in patients who are unresponsive (in terms of plasma homocysteine levels) because of the decreased risk of vascular disease associated with pyridoxine and betaine therapy [70].

Several drugs, including isoniazid and penicillamine, compete with pyridoxal phosphate and can thus lead to niacin deficiency.

Diagnosis
In pyridoxine deficiency, the following tests are used:

- Plasma pyridoxine (normal >40 nmol/l)

- Plasma pyridoxal phosphate (normal >30 nmol/l)

- Urinary excretion of pyridoxine (normal >20 μg per gram of creatinine)

- Urinary excretion of 4-pyridoxic acid (normal >0.8 mg/day)

- Activation coefficient of erythrocyte aspartate transaminase (normal >1.7)

Treatment
For convulsive disorders, infants should be given a single intravenous dose of 10 mg of pyridoxine or 10 mg/day orally for 1–2 weeks. Large doses of pyridoxine may be toxic to man and the synthetic analog deoxypyridoxine is highly poisonous.

Vitamin B$_{12}$ (cobalamin)
Cobalamin consists of a porphyrin ring containing a central cobalt atom. The two main reactions catalyzed by vitamin B$_{12}$ are the conversion of methylmalonyl CoA to succinyl CoA and the methylation of homocysteine to methionine, which is important in purine and pyrimidine metabolism.

Clinical aspects
Megaloblastic anemia arising from vitamin B$_{12}$ deficiency is rare in very early childhood because, in normal circumstances, the fetus has built up a store sufficient to last for the first year of life. However, infants of vegan mothers may be born with low stores. Vegan diets appear to supply insufficient vitamin B$_{12}$ for the growing infant after about 6 months, particularly if the mother is breastfeeding and takes a vegan diet [71]. There has been a

report of prolonged exclusive breastfeeding by a vegan mother leading to depletion of vitamin B_{12} stores and causing methylmalonic aciduria in an infant with a mild enzyme deficiency [72]. Children on a vegan or macrobiotic diet have been shown to have very low vitamin B_{12} levels [73]. Furthermore, disordered cobalamin metabolism has been described in adolescents some years after the discontinuation of a macrobiotic diet [74]. Parents who wish their children to follow a diet that excludes milk and egg as well as other animal products should be advised to give the child at least one pint of a modified infant soya formula daily until the age of 2 years. It is important to recognize vitamin B_{12} deficiency early in children receiving diets that exclude all animal products, in order to avoid long-term neurological sequelae [75] and to optimize growth [76].

Megaloblastic anemia has been described after terminal small-bowel resection in children, due to decreased absorption from the remaining distal ileum [77], and can be secondary to other diseases of the small intestine such as celiac enteropathy, Crohn's disease and bacterial overgrowth in the blind-loop syndrome. Other causes of impaired absorption of vitamin B_{12} include the long-term use of medications such as neomycin and p-aminosalicylate. The fish tapeworm *Diphyllobothrium latum* competes for available B_{12} in the gut lumen and gives rise to a megaloblastic anemia. Pernicious anemia is a megaloblastic anemia caused by failure of the gastric parietal cells to secrete adequate and potent intrinsic factor, resulting in malabsorption of vitamin B_{12}.

There are several congenital defects of cobalamin absorption and metabolism, which result in a number of conditions [78]. Hereditary absence or defective synthesis of intrinsic factor or of the specific transport protein transcobalamin II causes megaloblastic anemia that will manifest by the age of 3 years. In the rare congenital autosomal recessive Imerslund–Gräsbeck syndrome, there is defective transmembrane intestinal transport of vitamin B_{12} with benign proteinuria [79]. Some forms of the inborn errors homocystinuria and methylmalonic aciduria are responsive to pharmacologic doses of vitamin B_{12} [80].

Diagnosis
The blood smear and bone marrow film show a macrocytic megaloblastic anemia. In vitamin B_{12} deficiency, the serum level is less than 100 pg/ml (<75 pmol/1); the presence of antibiotics in patients may influence the microbiological assays. Vitamin B_{12} absorption tests will show if uptake is defective.

The Schilling test is used for the differential diagnosis of megaloblastic anemias. The test involves giving radioactive ^{57}Co-vitamin B_{12} (0.5–2.0 μg) orally, followed 2 h later by an intramuscular injection of 1000 μg of non-radioactive vitamin B_{12}. The latter saturates the vitamin B_{12}-binding protein and allows the oral radioactive vitamin to be excreted in the urine. Normal subjects excrete 10–35% of the administered labeled dose, whereas those with severe vitamin B_{12} malabsorption excrete less than 3%. The Schilling test can also be used to measure the availability of intrinsic factor and the intestinal phase of absorption.

Treatment
This comprises 25–100 μg of vitamin B_{12} as the initial therapy (intramuscular injection), followed by monthly injections of 50–100 μg for life.

Pantothenic acid

Pantothenic acid forms a part of the active form of CoA and as such is involved in lipid and carbohydrate metabolism, particularly the synthesis of fatty acids and steroid hormones plus gluconeogenesis.

Clinical aspects

Pantothenic acid is widely present in foods, hence human deficiency is rare. A clear clinical deficiency syndrome in infants and young children has not been described. In adults, symptoms may include paresthesiae, with 'burning feet'. In extreme conditions such as famine – or experimentally, using a pantothenate-free diet with a pantothenic acid antagonist – an isolated deficiency state can be produced.

There has been one report of improvement in cardiomyopathy secondary to type II 3-methylglucaconic aciduria after large doses of pantothenic acid [81].

Diagnosis

This is based on pantothenic acid levels in the blood or urine. Normal adult blood levels are greater than 1.57 μmol/l; in normal children and adolescents, lower values of 1.17 μmol/l have been reported. There are no data available for infants and young children. Urinary excretion is between 1 and 15 mg/day, dependent on dietary intake.

Vitamin C (ascorbic acid)

Ascorbic acid is L-xylo-ascorbic acid, and the major component of the molecule is a xylose sugar ring. Vitamin C functions as a strong reducing agent; it is an antioxidant and acts as a cofactor in hydroxylation reactions. Major roles of vitamin C include involvement in the synthesis of collagen and carnitine and in the metabolism of catecholamines. Delayed wound healing caused by impaired collagen synthesis is a feature of vitamin C deficiency. Vitamin C may be protective against heart disease and certain types of cancers; its role in reducing the incidence and severity of infections remains controversial. An important function of vitamin C in infant nutrition is its place in reducing dietary non-heme iron so that it can be absorbed. Ascorbate is a scavenger of free radicals yet under certain conditions may act as a pro-oxidant to generate hydroxyl radicals.

Deficiency of this water-soluble vitamin results in scurvy. A vivid description of this condition was recorded by Jacques Cartier in 1536 when his men were exploring the Saint Lawrence River:

> *'Some did lose all their strength and could not stand on their feet
> …Others also had their skins spotted with spots of blood …. Their
> mouths became stinking, their gums so rotten that all the flesh did
> fall off, even to the roots of the teeth.'*

Historically, long sea voyages in the sixteenth and seventeeth centuries were associated with ascorbic acid deficiency because of poor nutrition. In 1753, James Lind (1716–1794), who had been a naval surgeon, published *A Treatise of the Scurvy* and demonstrated how fresh fruit or lemon juice could prevent the disease.

Clinical aspects

In vitamin C deficiency, hemorrhages beneath the long-bone periosteum, usually at the knees and ankles, cause painful and tender swellings. The child is irritable and lies still ('pseudoparalysis'), because slight movement causes pain, and the thighs are positioned in abduction in the 'pithed frog position'. The costochondral junctions are prominent, forming a rosary from subluxation of the sternum. This is dissimilar to the rosary in rickets, in which there is expansion of the rib ends. In addition, hemorrhages may appear in the skin; the gums become spongy and swollen, but are less affected than in adults. Radiographs show a characteristic dense line of calcification at the metaphysis. The bones have a 'ground-glass' appearance and the epiphyses have a pencil outline or a ringed white margin. In advanced scurvy, red cells are found in the urine.

Vitamin C is destroyed by both heat and oxidation. Cow milk contains little vitamin C, and pasteurization and boiling of milk reduce levels further. Infantile scurvy has appeared in infants fed exclusively on cow milk [82]. Preterm infants have high requirements for all antioxidant nutrients, including vitamin C, although there are some concerns about intravenous administration of the vitamin as it may cause hemolysis [83]. Vitamin C is the major antioxidant present on the surface of lung tissue. An adequate vitamin C status appears to be important in the etiology of asthma, where it is positively associated with lung function and negatively associated with asthma symptoms [84]. In one study, consumption of fresh fruit and vegetables appeared to have a beneficial effect on lung function in children who wheezed, although there was little correlation with plasma vitamin C levels [85]. In children with cystic fibrosis, plasma vitamin C levels were negatively associated with markers of inflammation [86].

Diagnosis

Plasma levels below 6–11 μmol/l indicate vitamin C deficiency in adults. Levels in excess of 34 μmol/l are considered normal in infants and young children. Leukocyte ascorbic acid levels more closely reflect the vitamin C content of tissues: values below 20 μmol per 10^8 white blood cells are thought to indicate deficiency in adults and children.

Treatment

Vitamin C, 25 mg, is given four times a day for 4–5 days, then twice a day until healing occurs. Rarely, excessive vitamin C can cause renal oxalate stones.

Prophylaxis

According to USA recommendations, vitamin C should be given at a level of 30 mg/day for infants and 40–50 mg/day for preschool children. UK guidelines specify 25 mg/day for infants and 25–30 mg/day for preschool children.

Folic acid (pteroylglutamic acid)

Folic acid is the parent compound of the structurally related folates. Folate compounds consist of a double pteridine aromatic ring attached to *p*-aminobenzoate and glutamate. Tetrahydrofolates, the active forms of folic acid, act as coenzymes and serve as donors of one-carbon units in the biosynthesis of a variety of compounds such as amino acids, purines and pyrimidines. Folates are also important as methyl donors in methylation reactions involving homocysteine and methionine.

Clinical aspects

There has been a good deal of interest and research into folate metabolism since the discovery that depletion of plasma levels – to even moderately low values – during early pregnancy can increase the risk of neural tube defects [87]. There is also evidence that the incidence of some types of heart defects (transposition of the great arteries, tetralogy of Fallot and truncus arteriosus) and other congenital anomalies, including hypertrophic pyloric stenosis and orofacial clefts, may be decreased by periconceptional folic acid supplements [88]. In adults, mild folate deficiency, which is associated with elevated plasma homocysteine levels, is thought to increase the risk of vascular disease [89]. The metabolism of folic acid, pyridoxine and vitamin B_{12} are closely interrelated, and it is often difficult to ascribe deficiency syndromes to just one of these micronutrients alone.

Deficiency of folic acid (folate) is the commonest cause of megaloblastic anemia in childhood. Body stores of folate at birth are small and can be rapidly depleted as a result of growth, especially in small prematures [90].

Unlike vitamin B_{12}, which is not easily destroyed, folate is removed by oxidative processes such as cooking; boiling of milk reduces folate activity by about 50%. The folate content of goat milk is low ($< 6\,\mu g/l$) and the vitamin occurs in a bound form that renders it unavailable. Infants fed on goat milk without a folate supplement develop a megaloblastic anemia [91]. Human milk and cow milk contain approximately $50\,\mu g/l$. However, many formulas used in the USA are highly fortified with folate ($160\,\mu g/l$).

Malabsorption of folate resulting from a reduction in the surface area of the small bowel and/or mucosal damage (e.g. celiac disease, tropical sprue or extensive resection of the small bowel) increases requirements for the vitamin. Some anticonvulsants (e.g. phenobarbitone and carbamazepine) cause folate deficiency by the induction of liver enzymes [92]; however, large doses of folic acid, if given, antagonize the anticonvulsant drugs and cause more seizures. Malignancy, because of rapidly growing tissues, will increase the need for folic acid. Folate analogs such as methotrexate, pyrimethamine and trimethoprim inhibit dihydrofolate reductase, an enzyme required for the conversion of dihydrofolate to the active form [93].

There are a number of rare inherited disorders of folate absorption, transport and metabolism, which require pharmacologic doses of folic acid [80].

Clinical features of deficiency include anemia, irritability, failure to thrive and, in advanced cases, hemorrhages secondary to thrombocytopenia.

Diagnosis

Megaloblasts are present both in the bone marrow and in the buffy coat of centrifuged peripheral blood. A reduced red cell folate content (normal 160–640 ng/ml) is a better measure of the deficiency disorder than a low plasma folate level (normal 6–21 ng/ml).

Treatment

The therapeutic dosage for an established diagnosis is 0.5–1.0 mg of folic acid daily for 3 months. The maintenance dose is 0.1 mg/day.

MINERALS AND TRACE ELEMENTS

Many elements have a known or suspected role in nutrition, either as minerals or trace elements (Table 1.2).

Iron

Iron element has a number of vital functions in the body. Heme, an iron compound of protoporphyrin, constitutes the protein-free part of the hemoglobin molecule in erythrocytes and is responsible for its oxygen-carrying properties. Myoglobin, which is built like hemoglobin, acts as an oxygen store in muscle. Iron plays a pivotal role in the transport of electrons within the cell and, because of heme groups, also functions as part of several enzymes, including cytochromes. Iron is not only central to the transfer and release of energy in the body but is also involved in the metabolism of neurotransmitters, steroid hormones and in bile synthesis. Iron-containing enzymes are important in the detoxification of foreign substances in the liver.

Heme iron, from meats and fish, is relatively well absorbed from the gastrointestinal tract (25%); non-heme iron, from cereal and vegetable sources, is poorly absorbed (5–10%). Enhancers of non-heme iron absorption include meat and ascorbic acid; inhibitors include tea, soya and dietary fiber. Iron absorption is dependent on iron status: low iron stores or elevated erythropoiesis will increase the percentage of iron absorbed from the diet.

Phytates are salts of inositol hexaphosphates and in western diets 90% of the phytate content originates from cereals. Phytates strongly inhibit iron absorption, but sufficient ascorbic acid will counteract this inhibition.

Clinical aspects

Iron deficiency is one of the commonest global nutritional deficiency disorders. In infants and children, iron deficiency is generally defined as a hemoglobin value of less than 110 g/l [94] and a hematocrit of less than 33%. The major cause of deficiency is an insufficient dietary intake or a low bioavailability of dietary iron, but other factors such as blood loss through parasites (particularly hookworm) and malaria causing hemolysis are important in some environments. *Helicobacter pylori* infection may also result in gastrointestinal blood loss [95]. Iron interacts with a number of other nutrients. Vitamin A deficiency, for example, may contribute to the development of anemia [96]. Vitamin D deficiency has been shown to coexist with iron deficiency, although the cause of this relationship is not clear [97].

It is estimated that globally about 30% of the population suffer from anemia (but not all of these cases can be attributed to iron deficiency). The prevalence of anemia is considerably higher in less developed countries, and young children and adolescents are particularly vulnerable. It is estimated that over 50% of children under 5 years of age are anemic in less developed countries compared with about 10% in developed regions [98]. In the USA, the prevalence of iron deficiency is estimated at 9% for toddlers aged 1–2 years [99]. A national survey of British preschool children found that 12% of those aged 18–30 months had a hemoglobin value below 110 g/l (hematocrit <33%), though the prevalence decreased to 6% in children aged 30–54 months [100].

Name	Functions	Dietary sources
Iron	Hemoglobin and myoglobin; part of some enzyme systems	Liver and red meats, wholegrain cereals, fortified breakfast cereals, pulses (poorly absorbed from egg and dark-green vegetables)
Zinc	Part of >200 enzymes; involved in most areas of metabolism	Shellfish, meat, wholegrain cereals, nuts
Copper	Part of several enzymes – energy transfer and collagen synthesis	Green vegetables, fish and shellfish, liver, pulses, nuts
Selenium	Part of several enzymes – thyroid function; antioxidant	Wholegrain cereals, liver, meat, fish
Iodine	Part of thyroid hormones – metabolism and integrity of connective tissue	Fish and shellfish, meat, eggs, milk, vegetables
Chromium	Potentiates insulin action; involved in cholesterol metabolism	Yeast, beer, egg yolk, wholegrain cereals
Manganese	Part of several enzymes – glycolysis, polysaccharide synthesis	Tea, pulses, nuts, wholegrain cereals
Molybdenum	Part of several enzymes – uric acid metabolism, iron metabolism and sulfur metabolism	Wholegrain cereals, pulses, vegetables

Table 1.2 Trace elements – sources and functions.

The term infant has a store of iron that will last until the birth weight has approximately doubled. There is controversy as to whether infants actually require dietary iron intake before this time [101]. Starter formula infant milks in the UK are fortified with iron (approximately 0.5–0.6 mg/100 ml); elsewhere in Europe and in the USA, some starter formulas are not fortified (all standard iron fortified infant formulas in the USA contain 1.2–1.3 mg iron per 100 ml). When the birth weight has doubled or after the age of 6 months, breast milk contains insufficient iron to maintain adequate stores and additional sources must be obtained from weaning foods. However, infants fed on a formula fortified with iron, receive sufficient amounts and have less need of additional quantities from foods [102]. Introduction of cow milk (which is very low in iron) before the age of 1 year and the consumption of large volumes (>800 ml daily) of such are both risk factors for the early development of iron deficiency [103]. There is some evidence that unmodified cow milk causes gastrointestinal blood loss in infants, but this remains controversial [104]. The provision of iron-fortified drinks and cereals for low-income families in the USA has resulted in a decrease in the prevalence of iron deficiency [105].

Preterm infants are born with low body stores of hemoglobin. They have high requirements due to their rapid growth rate and require supplemental iron throughout the first year of life. The American Academy of Pediatrics and the European Society of Paediatric Gastroenterology and Nutrition recommend that preterm infants receive 2 mg/kg of iron daily from 8 weeks post delivery until 1 year of age [106,107].

Iron deficiency in infancy and early childhood is associated with developmental delay. The degree to which this is reversible by appropriate iron therapy is still unclear, but most studies have reported a favorable outcome [108]. Iron supplementation needs to be continued for sufficiently long to ensure that repletion of body stores has taken place, and at least 6 months therapy is recommended.

The adolescent growth spurt and menarche in girls increase iron requirements in the teenage years. This, coupled with a tendency to embark on slimming diets or to move away from family eating patterns, means that there is an increase in the prevalence of iron deficiency in adolescents. A Swedish study found that 40% of teenage girls had low levels of serum ferritin (a specific transport protein of iron), indicative of deficiency [109]. In a study in the USA, 9–11% of teenage girls and 1% of teenage boys were iron deficient [99].

Vegetarian diets should provide sufficient iron, although it is important that vitamin C is consumed with all non-heme iron sources. Studies have shown that the iron status of children on vegetarian diets – particularly vegan diets and others free of animal protein – is poorer than that in children consuming meat [76,110].

Immigrant populations are particularly at risk of developing iron deficiency. The children of immigrants to England, to other parts of Europe and to the USA have all been shown to have higher rates of anemia than the indigenous population [111–113]. The causes of this may lie in dietary or lifestyle patterns and/or have a genetic component.

Because of the high prevalence of iron deficiency and the prohibitive financial implications of individual supplementation, a large number of iron-fortification programs have evolved. Fortification programs must take into account the likelihood of iron overload in the population, as well as social and cultural issues. Fortification of common foodstuffs, for example cereal foods, has resulted in a reduction of the prevalence of anemia in many areas [114].

The thalassemia syndromes are a common cause of iron-overloading anemia, particularly in populations currently, or previously, living in areas with endemic malaria. Defective or inefficient erythropoiesis leads to anemia and increased iron absorption, which results in iron overload in later childhood. It is important to distinguish between hemoglobinopathies causing changes in red blood cells and those secondary to dietary iron deficiency. A number of other inherited disorders can also cause iron overload. In hemochromatosis, the absorption of dietary iron is increased, and, although this normally presents in adult life, it can be detected in symptom-free children. Other forms of iron overload appear earlier in infancy and childhood, and these conditions are often fatal [115].

Diagnosis
Parameters of iron status change during the first 6 months of life. Hemoglobin concentration falls by about 30% after birth to 110 g/l at 8 weeks, rising to 125 g/l at 4 months. Four stages or conditions of iron status have been described [116]:

- Iron sufficiency, where iron stores and erythropoiesis are normal

- Iron depletion, where erythropoiesis is normal but iron stores are reduced, with low ferritin levels

Indicator	Diminished iron stores	Low levels of iron transport	Iron-deficiency erythropoiesis	Iron-deficiency anemia
Serum ferritin	Low <7 mg/l	Low <7 mg/l	Low <7 mg/l	Low <7 mg/l
Transferrin receptors	Normal 3–7 mg/l or high >8.5 mg/l	High >8.5 mg/l	High >12 mg/l	High >12 mg/l
Serum iron	Normal 5–25 nmol/l	Low <5 nmol/l	Low <5 nmol/l	Low <5 nmol/l
Transferrin saturation	Normal 10–47%	Low <10%	Low <10%	Low <10%
Total iron-binding capacity	Normal 5–90 mmol/l	High >90 mmol/l	High >90 mmol/l	High >90 mmol/l
Hemoglobin	Normal 120–140 g/l	Normal 120–140 g/l	Normal/low 100–115 g/l	Low <110 g/l
Erythrocyte protoporphyrin	Normal 70 μg/100 ml RBC	Normal 70 μg/100 ml RBC	High >70 μg/100 ml RBC	High >80 μg/100 ml RBC
Mean cell volume	Normal 75–85 fl	Normal 75–85 fl	Low <70 fl	Low <70 fl
Red cell distribution width	Normal 11–16%	Normal 11–16%	High >16%	High >16%
Mean cell hemoglobin	Normal 23–31 pg	Normal 23–31 pg	Low <23 pg	Low <23 pg
Hypochromic cells	Normal 0.3–2.5%	Normal 0.3–2.5%	High >2.5%	High >2.5%

Table 1.3 Parameters of iron status. RBC=red blood cell.

- Iron-deficiency erythropoiesis, where some aspects of erythropoiesis are abnormal but hemoglobin levels may be within normal limits
- Iron-deficiency anemia

The progression of iron depletion is illustrated in Table 1.3. A number of indicators of iron status can be used. It is important that hemoglobin values are not used as the sole criterion for diagnosis, since anemia may be due to causes other than dietary iron deficiency [117].

Treatment

Medicinal iron, usually as a liquid preparation, is recommended for the treatment of iron deficiency. Ferrous iron is more readily absorbed than the ferric form, and ferrous sulfate is inexpensive and effective. Infants and children normally show a rapid response to iron, 4–6 mg/kg/day, during the early weeks of treatment. It is important to continue the dose of iron supplement for at least 3 months after the hemoglobin values have returned to normal, in order to ensure that body stores of iron are replenished. Temporary dental staining may appear. If iron deficiency recurs following treatment, occult blood loss must be considered.

Zinc

Zinc is a constituent of over 200 metalloenzymes and has diverse biological roles, including the structure of specific enzymes and the stabilization of membranes. It is involved in a large number of metabolic pathways and affects carbohydrate, lipid and protein metabolism and nucleic acid synthesis, repair and degradation. This metal is a cofactor for the superoxide dismutases and is important for the removal of free radicals. It is necessary for normal brain development, as well as cognitive function, immune defense systems, adequate weight gain in early infancy and longitudinal growth in childhood. The effects of zinc on growth are thought to be mediated through changes in insulin growth factor (IGF)-1. Zinc absorption is decreased by non-heme iron, and zinc supplements should be considered if supplemental iron is to be taken. Excessive intake of zinc can cause copper deficiency by competing for absorption sites.

Clinical aspects

Zinc, which is present in all the tissues and fluids of the body, is the element that is most likely to be deficient in childhood since it is needed in relatively large quantities compared with the other trace elements. Breast milk normally contains adequate zinc for the first 5 months of life; after this, additional zinc needs to be supplied from other foods in order to achieve optimal growth rates. There are a number of reports of term breastfed infants who developed deficiency because of low zinc concentrations in the breast milk [118,119]. Preterm infants have a high requirement for zinc and have been shown to develop deficiency if fed exclusively on breast milk [120,121].

Features of deficiency may include circumoral and acral (involving the extremities) dermatitis, diarrhea, alopecia, neuropsychiatric symptoms, failure to thrive, immune impairment and delayed sexual maturation.

In developing countries, the use of zinc supplements has been associated with a significant decrease of up to 25% in the prevalence of diarrhea and a 41% reduction in the incidence of childhood pneumonia [122]. Although there are some disadvantages, it would appear that zinc should be considered a routine part of any diarrheal control program in developing nations [123]. Zinc supplements may also have a role to play in the management of diarrheal disease in western society.

Inadequate zinc intake has been described in anorexia nervosa [124], and zinc supplementation can increase the rate of weight gain in such cases [125].

Increased zinc requirements during periods of rapid growth such as infancy and puberty may be a factor in some conditions in childhood in which deficiency is a feature. Low plasma zinc levels have been described in Down syndrome, and zinc supplementation has been shown to improve levels of thymulin (a zinc-dependent hormone) and apparently to decrease infection rates in children with this condition [126]. Increased turnover of zinc is thought to account for the low levels seen in celiac disease [127].

Increased losses of zinc from the urine (normal 0.5 mg/day), feces (normal 0.5–3 mg/day) and skin (normal 0.5 mg/day) are a further cause of depletion. Young infants diagnosed with cystic fibrosis showed low zinc levels, which were corrected when appropriate therapy was started [128]. Low plasma zinc values have been associated with short stature in thalassemia major [129]; desferrioxamine causes increased stool and urinary losses of zinc and other trace elements [130]. Adult patients treated with cisplatin have shown increased urinary losses of zinc and low plasma levels [131], and children with nephrotic syndrome have high urinary losses, leading to decreased plasma values [132]. Zinc deficiency has been described in Crohn's disease [133], celiac disease [134] and other chronic diarrheal states.

Acrodermatitis enteropathica is an inborn error of zinc absorption that results in severe deficiency, with skin lesions, diarrhea and neurological dysfunction [135]. Treatment with large oral doses of zinc (25–150 mg) improves this dermatological condition. However, excessive intakes of this metal can impede the absorption and utilization of other trace elements.

Diagnosis
There is no universally agreed functional test for zinc deficiency. Plasma and serum zinc levels are useful in determining frank deficiency but are not sensitive indicators of status. Normal values for children aged 0–5 years exceed 10.7 μmol/l; children aged 6–14 years appear to have higher levels (>11.6 μmol/l). Leukocyte zinc levels are thought to be a truer reflection of tissue values but there are no reference ranges for children.

Treatment
Infants should receive 1 mg/kg/day; children aged 1–10 years, 5 mg/day; and children aged over 10 years, 10 mg/day; all for 3 months.

For the treatment of diarrhea, doses of 20 mg/day have been used successfully in children with zinc deficiency.

Copper
This metal is widely distributed in the body and has a key role in many metalloenzymes. It is a constituent of most oxidase enzymes – including cytochrome oxidase and lysyl oxidase, which are necessary for proper cross-linking in collagen and elastin – and is involved in cholesterol, lipid and carbohydrate metabolism. Adequate copper status is necessary for the release of iron from stores, the incorporation of iron into plasma transferrin and the normal functioning of the immune system.

Clinical aspects
The most consistent features of deficiency are associated with both the hematopoietic and skeletal systems. These include microcytic hypochromic anemia which is unresponsive to iron, neutropenia and osteoporosis.

Term infants are not at risk of copper deficiency because they have stores that are adequate for approximately 5–6 months. After this age, a supplementary source from weaning foods is necessary to meet requirements. Unmodified cow milk is a poor source of dietary copper and has less than half the content of human milk. Infants fed on cow milk, or older children who consume large quantities of milk to the detriment of other foods, are likely to suffer from copper deficiency [136]. Copper accumulates in the fetus during the last trimester of pregnancy and infants born preterm have low liver stores which will last approximately 2 months. Plasma copper levels remain depressed for several months after preterm birth, unlike in term infants, where levels rise postnatally [137]. Low levels are likely to be the result of impaired ceruloplasmin synthesis.

Children exhibiting catch-up growth after malnutrition are particularly at risk from copper deficiency if they are fed a diet that is based on cow milk unless copper supplements are given. Poor growth and an increased rate of infection have been reported in such children [138,139]. Deficiency has also been observed in adults prescribed an enteral feed that was not supplemented with copper [140].

A number of other nutrients compete with copper for absorption. Iron, zinc, manganese and ascorbic acid can all potentially decrease absorption, and care should be taken to ensure that there is a sufficient copper intake when prescribing large supplements of any of these nutrients. Copper deficiency has been induced by large doses (16–24 mg daily) of zinc [141]. Acrodermatitis enteropathica requires the use of large oral zinc supplements, and poor copper status has been reported in this condition [142]. Large doses of zinc are used to block copper absorption in Wilson's disease [143]. A more important interaction may be that between iron and copper. Infant formulas containing high levels of both iron and vitamin C may interfere with copper status [144].

Increased losses of copper have been described in cystic fibrosis, celiac disease, burns, gut surgery, prolonged diarrhea, nephrotic syndrome and fat malabsorption [145]. A high fructose intake increases gut and urinary losses of copper, and has been shown to affect the status of this metal in adults [146,147]. Consequently, copper status may need to be checked in children receiving a high fructose or sucrose intake.

The main route of copper excretion is in the bile. Thus, patients receiving parenteral nutrition who have a degree of cholestasis and children with liver disease are at risk of raised plasma copper concentrations that may reach toxic levels [148]. Wilson's disease is an autosomal recessive inherited disorder resulting in abnormally high absorption and enhanced transport of copper. The element is accumulated in tissues and organs, and patients present with varying degrees of liver failure, hemolytic anemia and behavioral changes [149]. Treatment is with chelating agents for copper, including penicillamine and zinc. In children with liver failure, transplantation has been successful [150].

Menkes' steely-hair or kinky-hair syndrome is a rare X-linked recessive metabolic disorder in which there is impaired gastrointestinal transport of copper. First described by Danks [151], this abnormality results in low levels of copper in the brain and leads to severe neurological deterioration and death. The characteristic sign is the secondary growth of hair which lacks luster and breaks off easily, leaving stubble that feels like 'steely' hair. Other clinical features comprise skin and hair depigmentation, hypothermia, poor feeding, frequent infections, transient jaundice, seizures and death by the age of 5–6 years [152].

Diagnosis

Serum copper is low in term infants (5–8 μmol/l) and in early life, but rises to adult values of 10.1–24.6 μmol/l by the age of 4–6 months. Normal serum ceruloplasmin values are 200–400 mg/l after 4–6 months of age. Values of serum copper and ceruloplasmin below 10 μmol/l and 180 mg/l, respectively, are indicative of copper deficiency. Both serum copper and ceruloplasmin levels are insensitive to marginal copper deficiency. Ceruloplasmin acts as an acute-phase protein and increases during periods of infection or inflammation. Functional tests include erythrocyte copper/zinc superoxide dismutase and cytochrome oxidase activity.

Treatment

For treatment of deficiency, 400–600 μg of copper (2–3 mg copper sulfate as a 1% solution) should be given daily for 2 weeks or until blood values return to normal. The recommended intake for prophylaxis in low-birth-weight infants is 50–90 μg/kg/day.

Selenium

Selenium is an integral part of two enzyme systems:

- Glutathione peroxidase, which acts as an antioxidant and is important in the protection of membranes against lipid peroxidation

- Iodothyronine 5'-deiodinase, which catalyzes the conversion of the prohormone thyroxine (T_4) into the active form, triiodothyronine (T_3), and is therefore very significant in thyroid function

Selenium acts synergistically with vitamin E, and adequate selenium status protects against symptoms of vitamin E deficiency.

Clinical aspects

Keshan disease is an endemic cardiomyopathy that occurs mainly in young children and is responsive to selenium. It is almost entirely confined to selenium-depleted areas of China. Infants who are receiving breast milk appear to be protected against the condition, despite a low selenium intake during lactation [153]. Kashin–Beck disease, a degenerative osteoarthropathy seen in pre-adolescence and adolescence, also occurs in areas with very low soil levels of selenium [154]. The exact etiology of these two conditions is not clear, but selenium deficiency appears to interact with an infective agent in both situations. A cardiomyopathy similar to that found in Keshan disease has been reported in malnourished children with epidermolysis bullosa [155].

Selenium deficiency has been described in preterm and term infants , in children receiving long-term parenteral nutrition without supplementation [156–158] and in celiac disease [134]. Low selenium and glutathione peroxidase levels have been described in patients receiving protein-restricted diets for inborn errors of nitrogen metabolism such as phenylketonuria and maple syrup urine disease [153]. Selenium supplementation has been reported as modifying thyroid function in selenium-deficient children with phenylketonuria [159] and in cystic fibrosis [160].

Selenium excess (selenosis) has been reported with daily dietary intakes of 3.2–6.7 mg. Symptoms of excess include gastrointestinal upsets, hair loss, white blotchy nails, mild nerve damage, mottling of tooth enamel and a greater susceptibility to caries.

Diagnosis

A plasma selenium level less than 50 μmol/l is the most frequently used indicator of deficiency, although levels are age dependent. A decreased red cell glutathione peroxidase level may be a more reliable indicator – it is a valid index of reduced selenium intake and is easier to assay than the element itself. Levels below 80 nmol/mg Hb/min indicate deficiency in children.

Treatment

Treatment of selenium deficiency is by a daily dose of sodium selenite to provide 1–3 μg of selenium per kilogram body weight per day. Older children with deficiency have been successfully treated with a weekly dose of 150–300 μg of selenium from sodium selenite. Treatment should last until blood values return to normal (3–4 weeks). A maintenance daily dose of 1 μg/kg will prevent recurrence.

Iodine

Iodine was one of the earliest trace elements to be identified as essential. It is a constituent of the thyroid hormone thyroxine (T_4) and the more potent active form, triiodothyronine (T_3), a key regulator of cell processes. Adequate thyroid function is essential for normal growth and development. In adults, iodine deficiency is characterized by goiter, but deficiency in infancy and childhood has graver consequences. Many populations in developing countries are dependent on the iodine content of the local soil, and endemic iodine deficiency or iodine-deficiency disorders are still common in many parts of the world. Iodine can be leached from the soil by glaciation, high rainfall or flooding. Goitrogens (antithyroid compounds) in foods such as cassava, and some other cereals and vegetables, worsen the effect of iodine deficiency as they interfere with thyroid hormone formation. Iodine is rapidly absorbed from the gut and is equally easily excreted by the kidneys. Populations living close to the sea are less at risk of deficiency since the iodine content of seafood is high and fresh-water sources close to the sea also contain this element. In developed countries, milk is a major source of iodine, where it is mainly introduced as a contaminant from iodine-based disinfectants used during milking.

Clinical aspects

Deficiency of iodine or thyroid hormone *in utero* or in early life leads to increased perinatal mortality, severe stunting, skeletal abnormalities and retarded development. This condition was formerly described as cretinism. The WHO has described iodine deficiency as the most common preventable cause of brain damage in the world [161]. Older children who are iodine deficient develop goiter and have impaired academic performance and a lower IQ than iodine-sufficient children. In some western countries, mild-to-moderate iodine deficiency has been described [162]. There is also an interaction between iodine and selenium deficiency [163]. Children on vegetarian and vegan diets have been noted as having a lower iodine intake than omnivorous children [164,165]. Iodine deficiency has been described in an infant receiving a non-milk-based diet during infancy [166].

Iodine supplementation programs using iodized salt or iodized cooking oils are available in countries where iodine deficiency is endemic [167]. In the USA, where deficiency had been eradicated by public health measures such as iodized salt, iodine intakes have declined in recent years owing to changes in food habits. This may be of concern in women of reproductive age, who are likely to produce infants with mild-iodine deficiency [168].

Diagnosis
Because iodine is rapidly excreted in the urine, a 24-h urine sample is the optimal method for diagnosis of deficiency. An excretion level of less than 50 μg/day is indicative of a low iodine intake. In adults, the iodine:creatinine ratio in a single urine sample is used and values below 50 μg per gram of creatinine are considered abnormal. In general, infants and children have higher iodine:creatinine ratios, but few normal data are available. The level of serum thyroxine or thyroid-stimulating hormone (TSH) provides an indirect measure of iodine nutritional status.

Treatment
To prevent symptoms of iodine deficiency, a supplement of 100–300 μg/day is necessary. Treatment of hypothyroidism uses thyroxine tablets. An average dose is 100 μg/day, although this is age dependent: a daily dose of 6–10 μg/kg in infants aged under 1 year, 5–6 μg/kg in children aged 1–5 years, 4–5 μg/kg in those aged 6–12 years, and 2–3 μg/kg in those older than 12 years is sufficient. In iodine-deficient areas where tablets may not be available, a single intramuscular injection of 5 ml of iodized oil (providing 400 mg iodine/ml) should provide protection for about 4 years.

Chromium

This ultratrace element is essential in humans although no chromium-containing enzymes have been identified. The main physiologic function of trivalent chromium appears to be the regulation of insulin activity. The mode of action is thought to optimize the number of membrane insulin receptors, thus enhancing insulin binding to cells. The element also plays a direct or indirect role in the metabolism of lipids and nucleic acids. Stress, strenuous exercise and a diet high in refined carbohydrate tend to depress chromium status and increase requirements. Consumption from breast milk is 0.1–0.3 μg/day.

Clinical aspects
Although low chromium status has been frequently reported in type II diabetes in adults, this does not seem to have been investigated in the pediatric population. Plasma chromium values do not appear to be lower in preterm compared with term neonates [169]. Chromium deficiency is seen in protein–energy malnutrition, and the resulting impaired glucose tolerance can be corrected by supplementation [170].

Trivalent chromium is poorly absorbed and toxicity from dietary intakes is unlikely, but hexavalent chromium is more toxic. Chromium is a contaminant of parenteral nutrition solutions, and concerns have been expressed about possible excessive intakes from this source [171]. In one study of children receiving long-term parenteral nutrition, an inverse relationship was found between serum chromium values and glomerular filtration rate [172].

Manganese

Manganese is part of several enzyme systems and is necessary for mucopolysaccharide synthesis. It is important, therefore, in the metabolism of cartilage and prothrombin.

Clinical aspects

Deficiency in humans is rare; there is a theoretical risk of deficiency where there is excess bile loss, since ingested manganese is excreted in bile. Low levels of manganese have been described in children receiving synthetic diets or with a variety of conditions, including skeletal abnormalities and epilepsy [173]. Parenteral nutrition solutions containing high levels of this element have been shown to cause hypermanganesemia and deposition of manganese in the basal ganglia of the brain, with Parkinson-like symptoms [174]. Furthermore, mineworkers in Chile exposed to manganese have developed 'manganic madness' with psychosis and extrapyramidal features of parkinsonism. Manganese status should be checked in all children with cholestasis receiving long-term parenteral nutrition.

Molybdenum

Molybdenum, which is essential in humans, is a constituent of three enzyme systems: xanthine oxidase, sulfite oxidase and aldehyde oxidase. The element is therefore involved in the metabolism of purines and pyrimidines and in the regulation of sulfate metabolism.

Clinical aspects

The occurrence of molybdenum is widespread and no deficiencies have been noted in man. Formula-fed premature infants have been shown to have higher molybdenum requirements than breastfed infants, but the formula appeared to supply sufficient amounts [175]. In excess quantities, molybdenum interacts with iron and copper, impairing absorption of both of these nutrients, and molybdenum toxicity has been described in adults.

An inborn error of molybdenum metabolism – molybdenum cofactor deficiency – results in abnormal functioning of the three enzymes for which molybdenum is essential. Symptoms include severe disordered homocysteine metabolism, neurological abnormalities and dislocated lenses. Isolated sulfite oxidase deficiency gives rise to similar pathology. Both diseases are fatal and as yet there is no effective treatment [176].

REFERENCES

1. Beaton GH, Martorell R, Aronsen KJ et al. Effectiveness of vitamin A supplementation in the control of young child morbidity and mortality in developing countries. ACC/SCN Nutrition Policy Discussion Paper No. 13. Geneva: ACC/SCN, 1993.

2. Humphrey JH, Rice AL. Vitamin A supplementation of young infants. Lancet 2000;356:422–4.

3. Alnwick DJ. Combating micronutrient deficiencies: problems and perspectives. Proc Nutr Soc 1998;57:137–47.

4. Huet F, Semana D, Maingueneau C et al. Vitamin A deficiency and nocturnal vision in teenagers with cystic fibrosis. Eur J Pediatr 1997;156:949–51.

5. Verma RP, McColluch KM, Worrell L et al. Vitamin A deficiency and severe bronchopulmonary dysplasia in very low birthweight infants. Am J Perinatol 1996;13:389–93.

6. Ha TK, Sattar N, Talwar D et al. Abnormal antioxidant vitamin and carotenoid status in chronic renal failure. QJM 1996;89:765–9.

7.   Miller RK, Hendrickx AG, Mills JL et al. Periconceptional vitamin A use: how much is teratogenic? Reprod Toxicol 1998;12:75–88.

8.   Ott SM, Aitken ML. Osteoporosis in patients with cystic fibrosis. Clin Chest Med 1998;19:555–67.

9.   Challa A, Moulas A, Cholevas V et al. Vitamin D metabolites in patients with coeliac disease. Eur J Pediatr 1998;157:262–3.

10. Baer MT, Kozlowski BW, Blyler EM et al. Vitamin D, calcium, and bone status in children with developmental delay in relation to anticonvulsant use and ambulatory status. Am J Clin Nutr 1997;65:1042–51.

11. Holick MF. Sunlight "D"ilemma: risk of skin cancer or bone disease and muscle weakness. Lancet 2001;357:4–6.

12. Lawson DE. Dietary vitamin D: is it necessary? J Hum Nutr 1981;35:61–3.

13. Raghuramulu N, Reddy V. Serum 25-hydroxy-vitamin D levels in malnourished children with rickets. Arch Dis Child 1980;55:285–7.

14. Oginni LM, Worsfold M, Oyelami OA et al. Etiology of rickets in Nigerian children. J Pediatr 1996;128:692–4.

15. Clements MR. The problem of rickets in UK Asians. J Hum Nutr Diet 1989;2:105–16.

16. Meulmeester JF, van den Berg H, Wedel M et al. Vitamin D status, parathyroid hormone and sunlight in Turkish, Moroccan and Caucasian children in The Netherlands. Eur J Clin Nutr 1990;44:461–70.

17. Awumey EM, Mitra DA, Hollis BW et al. Vitamin D metabolism is altered in Asian Indians in the southern United States: A clinical research center study. J Clin Endocrinol Metab 1998;83:169–73.

18. Pillow JJ, Forrest PJ, Rodda CP. Vitamin D deficiency in infants and young children born to migrant parents. J Pediatr Child Health 1995;31:180–4.

19. Lawson M, Thomas M, Hardiman A. Dietary and lifestyle factors affecting plasma vitamin D levels in Asian children living in England. Eur J Clin Nutr 1999;53:268–72.

20. Alfaham M, Woodhead S, Pask G et al. Vitamin D deficiency: A concern in pregnant Asian women. Br J Nutr 1995;73:881–7.

21. Russell JG, Hill LF. True fetal rickets. Br J Radiol 1974;47:732–4.

22. Han P, Stacy D, Story C et al. The role of haemopoetic growth factors in the pathogenesis of early anaemia of premature infants. Br J Haematol 1995;91:327–9.

23. Fardy CH, Silverman M. Antioxidants in neonatal lung disease. Arch Dis Child Fetal Neonatal Ed 1995;73(Suppl.):F112–7.

24. Phillips PH, Repka MX. Current concepts in the treatment of retinopathy of prematurity. Semin Ophthalmol 1997;12:72–80.

25. Raju TN, Langenberg P, Bhutani V et al. Prophylaxis to reduce retinopathy of prematurity: a reappraisal of published trials. J Pediatr 1998;131:844–50.

26. Phelps DL. The role of vitamin E therapy in high-risk neonates. Clin Perinatol 1988;15:955–63.

27. American Academy of Pediatrics Committee on Nutrition. Commentary on breast feeding and infant formulas, including proposed standards for formulas. Pediatrics 1976;57:278–85.

28. Aggett P, Haschke F, Heine W et al. Comment on the content and composition of lipids in infant formulas. ESPGAN Committee on Nutrition. Acta Paediatr Scand 1991;80:887–96.

29. Aggett P, Bresson JL, Hernell O et al. Comment on the vitamin E content of infant formulas, follow-on formulas, and formulas for low birth weight infants. ESPGAN Committee on Nutrition. J Pediatr Gastroenterol Nutr 1998;26:351–2.

30. Peters SA, Kelly FJ. Vitamin E supplementation in cystic fibrosis. J Pediatr Gastroenterol Nutr 1996;22:341–5.

31. Sokol RJ, Butler-Simon N, Heubi JE et al. Vitamin E deficiency neuropathy in children with fat malabsorption: Studies in cystic fibrosis and chronic cholestasis. Ann NY Acad Sci 1989;570:156–69.

32. Kaufman SS, Murray ND, Wood RP et al. Nutritional support for the infant with extrahepatic biliary atresia. J Pediatr 1987;110:679–86.

33. Bousvaros A, Zurakowski D, Duggan C et al. Vitamins A and E serum levels in children and young adults with inflammatory bowel disease: Effect of disease activity. J Pediatr Gastroenterol Nutr 1998;26:129–35.

34. Keenan WJ, Jewett T, Glueck HI. Role of feeding and vitamin K in hypoprothrombinemia of the newborn. Am J Dis Child 1971;121:271–7.

35. von Kries R. Neonatal vitamin K prophylaxis: The Gordian knot still awaits untying. BMJ 1998;316:161–2.

36. Golding J, Greenwood R, Birmingham K, Mott M. Childhood cancer, intramuscular vitamin K, and pethidine given during labour. BMJ 1992;305:341–6.

37. Zipursky A. Vitamin K at birth. BMJ 1996;313:179–80.

38. Tripp JH, McNinch AW. The vitamin K debacle: Cut the Gordian knot but first do no harm. Arch Dis Child 1998;79:295–7.

39. American Academy of Pediatrics Vitamin K Ad Hoc Task Force. Controversies concerning vitamin K and the newborn. Pediatrics 1993;91:1001–3.

40. British Paediatric Association Expert Committee. Vitamin K prophylaxis in infancy. London: BPA, 1992.

41. Barton JS, Tripp JH, McNinch AW. Neonatal vitamin K prophylaxis in the British Isles: Current practice and trends. BMJ 1995;310:632–3.

42. von Kries R, Hanawa Y. Neonatal vitamin K prophylaxis: Report of scientific and standardisation subcommittee on perinatal haemostasis. Thromb Haemost 1993;69:293–5.

43. Logan S, Gilbert R. Vitamin K Prophylaxis for Haemorrhagic Disease of the Newborn: an Appraisal of the Effectiveness of Oral Regimens. London: Institute of Child Health, 1998.

44. Cornelissen M, von Kries R, Loughnan P et al. Prevention of vitamin K deficiency bleeding: efficacy of different multiple oral dose schedules of vitamin K. Eur J Pediatr 1997;156:126–30.

45. Friel JK, Andrews WL, Long DR et al. Thiamine, riboflavin, folate, and vitamin B12 status of infants with low birth weights receiving enteral nutrition. J Pediatr Gastroenterol Nutr 1996;22:289–95.

46. Hahn JS, Berquist W, Alcorn DM et al. Wernicke encephalopathy and beriberi during total parenteral nutrition attributable to multivitamin infusion shortage. Pediatrics 1998;101:E10.

47. Pihko H, Saarinen U, Paetau A. Wernicke encephalopathy – a preventable cause of death: Report of 2 children with malignant disease. Pediatr Neurol 1989;5:237–42.

48. Vasconcelos MM, Silva KP, Vidal G et al. Early diagnosis of pediatric Wernicke's encephalopathy. Pediatr Neurol 1999;20:289–94.

49. Chuang DT, Shih VE. Maple syrup urine disease. In: Scriver CR, Beaudet AL, Sly WS et al, editors. The Metabolic and Molecular Basis of Inherited Disease, Volume II, 8th ed. New York: McGraw-Hill, 2001:1971–2005.

50. Dagnelie PC, van Staveren WA, Verschuren SA et al. Nutritional status of infants aged 4 to 18 months on macrobiotic diets and matched omnivorous control infants: a population-based mixed-longitudinal study. I. Weaning pattern, energy and nutrient intake. Eur J Clin Nutr 1989;43:311–23.

51. Teran-Garcia M, Ibarra I, Velazquez A. Urinary organic acids in infant malnutrition. Pediatr Res 1998;44:386–91.

52. Lucas A, Bates CJ. Occurrence and significance of riboflavin deficiency in preterm infants. Biol Neonate 1987;52(Suppl. 1):113–8.

53. Porcelli PJ, Adcock EW, Del Paggio D et al. Plasma and urine riboflavin and pyridoxine concentrations in enterally fed very-low-birth-weight neonates. J Pediatr Gastroenterol Nutr 1996;23:141–6.

54. Ishii N, Nishihara Y. Pellagra encephalopathy among tuberculous patients: Its relation to isoniazid therapy. J Neurol Neurosurg Psychiatry 1985;48:628–34.

55. Virtanen SM, Aro A. Dietary factors in the aetiology of diabetes. Ann Med 1994;26:469–78.

56. Colletti RB, Neufield EJ, Roff NK. Niacin treatment of hypercholesterolemia in children. Pediatrics 1993;92:78–82.

57. Galadari E, Hadi S, Sabarinathan K. Hartnup disease. Int J Dermatol 1993;32:904.

58. Gillis J, Murphy FR, Boxall LB et al. Biotin deficiency in a child on long-term TPN. JPEN 1982;6:308–10.

59. Higuchi R, Noda E, Koyama Y et al. Biotin deficiency in an infant fed with amino acid formula and hypoallergenic rice. Acta Paediatr 1996;85:872–4.

60. Mock DM, Mock NI, Nelson RP et al. Disturbances in biotin metabolism in children undergoing long-term anticonvulsant therapy. J Pediatr Gastroenterol Nutr 1998:26:245–50.

61. Wolfe B. Disorders of biotin metabolism. In: Scriver CR, Beaudet AL, Sly WS, Valle D, editors. The Metabolic and Molecular Basis of Inherited Disease, Volume III, 8th ed. New York: McGraw-Hill, 2001:3935–56.

62. Dupuis L, Campeau E, Leclerc D et al. Mechanism of biotin responsiveness in biotin-responsive multiple carboxylase deficiency. Mol Genet Metab 1999;66:80–90.

63. Higgins JJ, Glasgow AM, Lusk M et al. MRI, clinical, and biochemical features of pyruvate carboxylase deficiency. J Child Neurol 1994;9:436–9.

64. Kang-Yoon SA, Kirksey A, Giacoia GP et al. Vitamin B6 adequacy in neonatal nutrition: Associations with preterm delivery, type of feeding, and vitamin B6 supplementation. Am J Clin Nutr 1995;62:932–42.

65. Heiskanen K, Siimes MA, Salmenpeera L et al. Low vitamin B6 status associated with slow growth in healthy breast-fed infants. Pediatr Res 1995;38:740–6.

66. Heiskanen K, Salmenpera L, Perheentupa J et al. Infant vitamin B6 changes with age and with formula feeding. Am J Clin Nutr 1994;60:907–10.

67. Baxter P. Epidemiology of pyridoxine dependent and pyridoxine responsive seizures in the UK. Arch Dis Child 1999;81:431–3.

68. Gospe SM. Current perspectives on pyridoxine-dependent seizures. J Pediatr 1997;132:919–23.

69. Mudd SH, Harvey HL, Kraus JP. Disorders of transsulfuration. In: Scriver CR, Beaudet AL, Sly WS, Valle D, editors. The Metabolic and Molecular Basis of Inherited Disease, Volume II, 8th ed. New York: McGraw-Hill, 2001:2007–56.

70. Wilcken DE, Wilcken B. The natural history of vascular disease in homocystinuria and the effects of treatment. J Inherit Metab Dis 1997;20:295–300.

71. Kuhne T, Bubl R, Baumgartner R. Maternal vegan diet causing a serious infantile neurological disorder due to vitamin B12 deficiency. Eur J Pediatr 1991;150:205–8.

72. Ciani F, Poggi GM, Pasquini E et al. Prolonged exclusive breastfeeding from vegan mother causing an acute onset methylmalonic aciduria due to a mild mutase deficiency. Clin Nutr 2000;19:137–9.

73. Dagnelie PC, van Staveren WA, Hautvast JG. Stunting and nutrient deficiencies in children on alternative diets. Acta Paediatr Scand Suppl 1991;374:111–8.

74. Van Dusseldorp M, Schneede J, Refsum H et al. Risk of persistent cobalamin deficiency in adolescents fed a macrobiotic diet in early life. Am J Clin Nutr 1999;69:664–71.

75. Graham SM, Arvela OM, Wise GA. Long-term neurological consequences of nutritional vitamin B12 deficiency in infants. J Pediatr 1992;121:710–4.

76. Sanders TA. Vegetarian diets and children. Pediatr Clin North Am 1995;42:955–65.

77. Davies BW, Abel G, Puntis JW et al. Limited ileal resection in infancy: the long-term consequences. J Pediatr Surg 1999;34:583–7.

78. Kapadia CR. Vitamin B12 in health and disease: Part 1 - inherited disorders of function, absorption and transport. Gastroenterologist 1995;3:329–44.

79. Gräsbeck R, Gordin R, Kantero I, Kuhlbäck B. Selective vitamin B12 malabsorption and proteinuria in young people. A syndrome. Acta Med Scand 1960;167:289–96.

80. Rosenblatt DS, Fenton WA. Inherited disorders of folate transport and metabolism. In: Scriver CR, Beaudet AL, Sly WS, Valle D, editors. The Metabolic and Molecular Basis of Inherited Disease, Volume III, 8th ed. New York: McGraw-Hill, 2001:3897–933.

81. Ostman-Smith I, Brown G, Johnson A, Land JM. Dilated cardiomyopathy due to type II X-linked 3-methylglucaconic aciduria: Successful treatment with pantothenic acid. Br Heart J 1994;72:349–53.

82. Evans PR. Infantile scurvy: The centenary of Barlow's disease. BMJ (Clin Res Ed) 1983;287:1862–3.

83. Bass WT, Malati N, Castle MC et al. Evidence for the safety of ascorbic acid supplementation to the premature infant. Am J Perinatol 1998;15:133–40.

84. Weiss ST. Diet as a risk factor for asthma. Ciba Found Symp 1997;206:244–57.

85. Cook DG, Carey IM, Whincup PH et al. Effect of fresh fruit consumption on lung function and wheeze in children. Thorax 1997;52:628–33.

86. Winklhofer-Roob BM, Ellemunter H, Fruhwirth M et al. Plasma vitamin C concentration in patients with cystic fibrosis: Evidence of association with lung inflammation. Am J Clin Nutr 1997;65:1891–2.

87. MRC Vitamin Study Research Group. Prevention of neural tube defects: results of the Medical Research Council Vitamin study. Lancet 1991;338:131–7.

88. Hall JG, Solehdin F. Folate and its various ramifications. Adv Pediatr 1998;45:1–35.

89. Scott JM, Weir DG. Homocysteine and cardiovascular disease. QJM 1996;89:561–3.

90. Worthington-White DA, Behnke M, Gross S. Premature infants require additional folate and vitamin B_{12} to reduce the severity of the anemia of prematurity. Am J Clin Nutr 1994;60:930–5.

91. Parry TE. Goats' milk in infants and children. BMJ (Clin Res Ed) 1984;228:863–4.

92. Kishi T, Fujita N, Eguchi T et al. Mechanism for reduction of serum folate by antiepileptic drugs during prolonged therapy. J Neurol Sci 1997;145:109–12.

93. Hum MC, Kamen BA. Folate, antifolates, and folate analogs in pediatric oncology. Invest New Drugs 1996;14:101–11.

94. WHO. Nutritional anemias. WHO technical report series, No. 503. Geneva: WHO, 1972.

95. Blecker U, Renders F, Lanciers S et al. Syncopes leading to the diagnosis of Helicobacter pylori positive chronic active haemorrhagic gastritis. Eur J Pediatr 1991;150:560–1.

96. Mejia LA, Chew F. Hematologic effect of supplementing anemic children with vitamin A alone or in combination with iron. Am J Clin Nutr 1988;48:595–600.

97. Lawson MS, Thomas M. Vitamin D concentrations in Asian children aged 2 years living in England: Population survey. BMJ 1999;318:28.

98. Baynes RD. Iron deficiency. In: Brock JH, Halliday JW, Pippard MJ, Powell LW, editors. Iron Metabolism in Health and Disease. London: WB Saunders, 1994:190–225.

99. Looker AC, Dallman PR, Carroll MD et al. Prevalence of iron deficiency in the United States. JAMA 1997;277:973–6.

100. Gregory JR, Collins DL, Davies PS et al. National diet & nutrition survey: children aged $1\frac{1}{2}$ to $4\frac{1}{2}$. London: HMSO, 1995.

101. Hemminki E, Nemet K, Horvath M et al. Impact of iron fortification of milk formulas on infants' growth and health. Nutr Res 1995;15:491–503.

102. Lawson MS. Iron in infancy and childhood. In: Iron, Nutritional and Physiological Significance. Report of the British Nutrition Foundation Task Force. London: Chapman & Hall, 1995:93–105.

103. Mills AF. Surveillance for anemia: Risk factors in patterns of milk intake. Arch Dis Child 1990;65:428–31.

104. Sullivan PB. Cows' milk induced intestinal bleeding in infancy. Arch Dis Child 1993;68:240–5.

105. Yip R, Binkin NJ, Fleshood L et al. Declining prevalence of anemia among low-income children in the United States. JAMA 1987;258:1619–23.

106. American Academy of Pediatrics Committee on Nutrition: Nutritional needs of low-birthweight infants. Pediatrics 1985;75:976–86.

107. ESPGAN Committee on Nutrition of the Preterm Infant. Nutrition and feeding of preterm infants. Acta Paediatr Scand Suppl 1987;336:1–14.

108. Lansdown R, Wharton BA. Iron and mental and motor behaviour in children. In: Iron, Nutritional and Physiological Significance. Report of the British Nutritional Foundation Task Force. London: Chapman & Hall, 1995:65–78.

109. Hallberg L, Hulten L, Lindstedt G et al. Prevalence of iron deficiency in Swedish adolescents. Pediatr Res 1993;34:680–7.

110. Donovan UM, Gibson RS. Iron and zinc status of young women aged 14–19 years consuming vegetarian and omnivorous diets. J Am Coll Nutr 1995;14:463–72.

111. Sargent JD, Stukel TA, Dalton MA et al. Iron deficiency in Massachusetts communities: Socioeconomic and demographic risk factors among children. Am J Public Health 1996;86:544–50.

112. Marx JJ. Iron deficiency in developed countries: Prevalence, influence of lifestyle factors, and hazards of prevention. Eur J Clin Nutr 1997;51:491–4.

113. Lawson MS, Thomas M, Hardiman A. Iron status of Asian children aged 2 years living in England. Arch Dis Child 1998;78:420–6.

114. Schumann K, Elsenhans B, Maurer A. Iron supplementation. J Trace Elem Med Biol 1998;12:129–40.

115. Halliday JW. Inherited iron overload. Acta Paediatr Scand Suppl 1989;361:86–95.

116. Oski FA, Hoing AS, Helu B et al. Effect of iron therapy on behavior performance in non-anemic iron deficient children. Pediatrics 1983;71:877–80.

117. Wharton B. Iron deficiency in children: detection and prevention. Br J Haematol 1999;106:270–80.

118. Mancini AJ, Tunnessen WW. Picture of the month. Acrodermatitis enteropathica like rash in a breast-fed full-term infant with zinc deficiency. Arch Pediatr Adolesc Med 1998;152:1239–40.

119. Stevens J, Lubitz L. Symptomatic zinc deficiency in breast-fed term and premature infants. J Paediatr Child Health 1998;34:97–100.

120. Obladen M, Loui A, Kampmann W et al. Zinc deficiency in rapidly growing preterm infants. Acta Paediatr 1998;87:685–91.

121. Heinen F, Matern D, Pringsheim W et al. Zinc deficiency in an exclusively breast-fed term infant. Eur J Pediatr 1995;154:71–5.

122. Bhutta ZA, Black RE, Brown KH et al. Prevention of diarrhea and pneumonia by zinc supplementation in children in developing countries: Pooled analysis of randomized controlled trials. Zinc Investigators' Collaborative Group. J Pediatr 1999;135:689–97.

123. Fuchs GJ. Possibilities for zinc in the treatment of diarrhea. Am J Clin Nutr 1998;68(Suppl.):480S–483S.

124. Van Voorhees AS, Riba M. Acquired zinc deficiency in association with anorexia nervosa: Case report and review of the literature. Pediatr Dermatol 1992;9:268–71.

125. Birmingham CL, Goldner EM, Bakan R. Controlled trial of zinc supplementation in anorexia nervosa. Int J Eating Disord 1994;15:251–5.

126. Licastro F, Mocchegiani E, Zannotti M et al. Zinc affects the metabolism of the thyroid hormones in children with Down's syndrome: Normalization of thyroid stimulating hormone and of reversal triidothryronine plasmic levels by dietary zinc supplements. Int J Neurosci 1992;65:259–68.

127. Crofton RW, Aggett PJ, Gvozdanovic S et al. Zinc metabolism in celiac disease. Am J Clin Nutr 1990;52:379–82.

128. Krebbs NF, Sontag M, Accurso FJ et al. Low plasma zinc levels in young infants with cystic fibrosis. J Pediatr 1998;133:761–4.

129. Fuchs GJ, Tienboon P, Linpisarn S et al. Nutritional factors and thalassaemia major. Arch Dis Child 1996;74:224–7.

130. De Virgillis S, Congia M, Turco MP et al. Depletion of trace elements and acute ocular toxicity induced by desferrioxamine in patients with thalassemia. Arch Dis Child 1988;63:250–5.

131. Sweeney JD, Ziegler P, Pruet C et al. Hyperzincuria and hypozincemia in patients treated with cisplatin. Cancer 1989;63:2093–5.

132. Perrone L, Gialanella G, Giordano V et al. Impaired zinc metabolic status in children affected by idiopathic nephrotic syndrome. Eur J Pediatr 1990;149:438–40.

133. Hendricks KM, Williams E, Stoker TW et al. Dietary intake of adolescents with Crohn's disease. J Am Diet Assoc 1994;94:441–4.

134. Varkonyi A, Boda M, Endreffy E et al. Coeliac disease: Always something to discover. Scand J Gastroenterol Suppl 1998:228:122–9.

135. Van Wouwe JP. Clinical and laboratory diagnosis of acrodermatitis enteropathica. Eur J Pediatr 1989;149:2–8.

136. Levy Y, Zeharia A, Grunebaum M et al. Copper deficiency in infants fed cow milk. J Pediatr 1985;106:786–8.

137. L'Abbe MR, Friel JK. Copper status of very low birthweight infants during the first twelve months of infancy. Pediatr Res 1992;32:183–8.

138. Castillo-Duran C, Uauy R. Copper deficiency impairs growth of infants recovering from malnutrition. Am J Clin Nutr 1988;47:710–4.

139. Castillo-Duran C, Fisberg M, Valenzuela A et al. Controlled trial of copper supplementation during the recovery from marasmus. Am J Clin Nutr 1983;37:898–903.

140. Tamura H, Hirose S, Watanabe O et al. Anemia and neutropenia due to copper deficiency in enteral nutrition. JPEN 1994;18:185–9.

141. Botash AS, Nasca J, Dubowy R et al. Zinc-induced copper deficiency in an infant. Am J Dis Child 1992;146:709–11.

142. Sandstrom B, Cederblad A, Lindblad B et al. Acrodermatitis enteropathica, zinc metabolism, copper status and immune function. Arch Pediatr Adolesc Med 1994;148:980–5.

143. Brewer GJ, Hill GM, Prasad AS et al. Oral zinc therapy for Wilson's disease. Ann Intern Med 1983;99:314–20.

144. Lonnerdal B. Copper nutrition during infancy and childhood. Am J Clin Nutr 1998;67(Suppl.):1046S–53S.

145. Taylor A. Detection and monitoring of disorders of essential trace elements. Ann Clin Biochem 1996;33:486–510.

146. Uauay R, Olivares M, Gonzales M. Essentiality of copper in humans. Am J Clin Nutr 1998;67(Suppl.):952S–959S.

147. Reiser S, Smith JC, Mertz W et al. Indices of copper status in humans consuming a typical American diet containing either fructose or starch. Am J Clin Nutr 1985;42:242–51.

148. Ohi R, Lilly JR. Copper kinetics in infantile hepatobiliary disease. J Pediatr Surg 1980;15:509–12.

149. Brewer GJ. Recognition, diagnosis, and management of Wilson's disease. Proc Soc Biol Med 2000;223:39–46.

150. Asonuma K, Inomata Y, Kasahara M et al. Living related liver transplantation from heterozygote genetic carriers to children with Wilson's disease. Pediatr Transplant 1999;3:201–5.

151. Danks DM, Cartwright E, Stevens BJ et al. Menkes' steely-hair (kinky hair) disease. Science 1973;179:1140–2.

152. Olivares M, Uauy R. Copper as an essential nutrient. Am J Clin Nutr 1996;63(Suppl.):791S–796S.

153. Litov RE, Combs GF. Selenium in pediatric nutrition. Pediatrics 1991;87:339–51.

154. Allander E. Kashin-Beck disease. An analysis of research and public health activities based on a bibliography 1849–1992. Scand J Rheumatol Suppl 1994;99:1–36.

155. Melville C, Atherton D, Burch M et al. Fatal cardiomyopathy in dystrophic epidermolysis bullosa. Br J Dermatol 1996;135:603–6.

156. Klinger G, Shamir R, Singer P et al. Parenteral selenium supplementation in extremely low birthweight infants: Inadequate dosage but no correlation with hypothyroidism. J Perinatol 1999;19:568–72.

157. Daniels L, Gibson R, Simmer K. Randomised clinical trial of parenteral selenium supplementation in preterm infants. Arch Dis Child Fetal Neonatal Ed 1996;74:F158–4.

158. Lipsky CL, Spear ML. Recent advances in parenteral nutrition. Clin Perinatol 1995;22:141–55.

159. Calomme M, Vanderpas J, Francois B et al. Effects of selenium supplementation on thyroid hormone metabolism in phenylketonuria subjects on a phenylalanine restricted diet. Biol Trace Elem Res 1995;47:349–53.

160. Kauf E, Dawczynski H, Jahreis G et al. Sodium selenite therapy and thyroid hormone status in cystic fibrosis and congenital hypothyroidism. Biol Trace Elem Res 1994;40:247–53.

161. Stanbury JB, Ermans AM, Hetzel BS et al. Endemic goitre and cretinism: Public health significance and prevention. WHO Chron 1974;28:220–8.

162. Valeix P, Preziosi P, Rossignol C et al. Iodine intakes assessed by urinary iodine concentrations in healthy children aged ten months, two years, and four years. Biol Trace Elem Res 1992;32:259–63.

163. Thilly CH, Vanderpas JB, Bebe N et al. Iodine deficiency, other trace elements and goitrogenic factors in the etiopathology of iodine deficiency disorders. Biol Trace Elem Res 1992;32:229–35.

164. Remer T, Neubert A, Manz F. Increased risk of iodine deficiency with vegetarian nutrition. Br J Nutr 1999;81:45–9.

165. Lightowler HJ, Davies GJ, Trevan MD. Iodine in the diet: Perspectives for vegans J R Soc Health 1996;116:14–20.

166. Kanaka C, Schutz B, Zuppinger KA. Risks of alternative nutrition in infancy: A case report of severe iodine and carnitine deficiency. Eur J Pediatr 1992;151:786–8.

167. Maberly GF. Iodine deficiency disorders: Contemporary scientific issues. J Nutr 1994;124(Suppl. 8): 1437S–1478S.

168. Lee K, Bradley R, Dwyer J et al. Too much versus too little: The implications of current iodine intakes in the United States. Nutr Rev 1999;57:177–81.

169. Bougle D, Bureau F, Voirin J et al. Chromium status of full-term and preterm newborns. Biol Trace Elem Res 1992;32:47–51.

170. Mertz W. Chromium in human nutrition: A review. J Nutr 1993;123:626–33.

171. Bougle D, Bureau F, Deschrevel G et al. Chromium and parenteral nutrition in children. J Pediatr Gastroenterol Nutr 1993;17:72–4.

172. Moukarzel AA, Song MK, Buchman AL et al. Excessive chromium intake in children receiving total parenteral nutrition. Lancet 1992;339:385–8.

173. Leach RM, Harris ED. Manganese. In: O'Dell BL, Sunde RA, editors. Handbook of Nutritionally Essential Mineral Elements. New York: Marcel Dekker, 1997:335–55.

174. Fell JM, Reynolds AP, Meadows N et al. Manganese toxicity in children receiving long-term parenteral nutrition. Lancet 1996;347:1218–21.

175. Bougle D, Foucalt D, Voirin J et al. Molybdenum in the premature infant. Biol Neonate 1991;59:201–3.

176. Johnson JL, Duran M. Molybdenum cofactor deficiency and isolated sulfite oxidase deficiency. In: Scriver CR, Beaudet AL, Sly WS, Valle D, editors. The Metabolic and Molecular Basis of Inherited Disease, Volume II, 8th ed. New York: McGraw-Hill, 2001:3163–77.

chapter *2*

Enteral and Parenteral Nutrition

The increased survival of severely ill patients has been made possible in part by the development of techniques that will secure their nutrition [1]. Whenever possible, the oral or enteral route is preferable; however, many patients are unable to receive appropriate calories in this manner and so require intravenous nutrition. This chapter describes these two techniques.

ENTERAL NUTRITION

Feeding by the enteral route is more physiologic than that by the parenteral route and consequently has fewer short-term and long-term complications. In addition, it is a less expensive option and easier to manage. The use of the gastrointestinal tract results in superior fluid homeostasis and – based on results from animal studies at least – function of the intestine is better-preserved [2]. Feeding also initiates the activity of non-luminal neuronal and hormonal factors, which stimulate the bowel [3]. Consequently, only if the enteral route is precluded through an inability to ingest, digest, absorb or propulse nutrients should parenteral nutrition be indicated. Before nutritional supplementation of any kind is implemented, the nutritional status of the patient should be assessed, the goals defined, and the risks and benefits explained to the parents and, if age-appropriate, to the patient. Introducing and maintaining in position a nasogastric tube may be of little relevance to a physician, but constitutes a major trauma to certain patients as well as their families.

Oral supplementation

Oral supplementation is feasible whenever the patient is capable and willing to swallow a liquid formula and retain it in the stomach. In infants, increasing the caloric density of liquid formulas can be achieved by the addition of glucose polymers, and/or fats, depending on the age and tolerance of the patient. In some instances, powder preparations can be dissolved in a smaller volume than that recommended by the manufacturer, thus providing hypercaloric formulas. However, it needs to be remembered that such modifications increase the osmolality of the preparation and so delay gastric emptying, which can cause vomiting and early satiety. Diarrhea and/or flatulence can also occur. At times, these complications will prevent the use of oral supplements even in patients willing to consume them. Children with prolonged caloric deprivation and consequent growth failure may be unwilling to take significant additional calories over baseline requirements. In this situation, a concentrated preparation may be indicated before tube feeding is initiated.

Recipes for high-protein, high-energy soups, milk shakes and fruit drinks are given on p. 392. The principles of feeding are the same as described for tube feeding.

The recommended daily allowances (RDAs) for protein, energy and fluid should be calculated and the amount of dietary sodium, minerals, vitamins and trace elements noted.

High-energy, high-protein drinks can be given in addition to food in an anorexic child or where nutrient requirements are particularly high. Supplements should be given 1–2 h before a meal or snack; they need to be emptied fairly rapidly from the stomach and therefore should not be too hot or cold or have an excess fat content in order to ensure the child retains his or her appetite.

Tube and gastrostomy feedings

There are many indications for tube feeding. The major ones include:

- Inability to coordinate suck and swallow (prematurity, brain injury, increased endocranial pressure)

- Debilitated newborn infants

- Orofacial malformations

- Severe respiratory illnesses

- Cardiopathies [4]

- Failure to thrive

- Gastroesophageal reflux [5]

In addition, tube feeding may be indicated in altered sensorium, renal disease [6], HIV infection [7], short-bowel syndrome [8], Crohn's disease [9], intestinal pseudo-obstruction [10], muscular dystrophy, anorexia nervosa, delayed gastric emptying, nutrient malabsorption, depression and inappropriate caloric intake.

If oral supplements to food or a complete liquid diet can be taken, then these approaches are preferable to a tube method. Moreover, there are obvious psychological advantages in maintaining oral feeds. Children who will require total or supplemental feedings for a prolonged time, and are dependent on a nasogastric tube for that purpose, are good candidates for the placement of a gastrostomy.

Tube feeding is contraindicated in the following conditions:

- Extreme prematurity

- Severe respiratory distress

- Severe cardiac failure

- Trauma, burns to the face

- Malnutrition in a severely immunocompromised host

- Severe vomiting, such as when chemotherapy is administered

Gastrostomy

In children, gastrostomies can be placed surgically, laparoscopically [11] or percutaneously [12,13]. A percutaneous gastrostomy can be performed under ultrasonic or fluoroscopic control [14], or endoscopically (push or pull technique) [15]. If the patient does not suffer from severe gastroesophageal reflux, a gastrostomy can be carried out without the need for a fundoplication [16], even in neurologically impaired children [17]. However, following placement of a gastrostomy, patients can develop gastroesophageal reflux or delayed gastric emptying.

The technique of percutaneous endoscopic gastrostomy (PEG) was introduced in 1980 as a method requiring neither a laparotomy nor general anesthesia [18]. The technique originally described – the pull method – involves puncturing the apposed gastric and abdominal walls under endoscopic control. A suture is then passed from the exterior into the gastric lumen and grasped with a snare. The suture is pulled out of the mouth, affixed to the end of a gastrostomy tube and then pulled back down into the stomach. The gastrostomy tube then exits the abdominal wall. Modifications of this technique have included pushing the gastrostomy tube over a guidewire (the push method) and direct puncture of the stomach under endoscopic control with an introducer and outer peel-away sheath. All of these options have been used with good results. The advantage of a percutaneous gastrostomy is that discharge from hospital occurs within 24 h. Although gastrostomies can be performed under conscious sedation and local anesthetic, when the procedure is undertaken in children, general anesthesia is often used.

The gastrostomy provides a transcutaneous and direct approach to the stomach. This method has several advantages:

- It frees the orofacial area from tubes, tape and manipulation
- It avoids accumulation of nasal secretions and obstruction of the internal ear canal
- It provides the patient with more privacy

Complications can occur with gastrostomy tubes either at the time of placement or subsequently, and include [19]:

- Skin infections
- Leakage
- Perforation of the colon
- Separation between the gastric and abdominal wall, with intraperitoneal leak
- Erosions of the gastric mucosa [20]
- Aspiration pneumonia
- Hemorrhage
- Necrotizing fasciitis

Children with neurological problems are at risk of aspiration, and tube feedings constitute an additional problem [21]. Contraindications for percutaneous gastrostomies comprise:

- Massive ascites

- Need for peritoneal dialysis

- Portal hypertension

- Severe coagulopathy

- Abdominal wall infection

Methods of tube feeding
Tube tips can be positioned in the stomach or duodenum, or surgically placed distal to an intestinal anastomotic site in the jejunum or ileum. The nutrients can be infused into the stomach by bolus (intermittent feeding regimen), which confers the benefit of simulating a normal pattern of feeding. Bolus feeding may be difficult in some very small preterm infants because of immaturity-associated delayed gastric emptying and poor antroduodenal motility [22]. Difficulties may also arise in those with gastroesophageal reflux or vomiting, as well as in patients receiving ventilatory support with high positive-end expiratory pressure (PEEP).

Alternatively, tube feeding can be used to provide a continuous infusion. Enteral feeding pumps are not as costly or as complex as those used for intravenous therapy. Constant infusions have the advantage of achieving a much higher fluid intake, less gastric distension and aspiration, as well as improved absorption of nutrients [23]. However, it may be better to have drugs infused as a bolus to prevent wastage and inaccuracies in dosages. Nocturnal infusions may interfere less with activity and daytime oral feedings.

Each anatomic position is associated with its own advantages and disadvantages. Tubes placed in the stomach are easy to replace, and feedings can be administered by bolus or gavage. In contrast, those sited in the small bowel can be dislodged and are difficult to reposition, and feedings may need to be administered as a constant infusion via a pump. Potential hazards include perforation of the stomach or intestine, and aspiration, which can prove fatal, especially in very young or compromised patients.

Bowel endocrine response to feeding
When selecting the method of enteral nutrition it should be remembered that the gut hormone profile, both in preterm and in term infants, is influenced by the feeding regimen [24]. Postprandial responses are greater when there has been bolus feeding of milk as opposed to continuous intragastric infusions [25–27].

It has been suggested that milk in the gut results in the release of a number of hormones inducing developmental changes in the bowel and pancreas. Hormonal responses to the first extrauterine feed are dissimilar in the preterm and term infant, as the mature neonate is primed to respond to the initial feed with metabolic and endocrine changes. It would seem that developmental changes arise in the final weeks of gestation that prepare the term baby for enteral feeding.

Studies in very small preterm infants (birth weight <900 g) have shown numerous advantages to priming using a nasogastric tube with progressive increments of feeds over 20 days [28,29].

Equipment for tube feeding

Feeding tubes are manufactured from polyurethane, silicone rubber (Silastic), polyethylene or polyvinyl chloride. Polyurethane and Silastic tubes are used more commonly than the other types as they are softer, cause less discomfort and can remain *in situ* for several weeks. However, they have a small internal diameter and hence are not suitable for all types of feeds. In addition, pumps are often required. Usually, it is difficult to aspirate from this type of product, and the unweighted tube is easily dislodged by coughing.

Polyethylene and polyvinyl chloride tubes generally have a wider lumen and can be used for blenderized whole diets or home-prepared feeds. They are more suitable for bolus feeding than the polyurethane or Silastic products, although they, too, can be used for continuous infusion. Furthermore, they are easier to introduce than the softer tubes; however, they harden *in situ* and have been reported to cause gut perforation unless they are changed frequently (every 3–5 days).

For tubes positioned in the small bowel, radiologic confirmation is useful. For those located in the stomach, air can be injected and the end of the tube auscultated at the presumed site of the opening to ensure that the bronchi have not been cannulated.

Various containers and gavage sets are available when tube feeding is by continuous infusion. All containers must be sterile when the feed is introduced and should be changed every 12–24 h in order to reduce the likelihood of introducing pathogens. Pumps are available to deliver the infusate at a predetermined rate.

Products for tube feeding

Enteral feeds can be classified into three categories:

- Chemically defined diets

- Specifically formulated diets

- Standard polymeric diets

Chemically defined or elemental diets contain nutrients that require little or no digestion and hence are easily absorbed. Their use is discussed more fully in Appendix IV.20. Specially formulated diets are those designed to overcome a specific problem in digestion such as lactose intolerance (see p. 109).

The standard polymeric diet has whole protein rather than amino acids as the nitrogen source and is appropriate where there is normal or near normal gastrointestinal function. Preparations suitable for tube feeding are of three types:

- Normal food that has been blenderized and sieved

- Reconstituted powder preparations which require the addition of water or milk

- Ready-to-feed products

Blenderized food has the disadvantage that it is difficult to achieve a uniform consistency that will readily pass through an enteric feeding tube. Home-prepared feeds will block the small lumen of polyurethane or Silastic tubes. Feeds of this type are usually low in energy unless modular fat and carbohydrate are used. Furthermore, liquidized preparations might become contaminated – from the food directly, its processing or from the use of unclean liquidizing equipment. For a child being fed at home via a gastrostomy, use of home-prepared foods may confer social and emotional benefits to the mother, child and family; however, these preparations have a limited role in tube feeding.

Complete feeds, either ready-to-use or reconstituted powders, should contain the RDA for all nutrients, including vitamins, minerals and trace elements. If the patient does not tolerate the required calories through the enteral route, supplementary minerals and vitamins will need to be given intravenously. Ready-to-feed products have advantages over reconstituted feeds in that they are sterile and less liable to preparation errors by hospital staff or parents. Unfortunately, they are both expensive and bulky for transport and storage. Products used for enteral feeding are described in Appendix III.1.

Modular products containing fat, protein or carbohydrate can be used to formulate an entire tube feed, thus allowing greater flexibility of content [30]. Details of modular products are given in Appendices IV.14 and IV.22.

Feeding different age groups
For those under 6 months of age, breast milk or a standard infant formula should be suitable. If nutrient requirements are high, it may be necessary to supplement with a milk fortifier in the case of breast milk, or with glucose polymers or fat in respect of an infant formula. In situations where an increased protein intake is indicated, formulas designed for preterm infants can be employed. After 6 months of age, infant formulas are generally used. However, beyond the age of 12 months, infant formulas fail to satisfy energy requirements if used as the sole source of nutrition. For infants and children over 12 months, specially designed complete pediatric formulas (see p. 381) are recommended. These formulas contain 1 kcal/ml (30 kcal/oz), equivalent to 1.48 kJ/ml (44.4 kJ/oz). The quantity of formula is determined by the fluid and energy requirements of the patient plus compensation for any energy deficit that may exist.

Energy supplements that provide over 1 kcal/ml can cause diarrhea and, in general, should be used only in patients requiring both an increased energy intake and fluid restriction. Hypercaloric formulas, if introduced too rapidly or used in large quantities, may result in diarrhea or gastric retention. Initiation of tube feedings as a constant infusion may be responsible for a small but increased number of liquid stools. However, this usually resolves within a few days.

Various products exist to meet the requirements of young children. Adult preparations usually supply more than the RDA for protein and sodium; however, provided levels of such are monitored, and vitamin and mineral deficits are supplemented, they offer an acceptable option if no pediatric formulas are available. Examples of tube feeds suitable for different age groups are shown in Appendix III.

Initiating tube feeding

Enteral feedings must be introduced gradually. Rapid increments can result in problems, particularly if the child has not been fed for more than 24 hours or has evidence of gastroesophageal reflux or malabsorption. Feedings should begin with a small volume given as regular bolus feeds or as an infusion over 20 or 24 hours. The volume can then be increased gradually until the child is on the full required volume to meet their nutritional needs. Increasing both the volume and concentration of the feed on the same day often provokes abdominal pain and diarrhea. When patients are also on intravenous regimes, decreases in parenteral fluids should be balanced with increases in enteral feeds.

Problems associated with tube feeding

Obstruction of the nasogastric tube may occur if it is inadequately rinsed after bolus feeding, especially if the tube is of the narrow-lumen polyurethane or Silastic type. A thick viscous tube feed containing discrete particles or a feed based on meat is the most likely to cause obstruction. Home-prepared feeds, whether derived from homogenized food or reconstituted powders, are more likely to cause obstruction than a commercially available ready-to-feed alternative. A solution with water and meat tenderizer or a cola drink injected through the tube may help resolve the obstruction.

The commonest problems are abdominal pain, flatulence and diarrhea. Sometimes these features can be resolved by advancing the regimen more gradually. If gastrointestinal symptoms occur the volume of feed should be decreased by 15–20%. The volume should gradually be increased over the next 2–3 days. If symptoms recur, administering the formula as a constant infusion should be considered; the rate can then be increased every other hour by 1–3 ml until the desired target – based on the condition and weight of the patient – is reached.

For young children, the carbohydrate concentration should not be above 10 g/100 ml (10%) and the fat content should not exceed 5 g/100 ml (5%). When such is tolerated, further increments in volume can be made. If the patient is receiving intravenous fluids and has good venous access, it may be easier to provide a low volume of full-strength enteral nutrition and increase the quantity progressively. This avoids wastage of formula if the patient does not tolerate a higher concentration, because the rate can be easily decreased. In contrast, in patients with poor intravenous access, it may be better to secure volume intake through the enteral route, followed by a gradual increase in the concentration.

Delayed gastric emptying may be due to decreased gut motility, as is seen in premature infants, in cases of intestinal inflammation and in the presence of primarily altered peristalsis. Alternatively, it may be the result of the bolus feeding of an over-concentrated hyperosmolar preparation. In such instances, a continuous infusion should be considered, and the volume of feeds decreased and subsequently gradually built up.

Overload of fluid and nutrients can occur if care is not taken in calculating the requirements of individual patients. RDAs for protein, fluid and sodium (Appendix I) should be particularly considered – excess protein, fluid retention and edema secondary to a high sodium intake will cause a raised level of blood urea, especially if the patient has hypoalbuminemia. In those on fluid restriction, the volumes of intravenous fluids and medications need to be added to the tally of fluids administered.

Weaning from enteral nutrition

The transition process varies depending on the age of the patient and the initial indications for the enteral feedings [31]. In premature infants, as their suck and swallow improves [32] and gut motility matures [33], the infant will progressively take more by mouth. In older children, periods of fasting may be necessary to elicit hunger and increase the amount of oral feedings. Tube supplements following the oral intake or nighttime supplementation may aid in the weaning process.

Monitoring

Growth, fluid intake, adjustments for differences in the seasonal ambient temperature and other nutritional parameters need to be supervised, particularly during the early phases.

Children on tube feeding require a team approach to ensure appropriate nutrition (nutritionist/dietician), continuation of development of oromotor skills and intake of nutrients by mouth whenever possible (speech therapist), appropriate support of the equipment and ostomy site (ileostomy/colostomy nurse practitioner) and psychological support whenever necessary [34].

PARENTERAL NUTRITION

Parenteral nutrition (PN) is one of the most innovative techniques to be introduced into pediatrics in the last 50 years. However, because of the development of enteral nutrition – using elemental diets and constant infusion techniques – PN is nowadays indicated less often than it has been. Although enteral nutrition is the preferred route of feeding, PN administered through a peripheral or central vein should be instituted without major delay whenever needs cannot be met by the enteral route. Advantages and disadvantages of intravenous nutrition are listed in Table 2.1.

Peripheral PN is sufficient in certain cases, while in others, central vein access, which allows for greater volumes and high glucose concentrations, is indicated (Table 2.2).

Total intravenous nutrition necessitates considerable clinical and pharmaceutical expertise and laboratory support to minimize biochemical, bacteriological and surgical complications. Infusates must be prepared aseptically. Experienced nursing care must be available to resolve problems related to the catheter, and the patient must be monitored closely.

Metabolic disturbances and/or dehydration must be corrected before PN is commenced.

Composition of infusions

The infusate should contain the following:

- Protein – crystalline amino acids

- Fat – lipids

- Carbohydrate – glucose

Advantages	Disadvantages
Guaranteed caloric intake	Risk of infection
Complete absorption	High cost
Relatively comfortable	Management requirements
Does not worsen gastrointestinal problems	Need for sophisticated infrastructure (nursing, medical, technical and laboratory)
High percentage of tolerance	
Socially acceptable (no visible tubing)	

Table 2.1 Advantages and disadvantages of intravenous nutrition.

Peripheral PN	Central PN
Nutritional status not severely compromised	Poor nutritional status
Patient able to tolerate some nutrition orally or enterally	Patient unable to tolerate any nutrition enterally
Recovery time predicted to be short	Expected prolonged need of nutritional support
Good venous access	Poor peripheral venous access

Table 2.2 Indications and requirements for total parenteral nutrition (PN).

- Electrolytes – sodium, potassium, chloride, calcium, phosphate and magnesium

- Metals/trace elements – zinc, copper, manganese, chromium and selenium (the role of iron in PN regimens is controversial)

- Vitamins – A, C, D, E, K, B_1 (thiamine), B_2 (riboflavin), niacin, pantothenic acid, B_6 (pyridoxine), B_{12}, biotin, choline (cofactor for enzymatic reactions) and folic acid

Acetate is used to correct metabolic acidemia.

Amino acids

Protein requirements can be met by providing the appropriate amounts of amino acids. The range in adults is from 0.5 to 3.5 g/kg/day. Blood urea, nitrogen and albumin should be monitored. To obtain information on recent protein synthesis, serum prealbumin, fibronectin or retinol-binding protein can be measured.

L-amino acids are preferred to D-amino acids because they are more effective in maintaining nitrogen balance and protein synthesis. There are a number of commercial preparations available. The latest amino acid solutions to be introduced, such as TrophAmine and Aminosyn PF, are formulated to meet the needs of premature infants. At times of specific nutritional needs, the non-essential amino acids may become essential or semi-essential. Furthermore, quite apart from the eight amino acids known to be essential for adults, histidine, proline and alanine are required by the young infant. Cystine and/or cysteine are also necessary for growth and so become semi-essential or essential, as opposed to non-essential, amino acids.

Nitrogen balance studies allow the clinician to ensure that the protein intake is at a safe level. The balance is the difference between nitrogen intake and nitrogen losses in the urine (as urinary urea), stools and sweat. Losses can also occur through the skin in burn patients. Starvation and infections result in a state of negative balance, and rapid growth a positive balance.

Lipids

Parenteral lipids provide high energy in a relatively small volume with a low osmolar load and are also a source of the essential fatty acids, linoleic and linolenic acids. Fat emulsion solutions are available as 10% or 20% preparations, with osmolalities of 280 mOsm/kg and 330 mOsm/kg, respectively. They are derived from soybean, safflower, or cotton-seed oil, with the fat mainly present as triglyceride. The ultimate total daily dose of parenteral lipid emulsion should not exceed 4 g/kg [35] and the infusion rate should be less than 0.25 g/kg/h. During the first week of life for low-birth-weight infants, the amount of lipids should not exceed 0.5–1 g/kg/day. The 20% emulsion provides approximately 2000 kcal/ml (8.4 MJ/l) and is cleared more rapidly than the 10% solution.

Lipid emulsions are contraindicated in the following chemical/biochemical circumstances:

- Serum bilirubin >100 μmol/l (6 mg/dl)

- Serum pH <7.25

- Serum triglycerides >7.8 mmol/l (300 mg/dl)

Free fatty acids may displace bilirubin from albumin in the neonate, with the risk of kernicterus [36]. Lipids may also interfere with platelet function and should be withheld if the count is less than $50,000 \times 10^9/l$ in the face of hypertriglyceridemia.

Infused lipid is hydrolyzed by lipoprotein lipase, an enzyme present in the endothelial cells of blood vessels. Lipids that are not cleared from the circulatory system are at greater risk of being deposited in the lung and brain, especially in the growth-retarded (IUGR) baby. Both the IUGR and the premature baby, as well as septic or severely stressed patients, are impeded in their ability to clear intravenous lipid particles.

Carbohydrate

Glucose is the sole monosaccharide used for intravenous nutrition. A solution with a glucose concentration of more than 10–12.5% is too hyperosmolar for peripheral use, while a concentration of up to 40% can be administered via a central line. The recommended amount of glucose to be infused is 10–20 g/kg/day. Urine must be closely monitored for glucose spillage. Patients who experience glucosuria, such as those who are infected, stressed or with cystic fibrosis, may benefit from the addition of insulin to the intravenous mixture (one unit of regular insulin per 10 g of glucose). Glycerol present in Intralipid is another source of carbohydrate. Other sugars such as fructose, galactose and sorbitol have been suggested, but fructose (via lactate and pyruvate) can cause a metabolic acidosis and hypoglycemia. In addition, sorbitol is metabolized to fructose.

Trace element	Infants*	Older children
Zinc	100–400 µg/kg	4,000 µg
Copper	10–40 µg/kg	1,600 µg
Chromium	0.1–0.4 µg/kg	16 µg
Manganese	2.5–10.0 µg/kg	400 µg
Selenium	1.5–2.0 µg/kg	8 µg
*weighing <2.5kg		

Table 2.3 Daily intravenous needs for some essential trace elements.

Vitamins

A multivitamin preparation, such as Multibionta Infusion (Merck) or MVI Pediatric (Amour), should be given daily. Multibionta given in dextrose saline at a rate of 0.15 ml/kg/day supplies all vitamin requirements. For MVI, the dose depends on the weight/age of the patient:

- ≤ 2.5 kg – 40% (2 ml) of an MVI Pediatric vial per kg per day

- >2.5 kg to 11 years – 1 vial (5 ml) of MVI Pediatric per day

- >11 years – 1 vial (10 ml) of MVI-12 + 20 µg of vitamin K per day

Minerals and trace elements

Iron is not part of the mineral preparation. Whenever needed, iron can be administered enterally, but if this is not tolerated most centers would give blood transfusions. To avoid leakage along the needle track with subsequent skin staining, a suitable injecting technique must be used. Because of the risk of allergic reactions, tolerance needs to be tested initially by giving small doses of iron under supervision.

Daily intravenous needs of some essential trace elements are listed in Table 2.3. Pediatric mineral supplements for addition to intravenous infusion are described on p. 378.

Aluminium toxicity is no longer a problem with current PN solutions in term infants and older children, but may still be of concern in preterm infants [37].

Technique of PN

Because there is a considerable risk of septicemia when using intravenous catheters, especially one that is centrally located, a peripheral or scalp vein should be used whenever possible. A 0.22-µm filter is recommended when using intravenous fluids.

Frequent repositioning of the infusion site (every 2 or 3 days) is advisable to avoid phlebitis. Ultimately, a catheter may need to be sited in a central vein under aseptic conditions.

Options include percutaneously inserted fine Silastic central venous catheters (0.64 mm inner diameter or 0.94 mm outer diameter) – longlines – and surgically placed Broviac catheters. Silicone catheters are inert, soft and radiopaque, and are thus less likely to cause thrombosis or

	Neonate		Child/Adolescent	
	Initial*	**Subsequently**	**Initial***	**Subsequently**
Strict I/O	Daily	Daily	Daily	Daily
Urinary glucose	Every void	Every shift	Every void	Every shift
Electrolytes, BUN	2–3 times per week	Every week	2–3 times per week	Every week
Ca, P, Mg	Every week	Every other week	2 times per week	Every week
Alkaline phosphatase, albumin	None	Every other week	Every week	Every other week
Triglycerides	4 h post initial infusion	With each change	4 h post initial infusion	With each change, then every week
Prealbumin	See below		See below	

*First 3–7 days, depending on the patient's stability
I/O = input and output; BUN = blood urea nitrogen

Prealbumin
Test 24–48 h post PN initiation to assess adequacy of protein intake. Monitor with any change in status or protein intake, or to assess adequacy of intake. May be falsely elevated with renal disease.

Triglycerides
If greater than 150 mg/dl (2 mmol/l), halve rate of infusion and retest to assess tolerance. Lipoprotein lipase is an inducible enzyme and tolerance to lipids will generally improve with time. Check baseline triglycerides in septic patients and in those with pancreatitis, renal disease or diabetes. If markedly elevated, the lipid infusion should be held for 12–24 h.

Ionized calcium
Check when serum calcium levels are altered by low albumin.

Zinc
Zinc status should be assessed in patients with increased gastrointestinal losses, inflammatory bowel disease, cystic fibrosis or fistulas.

Transaminases/bilirubin
Check monthly with patients on long-term PN (greater than 2 weeks) or PN-dependent patients.

Table 2.4 Monitoring of total parenteral nutrition (PN).

perforation. Furthermore, they inhibit fibrin formation. The site of the longline must be checked radiologically because, if the tip is within the heart, infusions could produce arrhythmias.

The use of peripherally inserted central venous catheters (PICCs) to provide prolonged intravenous access in children is increasing. PICCs have been shown to provide reliable and safe access for prolonged intravenous therapy in both neonates and children. In one study, 441 PICCs were inserted into 390 patients aged between 0 and 22 years [38]. No insertion complications occurred. Treatment of infectious disease was the most frequent reason (46%) for PICC insertion. The average catheter life was 13 ± 12 days. Similar complication rates with use in and out of hospital suggest that home intravenous therapy can be safely delivered with PICCs, thereby avoiding expensive hospitalization.

The concentrations of the nutrient solution in a PN regimen should be increased slowly over the first 4 days as follows:

Day 1. Provide necessary volume to cover fluid requirements. Use:

- Peripheral-strength (10–12%) glucose solution

- 20% Intralipid (or 10%) 0.5 g/kg

- Trophamine (or equivalent amino acid preparation)

Days 2–4. Increase progressively to provide total energy requirements, therefore:

- Double volume of Intralipid

- Double concentration of glucose

- Adjust concentration of amino acids

Some basic daily clinical measurements are essential whenever PN is initiated. The patient must be weighed, the total urine volume recorded and the quantity of any lost body fluids (e.g. via nasogastric or gastrostomy tubes) noted. A state of positive nitrogen balance should be attained because stools will be infrequent during PN, therefore there is little loss of nitrogen via the fecal route.

Lipids must be monitored by measuring serum triglycerides 4 h after initiation of the infusion, and also whenever the rate is increased or if the patient's clinical status deteriorates. Once a given rate of lipid infusion is well tolerated, serum triglycerides should be monitored less frequently (once a week to once a month).

Precautions and complications

Sepsis is the most frequent serious complication during PN, resulting in increased morbidity, mortality and healthcare costs [39]. A meticulous aseptic technique is essential when handling the infusion apparatus, particularly upon injecting into the system. Septicemia is more probable when central catheters are used. Common sources of infection include *Staphylococcus aureus*, *Staphylococcus epidermidis*, *Candida* species, *Pseudomonas* species and *Escherichia coli*.

Sudden termination of PN can cause hypoglycemia, particularly in malnourished patients. In patients on cyclic PN, the rate should be halved for 1 h prior to discontinuing it.

Cholestasis and, rarely, cirrhosis leading to liver failure are known hazards of PN in neonates and children with short-bowel syndrome [40]. There are data to suggest that intravenous amino acid mixtures play a role in the development of cholestasis in the very-low-birth-weight infant [41]. Oral administration of ursodeoxycholic acid (15–45 mg/kg/day divided into two or three doses) may improve cholestasis. Pancreatitis is a rare but possible complication [42]. There is a clear association between complete withdrawal of enteric feeding and intestinal mucosal atrophy as well as pancreatic hyposecretion. Non-enteral feeding causes a reduction in brush-border enzyme activity, therefore an early return to normal feeding is important. Small volumes of oral nutrients should be used whenever possible.

For details of monitoring during PN, see Table 2.4.

Regrading on to enteral nutrition

Oral feeds should be reintroduced very slowly with full PN back-up. Feeds should be given in small frequent doses. A suggested protocol for changing from PN to oral feeds is given in Appendix II.9.

REFERENCES

1. Ford EG. Nutrition support of pediatric patients. Nutr Clin Pract 1996;11:183–91.

2. Jenkins AP, Thompson RP. Enteral nutrition and the small intestine. Gut 1994;35:1765–9.

3. Lucas A, Bloom SR, Aynsley-Green A. Postnatal surges in plasma gut hormones in term and preterm infants. Biol Neonate 1982;41:63–7.

4. Vanderhoof JA, Hofschire PJ, Baluff MA et al. Continuous enteral feedings. An important adjunct to the management of complex congenital heart disease. Am J Dis Child 1982;136:825–7.

5. Ferry GD, Selby M, Pietro TJ. Clinical response to short-term nasogastric feeding in infants with gastroesophageal reflux and growth failure. J Pediatr Gastroenterol Nutr 1983;2:57–61.

6. Kuizon BD, Nelson PA, Salusky IB. Tube feeding in children with end-stage renal disease. Miner Electrolyte Metab 1997;23:306–10.

7. Miller TL, Awnetwant EL, Evans S et al. Gastrostomy tube supplementation for HIV-infected children. Pediatrics 1995;96:696–702.

8. Vanderhoof JA, Langnas AN. Short-bowel syndrome in children and adults. Gastroenterology 1997;113:1767–78.

9. Israel DM, Hassall E. Prolonged use of gastrostomy for enteral hyperalimentation in children with Crohn's disease. Am J Gastroenterol 1995;90:1084–8.

10. Di Lorenzo C, Flores AF, Buie T et al. Intestinal motility and jejunal feeding in children with chronic intestinal pseudo-obstruction. Gastroenterology 1995;108:1379–85.

11. Humphrey GM, Najmaldin A. Laparoscopic gastrostomy in children. Pediatr Surg Int 1997;12:501–4.

12. Behrens R, Lang T, Muschweck H et al. Percutaneous endoscopic gastrostomy in children and adolescents. J Pediatr Gastroenterol Nutr 1997;25:487–91.

13. Cosgrove M, Jenkins HR. Experience of percutaneous endoscopic gastrostomy in children with Crohn's disease. Arch Dis Child 1997;76:141–3.

14. Cory DA, Fitzgerald JF, Cohen MD. Percutaneous nonendoscopic gastrostomy in children. Am J Roentgenol 1988;151:995–7.

15. Marin OE, Glassman MS, Schoen BT et al. Safety and efficacy of percutaneous endoscopic gastrostomy in children. Am J Gastroenterol 1994;89:357–61.

16. Launay V, Gottrand F, Turck D et al. Percutaneous endoscopic gastrostomy in children: influence on gastroesophageal reflux. Pediatrics 1996;97:726–8.

17. Borowitz SM, Sutphen JL, Hutcheson RL. Percutaneous endoscopic gastrostomy without an antireflux procedure in neurologically disabled children. Clin Pediatr 1997;36:25–9.

18. Ponsky JL. Percutaneous endoscopic stomas. Surg Clin North Am 1989;69:1227–36.

19. Peters JM, Simpson P, Tolia V. Experience with gastrojejunal feeding tubes in children. Am J Gastroenterol 1997;92:476–80.

20. Kazi S, Gunasekaran TS, Berman JH et al. Gastric mucosal injuries in children from inflatable low-profile gastrostomy tubes. J Pediatr Gastroenterol Nutr 1997;24:75–8.

21. Strauss D, Kastner T, Ashwal S et al. Tubefeeding and mortality in children with severe disabilities and mental retardation. Pediatrics 1997;99:358–62.

22. Baker JH, Berseth CL. Duodenal motor responses in preterm infants fed formula with varying concentrations and rates of infusion. Pediatr Res 1997;42:618–22.

23. Belli DC, Seidman E, Bouthillier L et al. Chronic intermittent elemental diet improves growth failure in children with Crohn's disease. Gastroenterology 1988;94:603–10.

24. Berseth CL, Nordyke CK, Valdes MG et al. Responses of gastrointestinal peptides and motor activity to milk and water feedings in preterm and term infants. Pediatr Res 1992;31:587–90.

25. Lucas A, Bloom SR, Aynsley-Green A. Metabolic and endocrine events at the time of the first feed of human milk in preterm and term infants. Arch Dis Child 1978;53:731–6.

26. Aynsley-Green A, Adrian TE, Bloom SR. Feeding and the development of enteroinsular hormone secretion in the preterm infant: Effects of continuous gastric infusions of human milk compared with intermittent boluses. Acta Paediatr Scand 1982;71:379–83.

27. Cooke RJ, Embleton ND. Feeding issues in preterm infants. Arch Dis Child Fetal Neonatal Ed 2000;83:F215–8.

28. Schanler RJ, Shulman RJ, Lau C et al. Feeding strategies for premature infants: Randomized trial of gastrointestinal priming and tube-feeding method. Pediatrics 1999;103:434–9.

29. Silvestre MA, Morbach CA, Brans YW et al. A prospective randomized trial comparing continuous versus intermittent feeding methods in very low birth weight neonates. J Pediatr 1996;128:748–52.

30. Davis A, Baker S. The use of modular nutrients in pediatrics. J Parenter Enteral Nutr 1996;20:228–36.

31. Schauster H, Dwyer J. Transition from tube feedings to feedings by mouth in children: Preventing eating dysfunction. J Am Diet Assoc 1996;96:277–81.

32. Lemons PK, Lemons JA. Transition to breast/bottle feedings: The premature infant. J Am Coll Nutr 1996;15:126–35.

33. Tawil Y, Berseth CL. Gestational and postnatal maturation of duodenal motor responses to intragastric feeding. J Pediatr 1996;129:374–81.

34. Mascarenhas MR, Redd D, Bilodeau J et al. Pediatric enteral access center: A multidisciplinary approach. Nutr Clin Pract 1996;11:193–8.

35. American Academy of Pediatrics Committee on Nutrition. Pediatric Nutrition Handbook, 4th ed. American Academy of Pediatrics,1998.

36. Morris S, Simmer K, Gibson R. Characterization of fatty acid clearance in premature neonates during intralipid infusion. Pediatr Res 1998;43:245–9.

37. Bishop NJ, Morley R, Day JP et al. Aluminum neurotoxicity in preterm infants receiving intravenous-feeding solutions. N Engl J Med 1997;336:1557–61.

38. Thiagarajan RR, Ramamoorthy C, Gettmann T et al. Survey of the use of peripherally inserted central venous catheters in children. Pediatrics 1997;99:E4.

39. Yeung CY, Lee HC, Huang FY et al. Sepsis during total parenteral nutrition: Exploration of risk factors and determination of the effectiveness of peripherally inserted central venous catheters. Pediatr Infect Dis J 1998;17:135–42.

40. Misra S, Ament ME, Vargas JH et al. Chronic liver disease in children on long-term parenteral nutrition. J Gastroenterol Hepatol 1996;11:S4–6.

41. Brown MR, Thunberg BJ, Golub L et al. Decreased cholestasis with oral instead of intravenous protein in the very low birth weight infant. J Pediatr Gastroenterol Nutr 1989;9:21–7.

42. Dabbas M, Colomb V, de Potter S et al. Pancreatitis in children on long-term parenteral nutrition. Transplant Proc 1996;28:2782.

Acknowledgement

We would like to thank Claudia Conkin, MS, RD, LD, Director of the Dietary Department of Texas Children's Hospital, Houston TX for allowing us to use tables from the Pediatric Nutrition Reference Guide, 1999 Fifth Edition. Conkin C, Jennings H, Phillips S, Eds.

chapter 3

Protein–Energy Malnutrition

Public Health is purchasable. Within natural limitations any community can determine its own death rate.

Hermann M Biggs (1859–1923)

The first possibility of rural cleanliness lies in water supply.

Florence Nightingale (1820–1910)

Protein–energy malnutrition (PEM) includes marasmus, kwashiorkor and intermediate deficiencies. These disorders can be grouped together: indeed, some workers regard marasmus as successful adaptation to nutritional stress and kwashiorkor as representing the failure of an attempted adaptation. A comparison of marasmus and kwashiorkor is given in Table 3.1.

Worldwide, more than 15 million children die annually from malnutrition and associated infections. Mortality can be very high in underdeveloped countries except for those patients taken to specialized resuscitation centers.

PEM is a spectrum of disease ranging from life-threatening kwashiorkor and marasmus to deficiencies of specific dietary constituents such as zinc [1], folate or vitamin A. Most children with severe PEM who live in the developing world have parasitic infections, commonly due to *Giardia lamblia*, *Strongyloides stercoralis* or *Ascaris lumbricoides*. Immunological deficit secondary to malnutrition, combined with gastric achlorhydria and altered peristalsis, accounts for intestinal colonization and subsequent diarrhea.

PEM is not limited to non-industrialized countries. Fad and strict vegetarian diets, medically unsupervised elimination regimens and diseases such as uncontrolled gastroesophageal reflux, immunodeficiency syndromes, anorexia nervosa, congenital heart disease, inflammatory bowel disease, cystic fibrosis, neuromuscular disorders and cancer all have the potential for causing PEM. In congenital or acquired immunodeficiency, as well as malabsorption and increased intestinal losses, anorexia plays an important role in causing PEM. The loss of appetite can be the consequence of intercurrent infections [2], abdominal pain and distension secondary to bacterial and/or parasitic infestation of the bowel.

DEFINITION/CLASSIFICATION

Many classifications to delineate the syndromes of PEM have been suggested. The Wellcome Committee categorization, which is both simple and practical, is based on the presence of

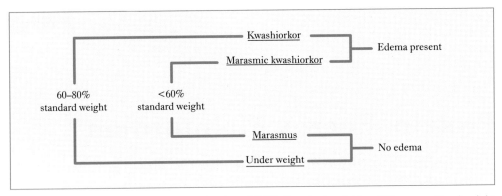

Figure 3.1 Wellcome Committee categorization of PEM. Standard weight = 50th percentile of weight for age (Harvard growth standards).

	Marasmus	Kwashiorkor
Weight	↓ ↓ ↓	↓ ↓
Edema	– – –	+ + +
Depigmentation	– – –	↑ ↑ ↑
Hair changes	±	+ +
Vitamin levels	↓ ↓ ↓	↓ ↓
Small intestine – villous atrophy	+ +	+ + +
Lactase/sucrase/maltase	↓ ↓	↓ ↓ ↓
Pancreatic enzymes	↓	↓
Fatty liver	+	+
↓ = slightly reduced; ↓ ↓ = moderately reduced; ↓ ↓ ↓ = markedly reduced.		

Table 3.1 Comparison of marasmus and kwashiorkor. Modified from Gryboski J, Walker WA. *Gastrointestinal Problems in the Infant*, 2nd ed. Philadelphia: WB Saunders, 1983.

edema and weight for age (Fig. 3.1) [3]. Alternatively, the severity of PEM can be determined by expressing the actual weight as a percentage of the expected weight of a healthy child of the same age using a standard:

- First degree (mild) – 89–75% of expected weight for age
- Second degree (moderate) – 74–60% of expected weight for age
- Third degree (severe) – <60% of expected weight for age

CHARACTERISTICS

Conditions such as reduced gastrointestinal motility, prolonged transit time and potassium depletion are common in PEM and can exacerbate this syndrome (Fig. 3.2). Bacterial overgrowth of the upper gastrointestinal tract can also occur.

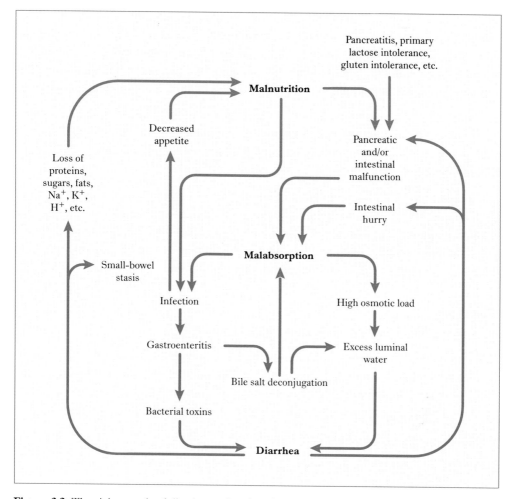

Figure 3.2 The vicious cycle of diarrhea and malnutrition. (Courtesy of WF Balistreri.)

Intestinal villous atrophy of various degrees is a common feature in PEM. Damage to the microvilli is more severe in protein-deficient children (kwashiorkor) than in those with energy deficiency (marasmus). In addition, the epithelial cells of the villi, bearing the brush-border disaccharidases, become injured, thereby resulting in carbohydrate malabsorption. Protein-losing enteropathy can occur as a consequence of small-bowel bacterial overgrowth. Iron deficiency, from intestinal bleeding, is well known, e.g. with hookworm infections (*Necator* species and *Ancylostoma* species). The loss of blood and mucus from the bowel (e.g. with *Entamoeba histolytica*) causes hypoproteinemia and this exacerbates PEM. Blood losses can also arise from vitamin K deficiency.

Hypercatabolism may develop as a consequence of systemic infections. Because immunocompetence is compromised in malnutrition, there is an increased susceptibility to infections. Tuberculosis and bronchopneumonia are important secondary problems. A major viral complication of PEM is measles, which has a high mortality in malnourished infants.

Some species of bacteria deconjugate bile acids and thus impair absorption of lipid-soluble and fat-soluble vitamins. A reduced bile acid pool results in decreased micelle formation and impaired fat absorption. There is also an atrophy of the pancreas in kwashiorkor. Abnormalities of the liver are common in PEM, and dietary toxins (e.g. aflatoxin) will increase hepatic deterioration. Infections and diarrhea are responsible for a decline in nitrogen absorption.

The absorption of simple carbohydrates by facilitated diffusion is impeded in severe PEM, and hexose absorption (active transport) is often reduced. There is edema of the gut, and many nutrients (including vitamin B_{12}) are malabsorbed. Atrophy of the gastric mucosa and hypochlorhydria are also seen.

During prolonged PEM, the decreased synthesis of insulin-like growth factor-1 (IGF-1) and the low level of insulin and/or its diminished effect, due to an insulin-resistant status in the presence of high circulating levels of growth hormone and cortisol, ensure substrate diversion away from growth toward metabolic homeostasis. Leptin appears to be an important signal in the process of metabolic/endocrine adaptation to prolonged nutritional deprivation [4].

TREATMENT

The main principles in the management of PEM are:

1. Correct dehydration and electrolyte imbalance (by enteric or intravenous route) (see Chapter 2). In the presence of wasting, it can be difficult to assess the severity of the dehydration. Mild dehydration can often be dealt with orally or by a nasogastric tube. Vomiting or persistent diarrhea is an indication for the intravenous route (see p. 44).

2. Treat underlying infection(s) and/or parasitic infestations.

3. Treat other deficiencies and associated conditions, for example:

   - Iron deficiency

   - Folate deficiency

   - Vitamin A deficiency

   - Vitamin K deficiency

   - Magnesium deficiency

   - Hypoglycemia

   - Candidiasis

   - Scabies

4. Nutritional rehabilitation ('catch-up' growth). Anthropometric measurements and the use of appropriate reference charts or standards are essential for the proper assessment of growth [5] (see Appendix I for standards). By the very simple act of measuring mid-upper arm circumference (MUAC), community health workers in Bangladesh could predict the 56% of children who would die within a month [6]. MUAC is a better screening technique than other anthropometric indices at identifying those at high risk

of death from invisible malnutrition in underprivileged communities. An MUAC of less than 110 mm denotes obvious malnutrition. The process of refeeding needs to be slow because potential fluid shifts in patients with severe hypoproteinemia may cause brain edema and death (see below) [7].

INFECTION

Pneumonia and septicemia (usually Gram-negative organisms) are the most common fatal infections. Some recommend antibiotics for severely malnourished infants even when the infection cannot be identified [8]. The catabolic effect of infections increases nutrient requirements and worsens the malnutrition.

DEFICIENCIES

Vitamin A (see page 2)

Vitamin A deficiency is one of the most common disorders seen in PEM. The WHO estimated, in 1991, that about six to seven million new cases of xerophthalmia occur every year and that three million children under the age of 10 years are blind at any one time. Even in the absence of xerophthalmia, vitamin A should be given according to the following regimen:

1. Infants aged 1 year or less should receive a single dose of vitamin A, administered either by intramuscular injection (15 mg) or orally (30 mg). Children aged over 1 year should be given 30 mg by intramuscular injection (single dose) or an oral dose of 60 mg/day for 2 days only.

2. Then, when patients have recovered from PEM, one oral dose of 30 mg should be given (infants aged ≤1 year) or 60 mg (those aged >1 year).

3. Finally, patients should take oral multivitamins providing 0.9–1.5 mg of vitamin A per day – in populations where deficiency is widespread this should be continued throughout childhood.

Anemia

Whole blood should be used where hemoglobin is under 4 g/dl (maximum volume 10 ml/kg over 3 h) [9].

REFEEDING – ACUTE PHASE

Once rehydration has been corrected, small milk feeds should be given slowly every 2 h. If the child is breastfeeding, every effort must be made to ensure this continues. It is preferable to use a cup and spoon for the non-breastfed child, but nasogastric feeding may be needed if an insufficient volume is consumed. A cautious and slow approach to refeeding is recommended. Initially, only half-strength feeds may be tolerated; a suggested schedule is shown in Table 3.2. Stabilization can be achieved on maintenance amounts of protein and energy; a suitable feed is given in Appendix III.11. Feeding in this way reduces the risks of cardiac and liver failure and lessens the probability of the child developing secondary lactose intolerance, hypoglycemia and hypothermia.

Day	Strength of feed	Number of feeds per day
1	Half	12
2	Half	8
3, 4	Two-thirds	8
5 and onward	Full	6

Table 3.2 Feeding schedule for a severely malnourished child based on 150 ml/kg/day. Adapted from Cameron M, Hofvander Y. Manual on Feeding Infants and Young Children, 3rd ed. Oxford: Oxford University Press, 1983.

As the appetite returns, the volume of full-strength feeds can be increased to 110 ml/kg/day, giving a daily intake, per kilogram, of 110 kcal (462 kJ) and 2 g of protein. Provided the child is passing urine, potassium (4 mmol/kg/day), magnesium (2 mmol/kg/day) and a multivitamin preparation should be given.

REHABILITATION

Once full-strength feeds are tolerated, intake can be stepped up to initiate weight gain. Administration of 150 ml/kg/day of a high-energy feed – supplying approximately 200 kcal/kg (840 kJ/kg) and 4.5 g protein/kg daily – divided into five or six parts, enables catch-up growth to take place over 4 to 6 weeks. Although fortification is needed to meet energy requirements, expensive protein preparations are unnecessary. If milk is both available and culturally acceptable, it can be fortified with sugar and oil to give a high-energy feed containing adequate protein (Appendix III.8). The staple cereal can form the basis of a feed, but, owing to its bulky nature, it has a low-energy density; hence, it needs to be fortified, preferably using local produce.

Weight-against-height should be plotted weekly, so that recurrent infection or inadequate intake can be identified. A record of food intake is valuable as it may explain poor weight gain. Mild diarrhea commonly persists. Unless the diarrhea is serious, the high-energy feed will not need diluting.

When fluids are reintroduced, the amounts initially need to be small. In nutrition rehabilitation centers, solids are introduced early in the recovery phase and the emphasis is on parental education to avoid recurrence of PEM.

An introductory regimen for cereals has to be carefully planned. High-energy feeds can be continued until normal weight-for-height has been achieved. The child is then given the usual diet, which will vary according to local custom, availability and preference for certain produce. A nutritionally adequate basic mix should contain a cereal, which might be rice or maize; a protein, for example pulses, beans, milk, chicken, fish or eggs; a vitamin and mineral source, for example dark leafy vegetables; and fat or oil for energy. Fruit juice and fresh fruit should be given at an early stage in the child's recovery.

Commercially processed weaning foods are widely available throughout the world but are too costly in less developed countries. Mothers need to be informed that their use is not essential and that a nutritionally adequate local mixture is satisfactory.

Hospitalized children with severe PEM should not be discharged until they have reached their target weight and can tolerate family food. This is of importance where facilities for monitoring progress are not available. The ability of children recovering from PEM to achieve full catch-up growth is unclear, because they commonly come from low socioeconomic groups and are likely to be shorter than infants from more affluent families. An increased growth velocity can be maintained for many months provided that an adequate energy intake is achieved.

Often, home conditions and standards of hygiene are such that the mother may be unable to follow any complex hospital regimen. Prevention through education is of prime importance if the high prevalence of PEM is to be reduced. Health workers must convey clear and concise information. Above all, education has to be appropriate to local economic/agricultural conditions and social circumstances.

Early intervention by parents can halt the development of PEM. Families need to know how to use, to their infants' optimal advantage, the locally available foods. Local household utensils and cooking methods should be supported as they have evolved in response to the prevailing conditions for that specific community.

REFERENCES

1. Doherty CP, Sarkar MA, Shakur MS et al. Zinc and rehabilitation from severe protein-energy malnutrition: Higher-dose regimens are associated with increased mortality. Am J Clin Nutr 1998;68:742–8.

2. Friedland IR. Bacteraemia in severely malnourished children. Ann Trop Paediatr 1992;12:433–40.

3. Waterlow JC. Classification and definition of protein-calorie malnutrition. BMJ 1972;3:566–9.

4. Soliman AT, El Zalabany MM, Salama M et al. Serum leptin concentrations during severe protein-energy malnutrition: Correlation with growth parameters and endocrine function. Metabolism 2000;49:819–25.

5. Motil KJ. Sensitive measures of nutritional status in children in hospital and in the field. Int J Cancer 1998;11(Suppl.):2–9.

6. Briend A, Wojtyniak B, Rowland MG. Arm circumference and other factors in children at high risk of death in rural Bangladesh. Lancet 1987;2:725–8.

7. Akinyinka OO, Adeyinka AO, Falade AG. The computed axial tomography of the brain in protein energy malnutrition. Ann Trop Paediatr 1995;15:329–33.

8. Gernaat HB, Dechering WH, Voorhoeve HW. Mortality in severe protein-energy malnutrition at Nchelenge, Zambia. J Trop Pediatr 1998;44:211–7.

9. Van Den Broeck J, Eeckels R, Vuylsteke J. Influence of nutritional status on child mortality in rural Zaire. Lancet 1993;341:1491–5.

chapter 4

Selected Inborn Errors of Metabolism

Currently, there are more than 300 known inborn errors of metabolism. However, only a relatively small proportion can be treated by dietary manipulation, and discussion in this chapter will be limited to these. Table 4.1 outlines the types of metabolic errors that may respond to nutritional intervention.

INITIAL DIAGNOSIS

The majority of disorders present in the neonatal period. Typically, the infant is normal at birth and gives no cause for concern for a period of several hours or even days. (A few conditions do not manifest until some weeks after birth, while intermittent types can remain undiagnosed until childhood or are only revealed during periods of metabolic stress such as an intercurrent infection.) The infant then deteriorates and does not respond to symptomatic treatment. The neonate has only a limited range of responses to overwhelming illness of any kind. Thus, the major features of undiagnosed metabolic disease are general or non-specific; they often include poor feeding, failure to gain weight, weight loss, vomiting, lethargy, seizures and hypoglycemia. The symptoms may resemble infection – indeed, sepsis often coexists initially with metabolic disease. For a full review of the management of neonates with suspected metabolic disease, see [1].

Intravenous feeding or clear feeds can reverse the situation as the harmful nutrient intake decreases. However, before such an improvement is achieved, it is essential to send blood and urine to the laboratory while there are sufficient metabolites to identify. A high index of suspicion of metabolic disease is of paramount importance. Some hospital laboratories provide thin-layer chromatography of amino acids but specialist biochemical help will be needed as many organic acids can only be identified by gas chromatography or mass spectrometry [1]. Table 4.2 summarizes the main investigations that should be carried out on all infants where there is unexplained deterioration or a family history of sudden and unexplained infant death(s) [2].

Feeds prior to diagnosis

Where a life-threatening condition is suspected, infants should be placed on a protein-free feed as a temporary measure after blood and urine samples have been appropriately stored to establish the diagnoses. The feed should consist of a high concentration of carbohydrate, preferably glucose polymers, with added vitamins and minerals. A suggested regimen is given

Nutrient	Type of disorder	Intervention
Amino acids	Metabolism of essential amino acid(s): • Phenylketonuria • Maple syrup urine disease	Restriction of one or more specific amino acids
	Metabolism of non-essential amino acids and carbon skeletons of amino acids: • Organic acidemias • Urea cycle defects	Restriction of precursor essential amino acids and/or restriction of total protein
Carbohydrates	Metabolism of complex carbohydrates (glycogen): • Glycogen storage diseases	Restriction of total carbohydrate and control of % energy from protein and fat
	Metabolism of monosaccharides: • Galactosemia • Hereditary fructose intolerance	Restriction of specific monosaccharides and disaccharides containing them
Fat	Metabolism of lipids: • Hyperlipidemias	Restriction of total fat and control of % energy from protein and carbohydrate
	Metabolism of fatty acids: • Fatty acid oxidation defects • Refsum's disease	Restriction of specific fatty acids

Table 4.1 Metabolic conditions that respond to nutritional treatment.

in Appendix V.13 and an energy intake of at least 100 kcal (420 kJ) per kilogram of body weight should be aimed for. In the initial stages, fat should be avoided as it can exacerbate ketosis.

DISORDERS OF NITROGEN AND AMINO ACID METABOLISM

The metabolic fate of protein and possible disorders are outlined in Figure 4.1. Dietary protein is digested into amino acids that form part of the body nitrogen pool. Amino acids are used to synthesize body protein; those in excess of requirements or the amount that is required to make up for an energy deficit are catabolized into the carbon skeleton, which is metabolized via the tricarboxylic acid (TCA) cycle to release energy and carbon dioxide. The nitrogen molecules resulting from the deamination of the amino acid are catabolized via the urea cycle to produce urea, which can be excreted in the urine. In defects involving specific amino acids, such as phenylketonuria, maple syrup urine disease and homocystinuria, the metabolic block occurs before catabolism of amino acids begins. Disorders of the carbon skeleton pathway cause the organic acidemias such as propionic acidemia and methylmalonic aciduria, whereas those of the nitrogen excretion pathway are responsible for urea cycle defects such as citrullinemia and ornithine transcarbamylase deficiency.

There are two major methods of dietary manipulation for the treatment of this type of inborn error. The first decreases the total nitrogen intake as in some organic acidurias and urea cycle defects where toxic products of protein metabolism accumulate but plasma levels of

	Test	Result indicative of metabolic disease
Urine	Smell and color	Abnormal smell or color
	Ketones	Present
	Acetone	Present
	pH	Acidosis
	Reducing substances	Present
	Organic acids	Present
Blood	Glucose	Hypoglycemia (<2 mmol/l)
	Liver function tests	Transaminases ⇑
	Electrolytes	Increased anion gap
	Lactate	>4 mmol/l
	pH	<7.3
	pCO_2	<30 mmHg
	HCO_3	<10 mmol/l
	Ammonia	>100 μmol/l
	Amino acids	Abnormal pattern

Table 4.2 Investigations for suspected metabolic disease.

amino acids remain normal. In contrast, the amino acid pattern of the diet can be altered if the metabolic error has resulted in elevated plasma levels of one or more essential amino acids or their direct metabolites. Furthermore, some amino acids may become essential because of a metabolic block and these must be added to the diet in adequate quantities. The diet must also contain sufficient nitrogen, minerals and vitamins for normal growth and development. Energy is particularly important in all these regimens, to prevent tissue breakdown and release of toxic metabolites.

PHENYLKETONURIA

Phenylketonuria (PKU) is a recessively inherited inborn error of metabolism with a prevalence of 1:10,000 in Caucasian populations. The gene is located on the long arm of chromosome 12 in the region of q22–q24.1 [3]. The disorder is normally caused by a deficiency or absence of the hepatic enzyme phenylalanine hydroxylase (PAH) (Fig. 4.2), and more than 300 mutations of the PAH locus have been identified. The enzyme defect varies from complete absence up to about 25% of normal values [4]. The hyperphenylalaninemias show a spectrum of clinical and biochemical phenotypes. In 'classic' PKU, plasma phenylalanine levels rise to in excess of 1000 μmol/l (16.5 mg/dl) and PAH activity is less than 1% of normal values. In persistent hyperphenylalaninemia or 'atypical' PKU, levels of plasma phenylalanine will reach 200–1000 μmol/l (3.3–16.5 mg/dl) and residual enzyme activity is usually 2–5% of normal. In the condition 'malignant' PKU or tetrahydrobiopterin (BH$_4$) deficiency – seen in 2% of infants with hyperphenylalaninemia – mutations of 6-pyruvoyl-tetrahydrobiopterin synthase (6-PTS) result in a lack of BH$_4$, a cofactor for phenylalanine, tyrosine and tryptophan hydroxylases, leading to a deficiency of dopamine and serotonin in the brain. This condition does not respond well to a restricted phenylalanine diet and the main treatment is the administration of BH$_4$, serotonin and L-dopa/carbidopa. For a full review of the biochemical background of the different forms of PKU see [5,6].

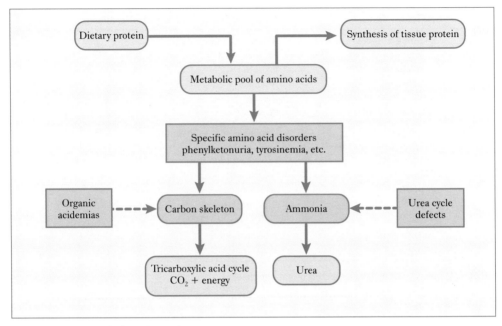

Figure 4.1 Metabolic fate of protein.

Diagnosis

PKU is detected by neonatal screening programs in many countries. Whole blood is obtained from a heelprick between 6 and 14 days of life and analyzed for phenylalanine. In the USA a heel prick test is usually done within the first 24–48 hours, whilst the infant is still in hospital. Blood for screening should be obtained after feeding proteins, to reduce the possibility of false-negative results. Diagnosis is based on the finding of persistent hyperphenylalaninemia of at least 400 μmol/l (6.6 mg/dl) on a normal diet and should be confirmed by a careful laboratory study of phenylalanine metabolites (phenylpyruvic and hydroxyphenylacetic acids) in freshly passed urine (see Fig. 4.2) as well as a BH_4 assay. It is recommended that treatment should begin by day 20 [7]. Prenatal diagnosis of classic PKU has been made by DNA analysis of amniotic fluid cells.

Clinical features

Infants with PKU, if untreated, present with severe mental retardation and may have an IQ of less than 30. Ultimately, only 3% of untreated PKU patients achieve an IQ above 50. Many are both fair-haired and fair-skinned with blue eyes and some have eczema. About one in four have seizures and approximately one-third are hypertonic; hyperactivity and autistic behavior are common [8]. Most children who have started a special diet early in life (<4 weeks old) have an IQ within the normal range, though there is evidence that the IQ of PKU children is about 0.5 standard deviations below that of the general population [9]. In older children, difficulties in information processing, organizational skills and abstract reasoning have been reported [10,11]. Cognitive function is related to the quality of blood phenylalanine control, particularly in the early years [12]. Older age at commencement of

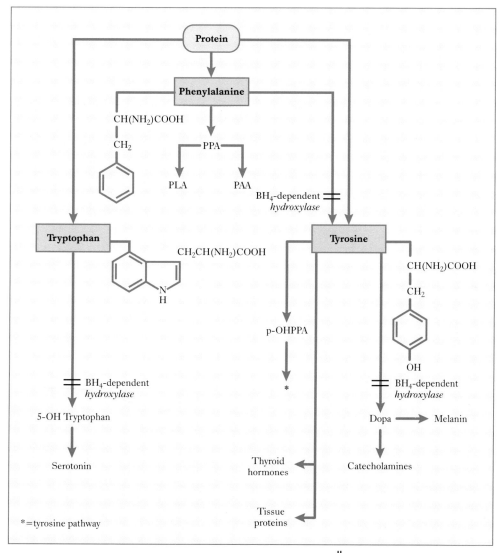

Figure 4.2 Metabolism of phenylalanine, tyrosine and tryptophan. ‡ is the enzyme dependent on biopterin cofactors (BH$_4$). PPA, PLA, and PAA represent phenylpyruvate, phenyl-lactate, and phenylacetate, respectively, metabolites from phenylalanine. *p*-OHPPA is the corresponding *p*-hydroxy metabolite from tyrosine.

diet, as well as a higher frequency and longer duration of episodes of blood phenylalanine concentrations above 400 μmol/l (6.6 mg/dl), are all associated with a reduction in IQ [13].

Dietary management

The nutrient requirements for a child with PKU are not significantly different from the normal recommendations. Phenylalanine tolerance will depend upon the nature and severity of the enzyme defect and the child's age and growth velocity. Requirements given in Table 4.3 are theoretical – the correct amount of phenylalanine for an individual is one that

Age	Phenylalanine (mg/kg body weight)	Protein from protein substitute (g/kg body weight)	Total protein* (g/kg body weight)
Premature infants	90†	3.5	4.0
0–3 months	50–90	3.0	3.6
3–6 months	50–80	3.0	3.5
6 months– 1 year	30–50	3.0	3.4
1–3 years	20–30	2.0–3.0	2.5–3.5
4–6 years	15–25	1.5–2.0	1.7–2.5
7–9 years	15–25	1.0–1.5	1.2–1.7
10+ years	10–20	1.0	1.5
Pregnancy	15–30	1.0	1.3

*Total protein consists of the natural protein plus the protein equivalent provided by the substitute as stated by the manufacturer.
†From [14]

Table 4.3 Nutrient requirements in phenylketonuria (PKU).

results in normal growth and development. Because of the nature of the enzyme deficiency, tyrosine becomes an essential amino acid and must be supplemented. The exact requirement for tyrosine in PKU is not known, but it has been shown to be a limiting amino acid in some regimens during periods of rapid growth [14].

Phenylalanine
Requirements for phenylalanine are monitored by regular and frequent estimations of plasma levels. Normal values are 30–70 μmol/l (0.5–1.2 mg/dl); it is customary to maintain levels slightly above this. From 0 to 4 years, plasma phenylalanine concentrations should be maintained between 120 and 360 μmol/l (2–6 mg/dl). From 5 to 10 years, the acceptable range is 120–380 μmol/l (2–6.3 mg/dl); and from 11 years onward, 120–700 μmol/l (2–11.7 mg/dl) [7]. The US recommendations for values of phenylalanine are <10 years 120–240 μmol/l (2–4 mg/dl) and >10 years 120–485 μmol/l (2–8 mg/dl). Average values for tolerance are given in Table 4.3. Children with classic PKU usually tolerate 200–500 mg of phenylalanine daily; in infants the tolerance per kilogram of body weight is higher than for children because of the high growth velocity at this age. It is recommended that blood is tested weekly for the first 4 years, once every 2 weeks between ages 5–10 years and once a month for children aged 11 and over and adults [7].

Protein
Protein requirements are shown in Table 4.3. Dietary protein intakes should be slightly higher than basic requirements, as the majority of protein is taken in the form of an artificial substitute. These products are fully described in Appendices V.7 and V.8. Because the

recommended dietary allowances (RDAs) are based on intact protein, it is important that the phenylalanine allowance is given at the same time as the protein substitute so that a full range of amino acids is taken. The substitute should be divided into at least three portions per day in order to improve utilization [15].

Energy

The provision of an adequate energy intake is vital in order to prevent catabolism of body tissues, with associated release of phenylalanine, into the circulation; hence, the recommendations for infants and children with PKU are a little above the RDA for the general population [16]. The rate of weight gain should be monitored to ensure that the intake is not excessive.

Other nutrients

The artificial nature of the diet is such that vitamins, minerals and trace elements will be inadequately supplied as a result of the limited amounts of natural foods allowed. Supplements are either integrated with the protein substitute or are recommended by manufacturers. It is important that the correct mineral, vitamin and trace element supplements are taken with the corresponding protein substitute (Appendix II.14 lists supplements). The optimal balance of micronutrients in such supplements has not been determined. Low bone mineral density and low serum calcium and magnesium levels have been described in children with PKU [17]. Low plasma zinc values [18], low ferritin and retinol values [19], vitamin B_{12} deficiency [20] and poor selenium status [21–23] have all been noted in PKU children receiving restricted phenylalanine diets.

Infants

The theoretical quantity of phenylalanine, protein and energy should be calculated for the individual infant. The type and amount of natural protein that will provide the phenylalanine is decided upon according to whether the mother wishes to breastfeed. The phenylalanine content of milks is shown in Table 4.4. The remaining protein and energy is derived from the selected protein substitute. Breastfeeding should be encouraged as there are advantages for the PKU infant: breast milk is naturally low in phenylalanine, thus breastfed infants are able to take a greater quantity of natural protein compared with those receiving formula milk. In addition, the benefits of breast milk for optimal cognitive development are particularly important. Infants with classic PKU will be unable to tolerate full breastfeeding and will need a protein substitute. The intake of breast milk must be varied in response to blood phenylalanine levels and this can be achieved by altering the quantity of protein substitute offered.

Formula feeding

The calculated volumes of protein replacement and milk are each divided into equal portions according to the feeding pattern. A whey-dominant, as opposed to casein-dominant, infant milk should be selected as the former is lower in phenylalanine (see Table 4.4). A certain amount of flexibility is allowed regarding the consumption of the protein substitute, because it is impossible to predict individual needs and energy requirements. The quantity of normal formula given is adjusted according to blood phenylalanine levels.

Product	Content per 100 g			
	Protein (g)	Phenylalanine (mg)	Energy	
			(kJ)	(kcal)
Human milk, mature	1.3	46	293	70
Cow milk	3.4	180	280	67
Casein-dominant baby milk (reconstituted liquid)	1.9	100	275	65
Whey-dominant baby milk (reconstituted liquid)	1.5	56	275	65

Table 4.4 Phenylalanine contents of milks.

Solid foods

Weaning foods or Beikost should be introduced at the normal time, i.e. from about 4–6 months of age. Initially, very small quantities of low-protein, low-phenylalanine foods such as fruits and vegetables can be offered; however, when larger amounts of solid food are consumed, the phenylalanine content must be counted as part of the daily allowance. In the USA it is usual to calculate all solid foods as part of the daily allowances of phenylalanine.

Older children

Because all protein-containing foods include phenylalanine, an exchange system similar to that used for diabetic diets has been developed. In the UK, the exchange system is based on 1 fluid ounce (30 ml) of milk, which contains 50 mg of phenylalanine; fruit and vegetables containing less than 1.5 g of protein per 100 g are usually allowed freely without being measured (Appendix V.9). In the USA, exchanges of food are based on 30-mg and 15-mg portions, and most fruit and vegetables are counted as exchanges (Appendix V.10). If the phenylalanine content of a food has not been determined, it can be calculated, provided the protein content is known, using the data listed in Table 4.5. Foods that are very high in protein, such as meat, fish, cheese and eggs, are not normally included in a low-phenylalanine diet. Some naturally occurring foods are low enough in protein to be included in the diet without their phenylalanine content being counted.

It is important in older children that the phenylalanine allowance and the protein substitute are given at the same time; the quantity of natural protein and its substitute should each be divided into at least three equal portions per day. There is evidence that consuming protein substitute on a 'little-and-often' basis results in a better blood phenylalanine profile [24].

For the older child receiving an amino acid preparation, it is important to include special proprietary products, based on wheatstarch or cornstarch, to achieve the energy requirements. Such products include low-protein breads, cookies and pasta, and are available in the USA, the UK and most other European countries.

Illness

It is most important to avoid weight loss and other catabolic states, because the breakdown of body protein will release phenylalanine into the body pool. Infection or intercurrent illness

Food	Phenylalanine content (mg/g of protein)
Milk, dairy products, meat, poultry, fish	
Cereals, pulses, peas, beans, lentils, nuts	50
Potato	
Dark-green leafy vegetables	40
Other vegetables, fruits	30
Mixed sources (e.g. manufactured foods)	50

Table 4.5 Phenylalanine content of proteins.

usually results in high serum phenylalanine levels. To minimize this, intake of high-energy, low-protein drinks should be encouraged (as described in Appendix V.3). If the protein substitute is rejected, it is safe to omit this for a few days, although continued consumption will minimize the rise in blood phenylalanine levels. Consumption of the phenylalanine allowance can continue, as it makes a relatively small contribution to the body pool compared with protein breakdown. The vitamin, mineral and trace element supplement may be safely omitted for a few days.

Derestriction of diet

Although former recommendations stated it was safe to discontinue the strict phenylalanine restriction in adolescence, subsequent research has indicated that this is not the case. The risk of intellectual deterioration decreases with age, but other neurological signs have been demonstrated in young people with PKU [10,25]. Some centers have found no intellectual deterioration several years after relaxing the diet in early childhood [26,27], while others have noted an effect on intelligence [28]. A compromise to discontinuing the diet is to allow the plasma levels to rise to 700 μmol/l (11.7 mg/dl). This permits the consumption of some normal foods, such as ordinary breads, and makes the diet more socially acceptable. However, it should be noted that plasma levels above 400 μmol/l (6.6 mg/dl) do cause brain abnormalities detectable on magnetic resonance imaging [13]. Continued consumption of the protein substitute at least once daily should be encouraged as there is evidence that it helps keep plasma phenylalanine levels low. This substitute will also provide tyrosine and tryptophan, precursors of neurotransmitters, which may become deficient because of the metabolic block. Poor nutritional status of vitamins and trace elements has been described in adolescents with PKU, and the protein substitute chosen should include a full range of micronutrients. It is particularly important for girls to continue with the substitute as they will need to recommence a strict low-phenylalanine diet prior to pregnancy [29].

Pregnancy

The other important dietary management issue relates to maternal PKU prior to and during pregnancy. By 1980, 110 PKU mothers in the USA had given birth to more than 200 damaged children, according to figures presented at a meeting of the US Collaborative Study [30].

More recent experience has shown that PKU mothers who begin a low-phenylalanine diet prior to conception and who maintain good control throughout pregnancy have better outcomes in terms of the infant's physical development [31,32], although there may still be some intellectual impairment in the offspring [33,34]. The UK Medical Research Council have recommended that blood levels should be 60–250 μmol/l (1–4.2 mg/dl) prior to conception and should remain at this level throughout pregnancy [12]. This requires a good deal of commitment by the woman, her family and her medical team.

Diet in tetrahydrobiopterin deficiency

A low-phenylalanine diet does not prevent abnormal features developing. Nevertheless, the diet is necessary because high phenylalanine concentrations limit neurotransmitter synthesis. Often, the plasma phenylalanine levels are not as elevated as in classic PKU and the infant has a high tolerance to the amino acid. The diet is the same as for classic PKU and the overall aim is to keep blood levels between 120–360 μmol/l (2–6 mg/dl). Phenylalanine tolerance improves with age: often, the child can accept a diet containing a moderate amount of protein (see Table 4.6) without the need for supplements by the age of 2 years [35].

UREA CYCLE DISORDERS AND HYPERAMMONEMIA

Catabolism of amino acids results in the formation of ammonia, which at high levels is toxic to the central nervous system (CNS). The synthesis of urea in the liver is the major route of its removal.

Known metabolic disorders are associated with each of the five hepatic enzymes involved in urea synthesis (Fig. 4.3). This group of disorders is characterized by the triad of encephalopathy, respiratory alkalosis and hyperammonemia [36]. These conditions may present acutely in the neonatal period or at any time in childhood or adult life, particularly during periods of stress such as intercurrent infection or weight loss. Clinical symptoms common to all urea cycle disorders may include vomiting, intermittent ataxia, irritability, lethargy, mental confusion, coma and aversion to a high-protein diet. Neonatal presentation is fairly rapid, with neurological symptoms, especially seizures and coma. Infants who present later generally show less acute and more generalized symptoms. Older children can exhibit acute or chronic neurological illness. The symptoms of arginase deficiency (hyperargininemia) differ from the other four conditions in having an insidious onset and more closely resemble cerebral palsy, although the neurological findings are progressive and may suggest a degenerative CNS condition. A number of other metabolic disorders, including organic acidemias, also present with hyperammonemia in the neonatal period, and urea cycle diseases may be wrongly diagnosed as Reye's syndrome [37]. Prognosis depends upon the age at presentation and the severity of the symptoms, and is generally poor in infants with encephalopathy. Frequent periods of decompensation are common and may be precipitated by infection, fasting or physical trauma. Prompt action is necessary as these episodes are life threatening.

The urea cycle has two major functions: to convert ammonia to the non-toxic nitrogen waste product urea and to synthesize the amino acid arginine (see Fig 4.3). All disorders of urea

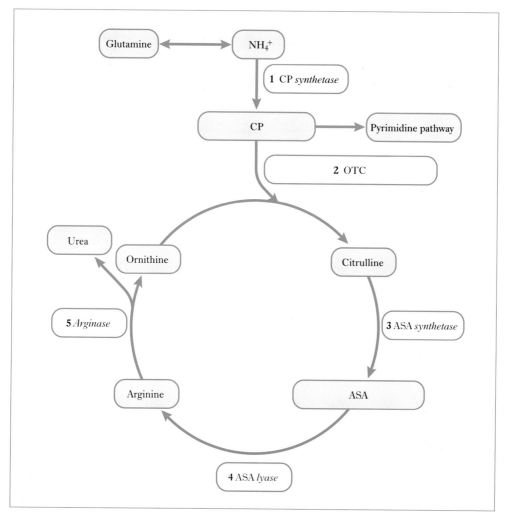

Figure 4.3 Enzymes in the urea cycle: (1) carbamyl phosphate (CP) synthetase; (2) ornithine transcarbamylase (OTC); (3) arginosuccinate (ASA) synthetase; (4) arginosuccinate lyase; (5) arginase.

synthesis cause ammonia intoxication, but this varies in proportion to the proximity of the block to the entry of ammonia into the cycle. Ammonia is toxic to the CNS because it increases the transport of tryptophan into the brain, which in turn leads to increased serotonin production [38]. Glutamine accumulates in plasma, as glutamate is the principal donor of nitrogen molecules into the urea cycle. Osmotic shifts caused by raised plasma glutamine levels are thought to be responsible for the cerebral edema that is seen in acute encephalopathy [39]. Disturbed levels of amino acids may be detected in the urine in arginosuccinate synthetase deficiency, arginosuccinase deficiency and arginase deficiency (see Fig 4.3).

In all defects of the urea cycle, except for arginase deficiency, arginine becomes an essential amino acid as it cannot be synthesized from precursors in the pathway. Therefore, it must be included as a supplement to the diet. Quantities required vary according to the disorder,

Age	Average minimum requirement* g protein/kg/day	Safe minimum intake[†] g protein/kg/day
0–1 month	1.99	2.69
1–2 months	1.54	2.04
2–3 months	1.19	1.53
3–4 months	1.06	1.37
4–5 months	0.98	1.25
5–6 months	0.92	1.19
6–9 months	0.85	1.09
9–12 months	0.78	1.02
1–1½ years	0.79	1.0
1½–2 years	0.76	0.94
2–3 years	0.74	0.92
3–4 years	0.72	0.90
4–5 years	0.71	0.88
5–10 years	0.69	0.86

	Girls		Boys	
	Average req.	Safe intake	Average req.	Safe intake
10–11 years	0.70	0.86	0.69	0.86
11–12 years	0.69	0.86	0.69	0.86
12–13 years	0.69	0.86	0.71	0.88
13–14 years	0.68	0.84	0.69	0.86
14–15 years	0.66	0.82	0.69	0.86
15–16 years	0.66	0.81	0.68	0.84
16–17 years	0.63	0.78	0.67	0.83
17–18 years	0.63	0.78	0.65	0.81

*Average minimum requirement – statistically will only meet the minimum requirements of approximately 50% of the population.
[†]Safe minimum intake – average minimum requirement + 2 standard deviations. Should meet the minimum requirements of approximately 97.5% of the population.

Table 4.6 Minimum protein requirements for infants and children. Adapted from [43].

but are usually within the range of 100–150 mg/kg in carbamyl phosphate synthetase deficiency and ornithine transcarbamylase deficiency, but may be as high as 700 mg/kg in arginosuccinate synthetase deficiency and arginosuccinase deficiency. The aim is to maintain plasma arginine levels within the normal range (50–200 μmol/l). For a full review of the biochemistry of the urea cycle disorders, see [39].

Most defects resulting in primary hyperammonemia respond to therapy with substances that increase nitrogen excretion by providing alternative pathways. For example, sodium benzoate is conjugated with glycine in the liver and each mole removes one molecule of nitrogen as hippurate from the metabolic pool. However, this is no longer commonly used because phenylbutyrate, which is oxidized to phenylacetate, conjugates with glutamine in the liver and removes two molecules of nitrogen in the form of phenylacetylglutamate. Doses range from 250–650 mg/kg/day [40].

The basis of dietary treatment is a low-protein diet, with the aim of decreasing plasma ammonia and glutamine levels. The plasma ammonia level should be kept below 80 μmol/l [39] and plasma glutamine less than 800 μmol/l [41]. The quantity of protein tolerated is monitored by assay of plasma ammonia, essential amino acid and glutamine levels.

Because of the poor prognosis and frequent episodes of decompensation, liver transplantation has been used to improve the condition of children with urea cycle disorders. Provided the procedure is carried out early, liver transplantation can be effective in correcting the hyperammonemia and preventing further neurological deterioration [42].

Dietary management of urea cycle disorders

Protein

Suggested protein requirements are given in Table 4.6 [43] according to age. These are lower than the dietary reference values (Appendix I.2) and can be regarded as the minimum safe intake level in order to achieve normal growth and development. As well as supplying an adequate amount of total nitrogen, the diet must also provide sufficient essential amino acids as these cannot be synthesized by the body. This is best achieved by giving the maximum amount of protein in the form of high biological value protein from meat, fish, eggs, cheese and milk. However, in practical terms, this may be difficult to achieve as children with inborn errors are typically poor and fussy eaters. A further drawback to the use of animal-protein foods is their relatively low energy content and bulk compared with vegetable and cereal-based foods. For example, 10 g of egg and 30 ml of cow milk both provide 1.0 g of protein and 15 and 20 kcal, respectively, whereas 70 g of potato is equal to 1.0 g of protein and 60 kcal.

Protein tolerance in urea cycle defects is normally in the region of 1.8–2.0 g/kg/day in infancy, decreasing to 1.2–1.5 g/kg/day during childhood and 0.5–1.0 g/kg/day after growth has stopped. If protein tolerance falls below the minimal suggested intake, the use of an essential amino acid mixture should be considered as a supplement to the diet to replace some of the natural protein; suitable products are listed in Appendix V.11. These supplements have an unpleasant taste and reduction of the natural protein intake renders the diet even more unpalatable. An increase in medication such as phenylbutyrate should be tried before this step is considered. Natural protein is measured in 1 g protein exchanges (Appendix V.2). In the USA the protein in minimal protein foods such as fats, fruits and vegetables is usually counted as part of the daily allowances for protein; however, in the UK a small variety of minimal protein foods are generally allowed freely.

Energy

Energy requirements are at least equal to those of children of similar age and size (Appendix I.1). An adequate and regular energy intake is essential in the management of inborn errors. Periods of fasting will cause breakdown of body tissue and the release of ammonia and glutamine into the system. Chronic undernutrition results in suboptimal growth, poor metabolic control and decreased protein tolerance. The amount of energy derived from natural foods and any amino acid supplement is insufficient to meet energy requirements. Supplements such as fat and carbohydrate (Appendices IV.16 and IV.17) and low-protein milk substitutes (Appendix V.3) provide important energy sources, while the inclusion of specialized low-protein products such as bread, biscuits and pasta adds variety as well as protein-free energy to the diet.

Minerals and micronutrients

The diet should provide at least the reference nutrient intake for minerals, vitamins and trace elements (Appendices I.3–I.7). The food contained in a restricted-protein diet such as this will be unlikely to supply sufficient minerals or micronutrients. Unless the child has a high tolerance for protein, it will be necessary to provide a complete mineral and micronutrient supplement (Appendix II.14). This should ideally be taken in a divided dose during the day to optimize nutrient utilization.

ORGANIC ACIDEMIAS

Organic acidemias comprise a heterogeneous group of disorders. The most common are those of propionate metabolism, methylmalonic acidemia and propionic acidemia. The enzyme blocks involved in these diseases occur widely throughout metabolism; disorders treatable by diet mainly involve the catabolism of a number of essential amino acids. The organic acid is not an amino acid but a substance that accumulates anywhere along catabolic pathways in fat, carbohydrate or protein metabolism; in fact, at any site in intermediary metabolism. Figure 4.4 describes the metabolic processes and disorders leading to organic acidemias. For a full review of the biochemistry of organic acidemias, see [44–46].

Presentation

Some will be ketotic (e.g. in methylmalonic acidemia, propionic acidemia, ketothiolase deficiency, maple syrup urine disease and isovaleric acidemia). Others, however, are not characterized by ketosis (e.g. 3-hydroxy-3-methylglutaric acidemia and acyl CoA dehydrogenase deficiency).

Many have an acute neonatal presentation with symptoms commonly including metabolic acidosis, dehydration as a result of acidosis, poor feeding, lethargy, vomiting, hypotonia, neutropenia and hypoglycemia. These symptoms may be misdiagnosed as acute gastrointestinal obstruction. Some conditions result in hyperammonemia, and the presenting picture may be very similar to urea cycle disorders. Typically, the rare glutaric aciduria type 1 has a less acute presentation, though infants are usually macrocephalic at birth. An increasing head circumference, ataxia and extrapyramidal symptoms develop more gradually. For all organic acidemias, the interval between birth and onset of symptoms may range from a few hours to several weeks, although some conditions only present in childhood, adulthood or during metabolic stress such as infection. Elevated plasma amino acids are not generally a feature of the organic acidemias, except in maple syrup urine disease, and diagnosis is generally by the identification of organic acids in the urine. In some of these disorders, diagnosis is established by assay of the relevant enzyme from leukocytes

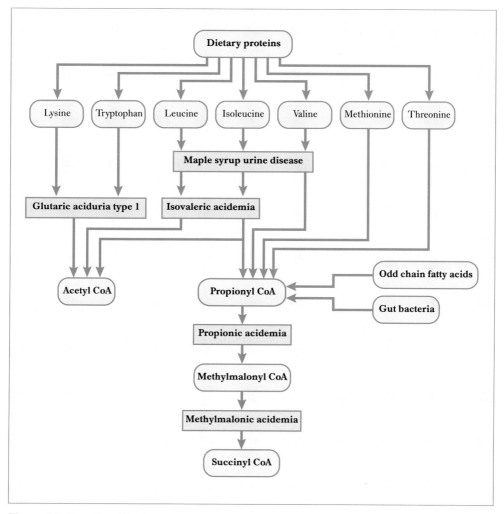

Figure 4.4 Organic acidemias.

and cultured fibroblasts. Prenatal diagnosis is sometimes possible by enzyme studies in aminocytes or chorionic villus samples. The subject is dealt with more fully by Saudubray et al. [47,48]. Other symptoms that develop later in individual conditions include renal lesions in methylmalonic acidemia and skin disorders, and alopecia and cardiomyopathy in methylmalonic and propionic acidemia. It is unclear whether or not some of these symptoms are due to dietary micronutrient deficiencies.

Infants and children who present with acute neurological symptoms suggestive of an organic acidemia should have protein removed from their feed and be given an emergency regimen as described in Appendix V.13. Because of the toxicity of a number of metabolites produced (e.g. isovaleric acidemia and β-ketothiolase deficiency), other means of reducing metabolite levels, such as hemofiltration, hemodialysis and exchange transfusion, should be considered [49]. Infants and children suffering from organic acidemias are prone to sudden episodes of decompensation which are life-threatening and appropriate therapy such as intravenous rehydration and withdrawal of protein from the diet should be instituted rapidly. Outcome depends upon the condition and its severity. Isovaleric acidemia has the best prognosis. Many patients with the other organic acidemias do not survive infancy, and most of those who do are left with a considerable degree of neurological and cognitive handicap [50]. Liver or liver plus kidney transplants have been successfully used in methylmalonic acidemia [51].

Many organic acid disorders have a vitamin-responsive and a non-responsive form. For example, methylmalonic aciduria can be due to a deficiency or mutation of methylmalonyl CoA mutase or cobalamin co-enzyme synthesis and improve with vitamin B_{12} therapy [52]. Propionic acidemia can be biotin responsive because this is the cofactor for propionyl CoA carboxylase, the defective enzyme in this disorder. Some forms of glutaric acidemia type I respond to riboflavin therapy [53].

Glycine can be used as an addition to the diet in isovaleric acidemia as it increases excretion of isovalerate. Carnitine supplementation (50–100 mg/kg/day) is used in a number of organic acidemias, partly to correct dietary deficiencies but also because it increases excretion of substances such as propionate and glutarate. Supplementation should be considered in all patients with a serum free carnitine less than 15 μmol/l. Gut bacteria are an important source of propionate in propionic acidemia and this can be suppressed by intermittent doses of an antibiotic such as metronidazole.

Dietary management of organic acidemias

Where the condition is not completely responsive to cofactor therapy, some form of dietary manipulation is required. A low-protein diet is the method used to control the metabolic disturbance. The aims of dietary treatment are to reduce the accumulation of toxic metabolites, to prevent catabolism and to provide sufficient nutrients for optimal growth and development. The amount of protein tolerated depends upon the patient's age, size, growth velocity and degree of responsiveness to cofactor therapy. The maximum tolerated amount of protein from natural foods should be allowed. If protein tolerance is below the minimum suggested intake (see Table 4.6), there are a number of synthetic amino acid mixtures that are free of the relevant precursor amino acids (Appendix V.11), although the routine inclusion of these in the diet has not been fully evaluated [54]. Children with isovaleric acidemia are usually able to tolerate sufficient natural protein to meet requirements without supplements. In methylmalonic and propionic acidemia, methionine, isoleucine, threonine and valine are restricted in the diet either by limiting total protein, ensuring adequate amounts of essential amino acids, or by use of a diet with measured amounts of methionine, isoleucine, threonine and valine and additional protein and essential amino acids provided by a special formula. In glutaric acidemia type I, lysine tolerance determines the natural protein intake and supplements of tryptophan may be necessary.

Plasma and urinary organic acids should be monitored to ensure that the protein intake is not excessive; plasma amino acid pattern and levels, and also weight and height velocity, should be studied to confirm the adequacy of protein for growth. Energy and micronutrient intakes should be as outlined in the management of urea cycle disorders (see p. 73). Deficiencies of essential fatty acids have been described [55]: blood levels must be monitored and appropriate supplements given where indicated.

Infants and children with organic acidemias often show poor appetite and hence frequently require the diet to be delivered by means of an enteral tube. Overnight feeding via a gastrostomy has been shown to improve nutritional status and symptoms in some of these disorders [56].

DISORDERS OF CARBOHYDRATE METABOLISM

Disorders of carbohydrate metabolism that respond to dietary intervention (excluding those whose primary feature is carbohydrate malabsorption) comprise those of monosaccharide metabolism – such as galactosemia, hereditary fructose intolerance and fructose-1,6-biphosphatase deficiency – and diseases of glycogen storage. The main aim of the dietary management of monosaccharide disorders is the elimination of the monosaccharide and replacement by an alternative carbohydrate, while providing a regimen that is adequate for all nutrients. In the glycogenoses, the purpose is to prevent excess glycogen storage and hypoglycemia. For a full review of carbohydrate disorders see [57–59].

DISORDERS OF FRUCTOSE METABOLISM
Deficiency of fructokinase (benign fructosuria)
This is an innocent and asymptomatic autosomal recessive condition, with a prevalence of 1:120,000. It is detected by the insignificant finding of a reducing sugar in the urine (positive Clinitest reaction) and a negative Clinitest response (as the urine carbohydrate is not glucose). The condition can be diagnosed by chromatography, which will reveal fructose in the urine.

Deficiency of fructose-1,6-biphosphate aldolase (aldolase B) (hereditary fructose intolerance)
This serious and potentially fatal disease may appear in early infancy with hypoglycemia and hepatomegaly. It presents when fructose, sucrose (table sugar – a disaccharide) or the artificial sweetener sorbitol is ingested.

Deficiency of fructose-1,6-biphosphatase
This condition affects gluconeogenesis and its main features are hypoglycemia and acidosis secondary to the accumulation of acetate and ketones.

Management
The diet of the infant normally does not contain fructose prior to the introduction of solid foods, although symptoms may present early in infants fed on a sucrose-containing soya milk. Sucrose is the main source of fructose in foods, and the diet should exclude all sources of added sugar. Some natural foods, particularly fruits, contain fructose and sucrose. The artificial sweetener sorbitol is converted to fructose in the liver. Appendix IV.27 describes the fructose content, and IV.28 the sucrose content, of foods.

In hereditary fructose intolerance, the aim is to exclude virtually all sources of fructose from the diet and to keep the intake below 2.0 g/day. Foods containing starch, lactose and glucose are allowed freely provided there is no added sucrose. Sucrose and sorbitol are often used in liquid medicines and to coat drugs in tablet form, therefore carbohydrate-free sources of drugs should be prescribed. Fructose, a monosaccharide, is not essential in a normal diet so the regime should be maintained for life.

In fructose-1,6-biphosphatase deficiency, the main aim is to reduce hypoglycemia by avoiding fasting and through frequent feeding using lactose during infancy, and starch during childhood. Strict avoidance of fructose is not necessary when the child is well, although concentrated sources of sucrose are likely to exacerbate hypoglycemia. During periods of illness, it is particularly important to avoid fasting and to provide a continuous or frequent (hourly) feed containing glucose. Furthermore, a diet containing minimal amounts of fructose and sucrose should be followed.

GALACTOSEMIA

Galactose is one of the constituent monosaccharides formed upon the hydrolysis of lactose. Galactosemia is the term used for three disorders caused by defects in the catabolic pathway of galactose. These are depicted in Figure 4.5. Without transferase (galactose-1-phosphate uridyl transferase), the infant cannot metabolize galactose-1-phosphate and so the substrate accumulates and damages the parenchymal cells of the kidney, liver and brain. Such damage may begin prenatally by transplacental transfer of galactose originating from the diet of a heterozygous mother. A diagnosis of transferase deficiency should be considered in a newborn with jaundice, hepatomegaly, failure to thrive, aminoaciduria and/or sepsis caused by *Escherichia coli*.

Deficiency of galactokinase is characterized by galactosemia, galactosuria and cataracts without mental impairment or aminoaciduria. Delayed diagnosis may result in cataracts being formed via galactose derived from lactose in the milk (breast or standard formula).

Classic galactosemia is the most common of the disorders, with an incidence of 1:60,000 in the USA and 1:45,000 in the UK. The gene is located on chromosome 9, and the most common mutation, $Q^{188}R$, exists in 72% of patients with classic galactosemia [60]. The condition presents in the first week of life with jaundice, liver failure, renal tubular defects and cataracts. Early diagnosis is essential in order to prevent irreversible liver damage and death. If galactosemia is suspected, it is important that the infant receives a lactose-free milk immediately, rather than awaiting a confirmatory test. Prior to stopping milk feeds, a urine sample should be tested for reducing substances and glucose. A positive test for reducing sugars and a negative reaction for glucose are indicative of galactosemia. Diagnosis is established by measuring the erythrocyte galactose-1-phosphate levels (>5 mg/100 ml or 150 μmol/l red cells). A Beutler test for galactose-1-phosphate uridyl transferase activity is often used now as an initial investigation. Both of these tests may yield false-negative results after a blood transfusion [61], but concentrations remain high for some weeks after milk feeds have ceased.

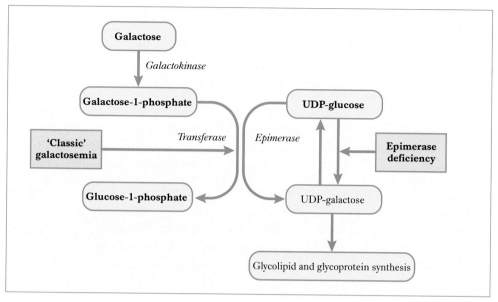

Figure 4.5 Galactose metabolism. UDP-glucose=urdine diphosphoglucose;
UDP-galactose=uridine diphosphogalactose.

Despite early diagnosis and good dietary compliance, the prognosis for galactosemia remains uncertain. Neurodevelopmental delay is common; speech and cognitive function are particularly affected, though most children manage attendance at a normal school [62,63].

In galactokinase deficiency, levels of galactose-1-phosphate uridyl transferase are normal. This condition is characterized by galactosemia, galactosuria and cataracts, but no mental retardation or hepatic enlargement. Galactitol formed from galactose is responsible for the cataracts.

The main aim of treatment is to exclude all dietary lactose, which is the main source of galactose. Other potential dietary sources are free and bound galactose found in a number of fruits and vegetables, galactosides and galactolipids in organ meats such as liver and kidney and galactose-containing oligosaccharides present in some leguminous vegetables (e.g. peas, beans and lentils). These sources are small compared with endogenous galactose production, although some pediatricians exclude these foods for the first 2 years of life. There continues to be some debate as to whether or not they should be restricted beyond that time. Most medicines that are in tablet form contain lactose as a filler, therefore lactose-free soy-based alternatives should be prescribed. The need for dietary restriction is lifelong and there is no justification for relaxing the dietary restriction at any age, as hepatic symptoms and cataracts will reappear. The galactose content of foods is described in Appendix IV.26. Starch, glucose and sucrose are allowed freely. For infants, breastfeeding is contraindicated since breast milk contains lactose. The formula of choice is an infant lactose-free preparation (Appendix IV.3), and not one with a reduced lactose content (Appendix IV.1) as even the residual lactose in these is harmful. In infants with liver damage, feeds initially may need to be a lactose-free protein hydrolysate containing medium-chain triglycerides (MCTs), such as Pregestimil (see Appendix IV.5). The diet in older children tends to be low in calcium, and poor bone mineralization as well as osteoporosis have been described [61]. A lactose-free calcium source and a vitamin D supplement should be considered in all children with galactosemia.

Dietary treatment needs to be lifelong because intellectual ability can deteriorate when the diet is derestricted. Furthermore, adolescents and adults should avoid alcohol, as galactose elimination is inhibited by ethanol. Monitoring of erythrocyte galactose-1-phosphate levels must be carried out regularly on all galactosemic individuals to ensure that dietary compliance is adequate. Levels of substrate must be maintained below 3 mg/100 ml.

A homozygous mother should receive a low galactose diet prior to her pregnancy and dietary advice ought to be reinforced. In addition, red cell galactose-1-phosphate levels must be checked early in pregnancy because free galactose and galctitol can damage the fetal eye. It is also thought that galactose in the heterozygous mother's blood can cause damage to a homozygous fetus; therefore many centers place the heterozygous mother on a low galactose diet. However, the value of this procedure has been questioned.

The long-term outcome of even early diagnosed and treated galactosemic children is disappointing in that impaired intellect and visual-perceptual difficulties may still be evident. The reasons for this may include damage occurring *in utero*, delayed neonatal diagnosis, poor dietary compliance that remains undiscovered due to infrequent biochemical monitoring and the possibility that galactose is a semi-essential nutrient in the neonate. Perhaps the current dietary management is too rigid or is not strict enough. Further research is needed to determine the optimum regimen for galactosemia.

GLYCOGEN STORAGE DISORDERS (GLYCOGENOSES)

These diseases (types 0–XI) can be classified according to the specific enzymatic defect or the presence of distinctive clinical features. Abnormal lysosomes are the hallmark of glycogen storage disorder (GSD) II (Pompe disease). Most, but not all, are characterized by the presence of hepatomegaly and hypoglycemia.

A number of secondary biochemical abnormalities are the result of hypoglycemia-induced disturbances of hormones regulating glucose homeostasis and these can cause significant morbidity in older children and adults [64]. There are many different enzyme defects resulting in a large number of types and subtypes of the condition. GSD I and III are the most common forms that present in childhood and are managed with nutritional intervention. Figure 4.6 outlines pathways of glycogen metabolism and associated disorders.

The presentation of GSD types I and III is similar, with hypoglycemia, hepatomegaly and failure to thrive being the major symptoms. Both tend to present within the first few months of life, although GSD III may become evident much later. Fasting hypoglycemia is pronounced in GSD I and rare in GSD III. In type I, where the defect occurs at the conversion of glucose-6-phosphate to glucose, blood glucose levels are entirely dependent on an exogenous glucose supply; in type III, glucose can be synthesized by gluconeogenesis and so a continuous exogenous source is not as important.

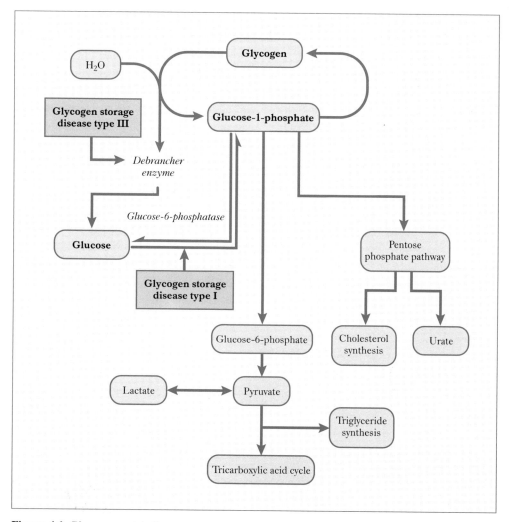

Figure 4.6 Glycogen metabolism.

Management

GSD type I

Frequent (2-hourly) feeds are required and continuous nasogastric tube infusions are necessary overnight. Glucose requirements are estimated at 0.5 g/kg/h in infants, and this is provided by the carbohydrate in a normal infant formula. If an insufficient volume of formula is consumed, a glucose polymer (Appendix IV.17) can be added. In older infants, starchy foods (Appendix IV.28) can replace the carbohydrate from formula milk and the volume can therefore be decreased. The use of concentrated sugary foods should be avoided, as rapid absorption of glucose leads to glycogen deposition.

Overnight feeds can be changed to a small volume of a solution containing 20 g of glucose polymer per 100 ml when the infant no longer requires a milk-based overnight preparation, although there may be some advantages in continuing with a protein-containing formula [65].

Glucose requirement decreases to 0.3–0.4 g/kg/h in childhood and to 0.2–0.25 g/kg/h in adolescents and adults. At about 2 years of age, uncooked cornstarch can be introduced into the diet. This is digested and absorbed more slowly than monosaccharides or disaccharides and helps maintain blood glucose levels for up to 4–6 h [66]. A dose of uncooked cornstarch is given mixed with water or diet drink after each meal of the day. This decreases the need for 2-hourly starch meals or glucose drinks and allows for a more normal meal pattern. A dose before bedtime in older children may permit termination of the continuous overnight feed, but the child would need to wake after 6 h to take a further cornstarch drink. Each dose of cornstarch should contain 2 g/kg for young children, 1.5 g/kg for older children and 1 g/kg for adults.

GSD type III

Treatment is very similar to that for type I in the early stages, although glucose intake does not need to be as precise. Two-hourly feeds during the day and a continuous overnight regimen are implemented, as in type I. The need for 2-hourly carbohydrate and continuous overnight feeds decreases as the child gets older. Between the ages of 4 and 9 years, the feed interval can be increased up to 6 h, depending on fasting tolerance, though a regular pattern is required. Because glucose can be synthesized from protein, it is usual in older children to give a diet that is relatively high in protein – usually comprising 20–25% of the normal energy intake. Carbohydrate should contribute 50–55% of the energy intake; fat remains relatively low, equaling 20–25% of the energy intake. After the age of 2 years, uncooked cornstarch can be introduced as for GSD I. In GSD III, uncooked cornstarch has been shown to be as efficacious in maintaining glycemia as a high-protein diet and has also resulted in improved growth [67].

DISORDERS OF LIPID AND FATTY ACID METABOLISM AND CARDIOVASCULAR DISEASE

There are several points in the metabolic pathway of lipids and fatty acids where defects give rise to pathologic conditions. Dyslipidemias result from abnormalities in the formation, modification and removal of lipoproteins, while fatty acid oxidation disorders are the consequence of defects in mitochondrial oxidation to yield energy. Figure 4.7 outlines lipid metabolism and its disorders.

FACTORS ASSOCIATED WITH CARDIOVASCULAR DISEASE

Atherosclerosis is a generic term for different patterns of occluding arterial disease seen in developed countries; it is common in North America, Europe and Russia. Events leading to the development of atherosclerotic vascular deposits are outlined in Figure 4.8. There are two major sets of factors involved: the formation of the intimal plaque and the adhesion of cells to the atheroma. Histologically, the initial phase is an accumulation of groups of foam cells (macrophages filled with cholesterol ester). Although total serum cholesterol is one of the major determinants of coronary heart disease, it is the amount carried in the low-density lipoprotein (LDL) fraction that appears to be the most important. Raised values of LDL cholesterol are a strong risk factor for cardiovascular disease, whereas elevated levels of high-density lipoprotein (HDL) are associated with a reduced likelihood of disease. Synthesis and

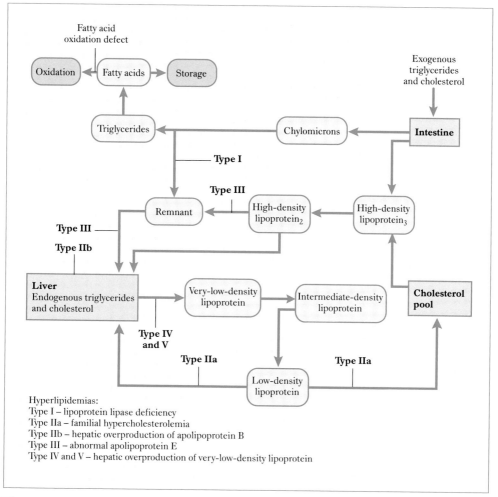

Figure 4.7 Lipid metabolism and its disorders.

metabolism of lipoproteins are controlled by apoproteins, and plasma levels of these are mainly genetically determined. Apolipoprotein B (apoB) comprises 90% of the protein content of LDL and is a major component of very-low-density lipoprotein (VLDL), also associated with an increased risk of cardiovascular disease independent of cholesterol levels. Apolipoprotein A (apoA) is the main protein in HDL. Intermediate-density lipoprotein (IDL) is a transient product formed during the conversion of VLDL to LDL – it is not detectable in normal plasma.

The LDL cholesterol fraction may be modified by oxidation or glycosylation, taken up by macrophages and deposited in the atheromatous plaque. HDL can reverse the process by transporting cholesterol to the liver for excretion in bile. Modification of LDL cholesterol can be inhibited by several factors, including dietary antioxidants.

Endothelial physiology, thrombogenesis and platelet dysfunction have been identified as significant factors in the pathogenesis of cardiovascular disease. The type of dietary fat can

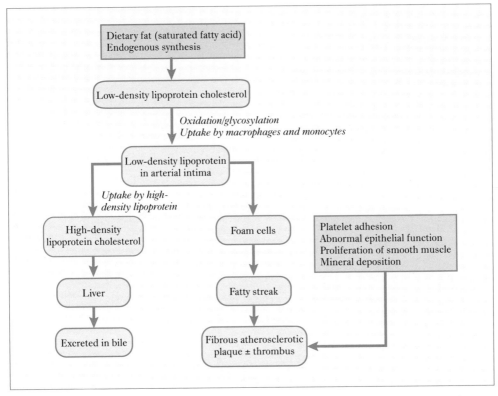

Figure 4.8 Development of atherosclerosis. LDL=low-density lipoprotein; HDL=high-density lipoprotein.

influence thrombogenesis as well as platelet adhesiveness. Furthermore, raised plasma homocysteine levels have been shown to be associated with an increased risk of cardiovascular disease. The role of homocysteine is thought to be in promoting procoagulant activity and increasing platelet aggregation. Platelet aggregation is largely controlled by a balance between the pro-aggregatory compound thromboxane A_2 and the anti-aggregatory prostacyclin (PGI_2) both of which are synthesized from arachidonic acid. For a full review of the biochemistry and physiology of the development of atheroma, see [68].

Dietary factors affecting lipoprotein and cholesterol metabolism

A number of dietary factors affect plasma lipoprotein and cholesterol values and the distribution of total cholesterol into its constituent fractions.

Fats and lipids

Much of the plasma cholesterol is endogenous, although dietary cholesterol intake does influence plasma values. Since sources of saturated fatty acid (SFA) and cholesterol tend to be similar (mainly foods of animal origin), it is difficult to separate the effects of each component [69], although there is some evidence that a high-cholesterol diet increases the risk of cardiovascular disease independent of the fatty acid consumed [70]. The intake of saturated fatty acids, monounsaturated fatty acids (MUFA), and polyunsaturated fatty acids

Fat type	Dietary sources	Effects
Saturated		
Short chain (C<10)	Butterfat, coconut oil	Little effect
Long chain (C12–18)	Meat and animal fats	Increase total and LDL cholesterol and triglycerides
Very long chain (C>20)	Some vegetable fats	Increase platelet aggregation
Trans fatty acids	Hydrogenated fats Milk and meat	Decrease HDL cholesterol; increase total cholesterol, triglycerides and lipoprotein A
Unsaturated		
Monounsaturated fatty acids	Olive, rapeseed, canola oils	Decrease total and LDL cholesterol; no effect on HDL cholesterol
Polyunsaturated fatty acids	n-6/omega 6 – corn, sunflower, safflower, soy oils	Decrease total, LDL and HDL cholesterol; also decrease triglycerides
	n-3/omega 3 – fish and marine oils	No effect on lipids; antithrombotic effects

LDL = low-density lipoprotein; HDL = high-density lipoprotein.

Table 4.7 Dietary fats and cardiovascular risk factors.

(PUFA) all affect blood levels of cholesterol components [69]. The roles of various types of fats are outlined in Table 4.7. *Trans* fatty acids, mainly derived from food-processing procedures, have a similar effect to SFAs [71]. The P/S ratio, or the proportions of PUFA to SFA in the diet, was advocated as an indication of the cholesterol-lowering potential of the diet. Diets with a low P/S ratio (0.2) are associated with raised plasma cholesterol values and high-risk populations, while a high P/S ratio (0.8), as seen in Mediterranean countries, is associated with a lower plasma cholesterol and a reduced risk of cardiovascular disease. Very high ratios (>1.0) may decrease HDL levels. However, with the realization of the role of other factors such as thrombogenesis, the P/S ratio is now thought to be an oversimplification and no ideal method for summarizing the atherogenic potential of diets has been suggested. Raised levels of plasma triglycerides are independently associated with an increased risk of cardiovascular disease if associated with low values of HDL. Hypertriglyceridemia is significant in determining cardiovascular risk in diabetics.

Carbohydrates and non-starch polysaccharides
Carbohydrates have little effect on total cholesterol levels (Table 4.8); simple sugars tend to decrease HDL levels, although consumption has not been linked with cardiovascular risk. Starches can depress HDL levels if taken in large quantities. Soluble fiber or non-starch polysaccharides has some effect in lowering total and LDL cholesterol values, mainly by reducing absorption of fat, bile acids and biliary cholesterol. Insoluble fiber (from wheat, rice and other grains) does not influence lipoprotein or cholesterol levels [72].

Carbohydrate type	Dietary sources	Effects
Free sugars (mono- and disaccharides)		
Glucose, fructose	Fruits and vegetables	Increase triglycerides; associated with high blood sugar and insulin levels; effect modified by presence/absence of starch and NSP; little effect on cholesterol
Sucrose	Fruits and vegetables Added sugar Sweet processed foods and drinks	
Lactose	Milk, yogurt, ice cream	Moderate effect on blood sugar and insulin
Complex carbohydrates		
Rapidly digested starch	Processed cereal foods – bread, cakes, potatoes, rice, root vegetables, sweetcorn, rice-based breakfast cereals	Similar effects to free sugars; modified by the presence/absence of slowly digested starch and NSP
Slowly digested starch	Wholegrain breakfast cereals Pulses (beans, peas and lentils) Pasta, wholegrain biscuits	Decrease HDL and LDL cholesterol; little effect on triglycerides, blood sugar and insulin levels
NSP/dietary fiber	Wholegrain cereals, potatoes, root vegetables, some fruits Pulses (beans, peas and lentils)	Decrease total and LDL cholesterol (particularly soluble fiber – oats, peas and beans)
HDL = high-density lipoprotein; LDL = low-density lipoprotein; NSP = non-starch polysaccharides		

Table 4.8 Carbohydrates and cardiovascular risk factors.

Energy

Excess energy, whether derived from fat, carbohydrate or protein, will lead to the development of obesity. Blood lipid levels have been shown to be higher in overweight children than in lean children, and obesity and insulin resistance have been linked to the early development of atheroma in young adults [73]. Furthermore, there is evidence that weight loss in obese children decreases plasma lipid levels [74].

Dietary factors affecting endothelial health and thrombogenesis

PUFAs of the n-3 series, mainly derived from fish oils, have a powerful antithrombotic effect [75]; PUFAs from the n-6 series, derived from seed oils and MUFAs (from olive, canola and peanut oil) reduce platelet aggregation. A high-fat diet, particularly one that is rich in SFAs, increases thrombogenicity [76]. Diets that are low in folic acid and vitamin B_6 (both found in vegetables and wholegrain cereals) and vitamin B_{12} (found in animal foods) are associated with raised plasma homocysteine levels [77]. Plant sterols and flavenoids (which supply B vitamins) may have an independent and positive effect on endothelial health [78]. Consumption of antioxidants (found mainly in fruits, vegetables and whole grains) inhibits proatherogenic and prothrombotic oxidative reactions in the artery wall [79].

	Mean		5th percentile		95th percentile	
	mmol/l	mg/dl	mmol//l	mg/dl	mmol/l	mg/dl
USA[†]						
Males						
0–4 years	4.11	159	3.02	117	5.40	209
5–9 years	4.27	165	3.32	125	5.40	209
10–14 years	4.19	162	3.18	123	5.38	208
15–19 years	3.98	154	3.00	116	5.25	203
Females						
0–4 years	4.16	161	2.97	115	5.33	206
5–9 years	4.37	169	3.36	130	5.46	211
10–14 years	4.24	164	3.31	128	5.35	207
15–19 years	4.19	162	3.20	124	5.40	209
UK						
Males + females[‡]						
$1^1/_2$–$2^1/_2$ years	4.39	170	3.01	116	5.72	222
$2^1/_2$–$3^1/_2$ years	4.42	171	3.18	123	5.68	220
Males						
$3^1/_2$–$4^1/_2$ years[‡]	4.36	169	3.23	125	5.46	211
$4^1/_2$–6 years[¶]	4.11	160	2.94	114	5.11	198
7–10 years	4.40	170	3.00	116	5.59	216
11–14 years	4.13	160	2.54	98	5.50	213
15–18 years	3.95	153	2.85	110	5.08	196
Females						
$3^1/_2$–$4^1/_2$ years[‡]	4.45	172	3.06	118	5.67	219
$4^1/_2$–6 years[¶]	4.61	178	2.87	111	6.22	240
7–10 years	4.43	171	2.72	105	6.02	233
11–14 years	4.26	165	2.99	116	5.49	212
15–18 years	4.20	162	2.90	112	5.44	210

*Serum values = plasma levels × 1.03
[†]Adapted from [87].
[‡]Adapted from Gregory JR, Collins DL, Davies PS, Hughes JM, Clarke PC. National Diet & Nutrition Survey: children aged $1^1/_2$-$4^1/_2$ years. London: HMSO, 1995.
[¶]Adapted from Gregory JR, Lowe S. National Diet & Nutrition Survey: young people aged 4 to 18 years. London: The Stationery Office, 2000.

Table 4.9 Normal serum* cholesterol levels in childhood and adolescence/early adulthood.

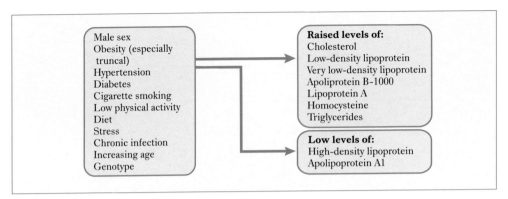

Figure 4.9 Risk factors for adult cardiovascular disease.

Dietary factors affecting blood pressure

The major dietary component affecting blood pressure is sodium, and a number of large epidemiological surveys have shown a positive relationship between sodium intake and blood pressure. In adults, a combination of high sodium and low potassium excretion, high alcohol intake and obesity increases the risk of hypertension [80]. In children, studies on intakes of potassium, calcium, magnesium and other dietary components are inconclusive, though the relationship with sodium described in adults has been shown to be valid for children and adolescents [81].

CARDIOVASCULAR RISK FACTORS IN CHILDHOOD

The processes that lead to atherosclerosis (see Fig. 4.8) begin in childhood with the development of fatty streaks in the arterial intima, although the presence of such streaks in itself is not a predictor of adult cardiovascular disease [82]. Thickened layers of the coronary artery have been noted in infants from populations with an increased prevalence of coronary heart disease [83]. Risk factors such as high plasma cholesterol concentrations and hypertension in childhood are predictive of adult cardiovascular health [84]. A number of agencies have recommended that primary prevention of coronary heart disease should begin in childhood since not only do cholesterol, blood pressure and obesity track from late childhood, but lifestyle factors such as physical activity, diet and smoking habits are learned early on and set the pattern for adult behavior [85]. Risk factors for adult cardiovascular disease are shown in Figure 4.9.

DETECTION OF RAISED CHOLESTEROL LEVELS

Raised serum cholesterol is the most frequently identified risk factor for cardiovascular disease in most western populations [86]. Normal values for plasma cholesterol levels in the USA and in the UK are shown in Table 4.9 and interpretation of results in Table 4.10.

Two approaches to detection have been suggested: population screening, where all children are tested for cholesterol levels; and selective testing, where only individuals known to be at increased risk are studied.

Cholesterol level mmol/l	Sex	Family history of premature heart disease	Risk category
5.3–6.9	M & F	No family history	Low
	F	History of early CHD in men only	Low
	M	History of early CHD	Moderate
	F	History of early CHD	Moderate
7.0–9.9	F	No family history	Low
	M	No family history	Moderate
	M & F	History of early CHD	High
≥10.0	F	No family history	Moderate
	M	No family history	High

CHD = coronary heart disease.

Table 4.10 Risk categories for premature heart disease in children. Adapted from [94].

Both in the USA and in the UK, selective vetting of the pediatric population is recommended. In the US National Cholesterol Education Program, it is recommended that all persons aged 20 years and over are tested at least once [87]. Children over the age of 2 years should be checked if they have parents or grandparents who, at 55 years of age or younger, were found to have coronary atherosclerosis diagnosed by arteriography or suffered documented myocardial infarction, angina, peripheral or cerebrovascular disease or sudden cardiac death. Children with a parent who has a cholesterol level exceeding 6.2 mmol/l (240 mg/dl) should also be screened [87]. Recommendations in the UK are slightly different, and testing is only recommended for children beyond 2 years who have a first-degree relative with familial hypercholesterolemia or with a history of premature-onset coronary disease. The cut-off for the definition of 'premature' disease is earlier than 50–55 years in men and 55–60 years in women [88].

For most children, the initial test should be a non-fasting measurement of total cholesterol. If levels are high – above 5.2 mmol/l (200 mg/dl) in the USA and above 5.5 mmol/l (210 mg/dl) in the UK – a fasting test should be arranged. Those with a total cholesterol level between 4.4 and 5.2 mmol/l (170–200 mg/dl) should have a repeat non-fasting sample measured. If the average of these two non-fasting measurements is greater than 4.4 mmol/l (170 mg/dl), a lipoprotein and triglyceride analysis should be carried out [87]. To obtain an estimate of LDL cholesterol, the following equation can be used [88]:

$$\text{LDL cholesterol} = \frac{\text{total cholesterol} - \text{HDL cholesterol} - \text{triglycerides}}{2.19}$$

NUTRITION AND THE PREVENTION OF CORONARY HEART DISEASE IN THE GENERAL PEDIATRIC POPULATION

Dietary recommendations are made for the whole pediatric population because there is evidence to suggest that nutrition in childhood affects adult levels of plasma lipids and that an improved diet may slow the progress of atherosclerosis. Dietary habits are formed in childhood, largely through home experience, and any changes should be adopted by the whole family if the future eating customs of the child are to be refashioned.

	USA*	UK†	ESPGAN‡
Age at which recommendations apply	>2 years	>2–5 years	>2–3 years
Total fat as % of energy	30%	35%	30–35%
Saturated fats as % of energy	8–10%	10%	8–12%
Polyunsaturated fats as % of energy	Not >10%	Not >10%	Not >10%
Monounsaturated fats as % of energy	10–15%	–	No restriction
Trans fatty acids as % of energy	–	Not >2%	Low intake
Cholesterol mg/day	<300	Not >165 mg/1000 kcal	Not >300
Protein as % of energy	15–20%	–	–
Carbohydrate as % of energy	55%	–	–
Dietary fiber g/day	Age + 5 g (max. age + 10 g)	–	–

*From [87].
†From [89].
‡European Society for Paediatric Gastroenterology and Nutrition guidelines. From [82].

Table 4.11 Recommendations for lowering cholesterol in the general population.

A summary of the recommendations for healthy children and adolescents in the USA [87], the UK [89] and Europe [82] is given in Table 4.11. In all reports, dietary modification is not recommended for children under the age of 2 years, since infants and young children require a diet with a low bulk and high energy density (supplied by fat) in order to achieve optimal growth and development. By the age of 5 years, children should be able to tolerate a diet with a moderate intake of fat that is low in SFAs, and an emphasis on cereal, fruit and vegetable foods to replace some dairy products. Between the age of 2 and 5 years, most bodies recommend a gradual change from the high-fat milk-based diet to one that more closely follows adult recommendations.

High and low fat foods are shown in Appendix IV.30 and the fat content of foods in Appendix IV.31. Dietary fat can be reduced by decreasing the amount of fried foods and high-fat snacks such as crisps/potato chips, and by keeping processed items to a minimum, e.g. burgers, sausages, cookies and cakes, all of which contain large quantities of saturated fats. White meats (i.e. chicken and turkey) are lower in total fat and cholesterol than red meats and eggs. The inclusion of white fish is advantageous because it is very low in fat, and the consumption of fish oils found in the fatty fish may have a protective role against the development of atheroma. Low-fat yogurt can be substituted for pouring cream in desserts, sauces and dressings, and homemade ice cream can be prepared from skimmed milk.

The benefits of substituting a PUFA or MUFA margarine for butter are not clearly established; the use of any type of butter or margarine should be restricted to spreading on bread etc. and should not be added to vegetables or applied as a decoration. Although fried foods should be kept to a minimum, when foods are prepared in this way an oil that is rich in PUFA or MUFA is preferable to one high in saturated fat.

Consumption of additional complex carbohydrate in the form of starch should gradually replace energy derived from fats. Useful foods include pasta, potato, rice, legumes, root vegetables, cereals and breads. Fruits and vegetables contain mainly simple sugars and should be consumed as well as starchy foods, since they represent a source of dietary fiber, antioxidant vitamins and other beneficial substances. It is recommended that children eat a minimum of five portions of fruit and vegetables each day (excluding potato which is considered a starch).

Infants

A number of studies have suggested a relationship between breastfeeding and consequent cholesterol levels, and that breast milk is protective against coronary heart disease [90]. Breastfed infants have a higher plasma cholesterol level than those given formulas that include vegetable oils, but the difference disappears when solid foods are introduced. Furthermore, in older children, there appears to be no correlation between breast or bottle feeding and cholesterol levels. Findings at birth are not predictive for infancy or childhood, although, after the age of 1 year, plasma cholesterol is indicative of the probable subsequent percentile. At weaning, very fatty foods are best avoided because infants often find difficulty in digesting them. They are also very energy dense and their use may cause satiety and deter consumption of other more beneficial foods. Low intakes of salt and sugar should be encouraged.

Children up to the age of 5 years

Whole cow milk can be introduced in place of breast milk or formula after the age of 1 year. The milk should be a full-fat product because in infants and young children it is the major source of energy as well as of other nutrients. Beyond 2 years, a low-fat or semi-skimmed milk can be introduced, but most children do not obtain an adequate energy intake if skimmed milk is used. Fully skimmed milk is safe for most children over the age of 5 years. For preschool children with a small appetite or who are fussy eaters, it is advisable to continue with a full-fat milk or one in which vegetable oil has been substituted for butterfat.

Children over the age of 5 years

With the proviso that the child can obtain an adequate energy intake, the recommendations are as for adults.

Adolescents

This group may be reluctant to change their dietary customs. Unfortunately, many of the popular 'fast foods' are high in both total and saturated fat. Adolescents have a large energy requirement so will need to consume a diet fairly high in fat. For example, a daily

Disorder	Biochemistry	Clinical features
Lipoprotein lipase deficiency (Type I)	Cholesterol N or ⇑ Triglycerides ⇑⇑ Chylomicrons ⇑ VLDL N HDL & LDL ⇓	Rare autosomal recessive disease Abdominal pain, recurrent acute pancreatitis, hepatosplenomegaly, xanthoma, lipemia retinalis, creamy serum No premature atherosclerosis or ischemic heart disease
Familial hypercholesterolemia (Type IIa)	Cholesterol ⇑⇑⇑ Triglycerides N or ⇑ LDL ⇑	Autosomal dominant *Heterozygous form*: tendon xanthomas, xanthelasma, arcus senilis, premature atherosclerosis *Homozygous form*: very rare, poor prognosis; death from atherosclerosis before age 20 years unless liver transplant
Familial combined hyperlipidemia (Type IIb)	Cholesterol ⇑ (not all) Triglycerides ⇑ (not all) VLDL ⇑	Autosomal dominant No xanthomas; no acute pancreatitis Increased risk of early atherosclerosis
Broad-beta disease (Type III) (remnant hyperlipidemia)	Cholesterol ⇑ or ⇑⇑ Triglycerides ⇑ or ⇑⇑ IDL ⇑	Autosomal recessive Skin xanthomas are deep-orange and prominent on palms and fingers; arcus senilis, abnormal glucose tolerance test and hyperuricemia; obesity is common Increased risk of early atherosclerosis and peripheral vascular disease
Familial hypertriglyceridemia (Type IV)	Cholesterol N or ⇑ Triglycerides ⇑⇑ LDL N VLDL ⇑	Autosomal dominant No xanthomas; obesity, hyperuricemia, abnormal glucose tolerance test and acute pancreatitis Slightly increased risk of atherosclerosis
Apolipoprotein C-II deficiency (Type V) (familial type-5 disease)	Cholesterol ⇑ or ⇑⇑ Triglycerides ⇑⇑⇑ Chylomicrons ⇑ VLDL ⇑	Autosomal dominant Acute pancreatitis/abdominal pain; often secondary to diabetes, obesity, alcoholism Variable risk of premature atherosclerosis

N = normal; ⇑ = slight increase; ⇑⇑ = moderate increase; ⇑⇑⇑ = very high; ⇓ = decrease.
HDL = high-density lipoprotein; IDL = intermediate-density lipoprotein; LDL = low-density lipoprotein; VLDL = very-low-density lipoprotein.

Table 4.12 Hyperlipidemias.

requirement of 3000 kcal (12.5 MJ) is not unusual for an active teenager and, if 30% of the energy is derived from fat, this will mean an intake of some 90 g of fat daily. Hence, the consumption of moderate quantities of fried foods is not unreasonable.

HYPERLIPIDEMIAS

The hyperlipoproteinemias were categorized by Fredrickson and colleagues in 1967 [91]. However, this classification has since been amended (Table 4.12). Elevated lipoprotein may be due to genetically heterogeneous determined disease or occur secondarily to another disorder (e.g. nephrotic syndrome, diabetes mellitus).

Treatment of hyperlipidemias

Familial hypercholesterolemia

Children who are screened because of a positive family history and have a total blood cholesterol level less than 4.8 mmol/l (185 mg/dl) should be given advice in line with national recommendations (see Table 4.10). Those with levels of total cholesterol above 4.4 mmol/l (170 mg/dl) and LDL cholesterol greater than 2.8 mmol/l (85 mg/dl) should be advised to follow a diet that is low in saturated fat or a Step 1 diet (as recommended by the American Heart Association). In this diet, total fat contributes not more than 30% of energy and saturated fat not more than 10%. In the USA, the daily intake of cholesterol is limited to less than 300 mg, or less than 100 mg per 1000 kcal (4200 kJ). The cholesterol content of foods is shown in Appendix IV.32.

If a significant reduction of total cholesterol to 5 mmol/l or less (≤193 mg/dl) and a reduction of LDL cholesterol to 3 mmol/l or less (≤116 mg/dl) is not achieved after at least 3 months compliance with this dietary regimen, progression to a stricter practice is recommended. Known as a Step 2 diet in the USA recommended by the American Heart Association, this reduces saturated fat to less than 7% of energy and cholesterol to less than 200 mg/day [87].

It is important that these low-fat diets are individually constructed and that clear instructions and counseling are given by a dietitian to ensure an adequate intake of energy, protein, minerals and micronutrients. Dietary manipulation should reduce total and LDL cholesterol by 10–20%, although compliance with this type of regimen is often poor [87]. Regular monitoring of plasma cholesterol and frequent counseling about the diet are essential.

Two main types of drugs are available for the treatment of hypercholesterolemia if dietary therapy alone does not achieve the desired reduction. Bile-acid sequestrants such as cholestyramine and colestipol act by binding bile acids in the gut lumen. This interruption of the enterohepatic circulation promotes increased synthesis of bile acids from cholesterol and thus increases excretion. They are considered safe to use in children as they are not absorbed from the intestine [87]. The dose used is dependent on the LDL cholesterol level at the beginning of treatment, but all children should begin with the smallest dose of 8 g/day [92]. Compliance with bile-acid resin therapy is often poor because of the unpalatability of the powders used and the side effects such as constipation, nausea and bloating. In addition, it is important that a supplement of fat-soluble vitamins and folic acid are prescribed as these are poorly absorbed as a result of the drug therapy.

Drugs that inhibit the enzyme hydroxymethylglutaryl (HMG) CoA reductase, known as statins, reduce total and LDL cholesterol by inhibiting synthesis of LDL and VLDL. They have been shown to reduce LDL cholesterol by up to 40% in children and adolescents [93]; however their widespread use in children is not generally approved by most authorities. Other cholesterol-lowering agents such as nicotinic acid, plant sterols and fibrates may have a limited role in drug therapy for the pediatric population, but their long-term safety has not been evaluated.

Medication should only be considered where a trial of a low-fat diet with appropriate counseling and help has been followed for a year without the desired reduction in total or LDL cholesterol [87]. Initiation of resin therapy in children with familial hypercholesterolemia should not normally begin earlier than the age of 10 years except in boys who are at high risk (see Table 4.10), where it may be considered from the age of 7 years. Boys with hypercholesterolemia who are at moderate risk and girls who are at high risk can begin resin medication from the age of 12 years. From the age of 15–18 years, both boys and girls with cholesterol levels above 5.2 mmol/l (200 mg/dl) should be considered for resin. Statins can be used in this age group for boys at high or moderate risk and for girls at high risk [94].

Lipoprotein lipase deficiency
This is a very rare (<1:10,000) autosomal recessive disorder. Patients have a striking chylomicronemia with eruptive xanthomas over the trunk, lipemia retinalis and recurrent pancreatitis.

All fat should be restricted. If the child suffers from acute abdominal pain and vomiting, fat ought to be reduced temporarily to less than 5 g daily. Once the acute episode has passed, fat can be reintroduced slowly. Usually only about 20–30 g daily can be taken without abdominal symptoms recurring. Only foods that have a low or moderate fat content should be selected (Appendices IV.30 and IV.31). Because MCTs are not absorbed through the chylomicron route, they may provide a useful alternative source of energy. They should be introduced with caution, as described in the section on MCTs in Appendix IV.9. Care must be taken to ensure that the child receives adequate energy from carbohydrate and protein foods and that supplements of the fat-soluble vitamins are given. If dietary carbohydrate includes unrefined sources such as fruit, vegetables and wholemeal cereals, the abdominal discomfort associated with fat ingestion seems to be improved, possibly due to delayed or reduced fat absorption. However, this type of regimen may not be possible in younger children because they need a diet with a high energy density. As this condition is not associated with premature atherosclerosis, the diet only serves to relieve symptoms and, although plasma triglycerides often remain raised, there appears to be no advantage in correcting the hypertriglyceridemia.

Familial combined hyperlipidemia (FCHL)
This is the most frequent inherited form of dyslipoproteinemia in adults. The risk of premature heart disease is significant; therefore, children in these families must be identified. The need for strict dietary intervention in children with this disorder has yet to be established because plasma lipid patterns are dissimilar from those in adults. If there is obesity, a weight-reducing program is necessary; otherwise, a prudent diet as recommended for the general pediatric population (see p. 2) should be followed.

Broad-beta disease
Dietary recommendations are similar to those for the general pediatric population (see p. 2), with particular emphasis on the maintenance of a normal weight.

Familial hypertriglyceridemia (FHTG)
Hypertriglyceridemia is not known to cause coronary heart disease, but it may prove to be an important independent risk factor. This condition in adults is often associated with a high intake of refined carbohydrate and obesity. Although the disorder rarely manifests before puberty, children who are affected should restrict their carbohydrate intake to unrefined

sources as far as possible and avoid added sucrose. Dietary saturated fats should be restricted and polyunsaturated or monounsaturated fats used in their place. Drug therapy is not usually indicated.

Familial type V hyperlipidemia

This rare disorder (<1:5000) is characterized by marked elevations of chylomicrons and VLDL triglycerides. In children, the symptoms are akin to those of lipoprotein lipase deficiency, with acute attacks of abdominal pain and pancreatitis. Dietary management is also similar; in addition, particular care is necessary to avoid high intakes of refined sugars and to maintain weight within the normal range. Marine oils rich in eicosapentenoic acid (EPA) and decosahexenoic acid can decrease hypertriglyceridemia. A concentrated fish oil preparation, Maxepa, may prove beneficial in type V hyperlipidemia.

HYPOLIPIDEMIAS

Familial HDL deficiency or Tangier disease is characterized by large yellowish tonsils and adenoids, caused by the presence of cholesterol esters. Most patients show symptoms of peripheral neuropathy, which may be intermittent or progressive. There is a severe deficiency of normal HDL and apoA-1 in plasma; cholesterol levels are low and triglycerides may be raised [95]. There is no specific treatment, although a moderate reduction in fat intake is usually recommended.

Familial lecithin-cholesterol acyltranferase (LCAT) deficiency and fish eye disease (partial LCAT deficiency) are both characterized by corneal opacities. Additionally, anemia and proteinuria with eventual renal failure develop in LCAT deficiency. The cholesterol esters, lysolecithin and apoA-1 are reduced. In LCAT deficiency, there is a characteristic low ratio (<0.7) of cholesterol ester to total cholesterol. There is no specific treatment apart from reducing other cardiac risk factors in adult patients, who often show premature atherosclerosis [95]. Abetalipoproteinemia is discussed on page 124.

FATTY ACID OXIDATION DISORDERS

A number of disorders of mitochondrial fatty acid oxidation have been reported; Figure 4.10 describes the metabolic pathways and defects involved. Medium-chain acyl CoA dehydrogenase (MCAD) deficiency is the most common, with an estimated prevalence of 1:13,000 in northwest Europe and populations that derive from there [96]. Disorders of the three stages of fatty acid oxidation – carnitine cycle defects, acyl CoA dehydrogenase deficiencies and long chain 3-hydroxyacyl CoA dehydrogenase (LCHAD) deficiencies – appear with varying degrees of severity in infancy or later, including adult life. The major presenting feature is hypoglycemia without ketosis; in infancy, encephalopathy may be an important initial symptom. The clinical picture is the result of an inability to metabolize sufficient fatty acids for energy, leading to the accumulation of toxic intermediate metabolites. In defects of the carnitine cycle, infants often have a cardiomyopathy and older children muscle problems. In some disorders the appearance of symptoms may be episodic and is usually precipitated by intercurrent infections or periods of fasting since fat is unable to be mobilized and glycogen stores are rapidly exhausted. For a full review of the

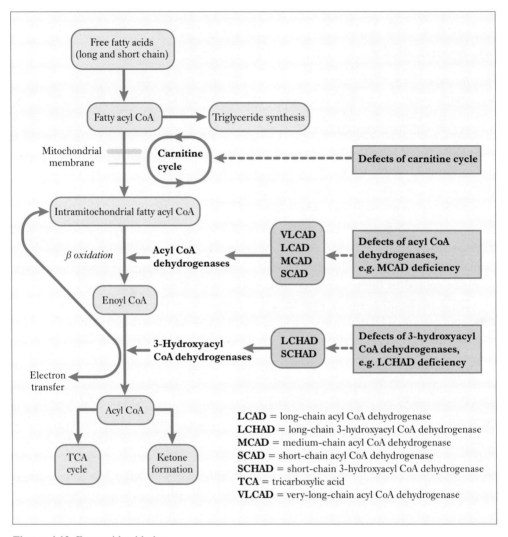

Figure 4.10 Fatty acid oxidation.

biochemistry of these disorders, see [97]. LCHAD deficiency in the fetus gives rise to maternal liver disease and pre-eclampsia [98]. Fatty acid oxidation defects may be a cause of unexplained death in undiagnosed infants [99]. Conditions that present later, particularly MCAD deficiency and glutaric acidemia type II, may be misdiagnosed as cyclical vomiting syndrome [100]. The prognosis for MCAD deficiency is fairly good, providing that the diagnosis is made before the brain is damaged by frequent hypoglycemic episodes. The prognosis for the less common conditions is more uncertain [99].

Diagnosis

Fatty acid oxidation disorders may not be picked up by routine screening for organic acids in urine, since these only appear in the urine when the infant is hypoglycemic or decompensated. This may be important, as many of the symptoms are similar to those of organic acidemias. Investigations should include urinary organic acids, plasma free and total carnitine, acyl carnitine (if the test is available), glucose, ketone bodies, lactate and non-esterified fatty acids. Several disorders, including MCAD deficiency, result in a low ratio of ketone bodies to non-esterified fatty acid [37].

Management

Some patients with glutaric aciduria type II respond to riboflavin and carnitine therapy. Carnitine at a dose of 50–100 mg/kg/day is beneficial in carnitine transporter defects but its routine use in other fatty acid oxidation defects is unclear. It may be useful during periods of decompensation, as it helps remove toxic metabolites [101].

The degree of dietary restriction varies according to the condition. The overall aims of dietary management of this type of disorder are to prevent fatty acids being required as a main fuel, thus avoiding fasting, and to restrict the intake of fatty acids that may result in the accumulation of toxic metabolites. During periods of illness, it is vital that carers have an emergency regimen available in order to stimulate insulin secretion and prevent lipolysis. This is usually a glucose polymer solution (see Appendix V.13), which may need to be concentrated to 25% glucose in older infants and children. The feed is given at frequent intervals (every 2–3 h) day and night.

Infants with MCAD deficiency require frequent (every 3–4 h) feeding day and night. They can be breastfed but may require a supplemental glucose polymer if they are slow feeders and become hypoglycemic. Older children can take a normal diet when they are well, and fat does not need to be restricted. Starchy foods should be taken at every meal and children should have a minimum of three meals plus a bedtime snack each day. Long periods without food should be avoided and the maximum overnight fast that is tolerated by older children is about 12 h. Although MCTs are not metabolized in MCAD deficiency, the small amount of MCT present in the normal diet does not usually present a problem. Coconut and coconut oil are the richest source of MCT; although small quantities of coconut can be tolerated, large amounts should be avoided. All dietary fat should be restricted during periods of intercurrent infection or other stress.

In contrast, disorders of long-chain oxidation require a diet that is very low in long-chain fat. MCT can be used to supply additional energy in some conditions, but is contraindicated in certain disorders of the carnitine cycle. Breast milk is not suitable for these infants and a complete minimal-fat infant feed must be substituted. If MCT can be oxidized, a feed such as Monogen (Appendices IV.7 and IV.8) or a modular feed (Appendix IV.12) can be used. If MCT is contraindicated, a minimal-fat modular feed (Appendix IV.11) is suitable. A modular feed will contain inadequate quantities of essential fatty acids (although Monogen is sufficient in these) and a supplement of walnut oil is necessary (Appendix IV.10). Infants require frequent feeding during the day and an overnight continuous feed delivered by a nasogastric tube or gastrostomy. Older children with long-chain disorders should remain on a minimal-fat diet.

The diet is based on starchy foods, and low-fat sources of protein such as white fish can be used (see Appendices IV.30 and IV.31). A source of fat-soluble vitamins must be included unless 500 ml of Monogen is taken each day. Prolonged periods without food must be avoided. Meals that are missed should be replaced with a glucose drink in order to stimulate insulin secretion and reduce lipolysis. Uncooked cornstarch may be useful in older children (for dosage and use, see glycogen storage disorders, p. 80) as a source of slow-release carbohydrate to reduce the need for overnight continuous feeds. If MCT is tolerated, oil can be used to provide additional energy and variety. The use of MCT in cooking is discussed in Appendix IV.9.

REFERENCES

1.   Walter JH. Investigation and initial management of suspected metabolic disease. Curr Pediatr 1997;7:103–7.

2.   Leonard JV, Morris AA. Inborn errors of metabolism around time of birth. Lancet 2000;356:583–7.

3.   Kwok SC, Ledley FD, DiLella AG et al. Nucleotide sequence of a full-length complementary DNA clone and amino acid sequence of human phenylalanine hydroxylase. Biochemistry 1985;24:556–61.

4.   Guttler F, Guldberg P. The influence of mutations on enzyme activity and phenylalanine tolerance in phenylalanine hydroxylase deficiency. Eur J Pediatr 1996;155(Suppl. 1):S6–10.

5.   Scriver CR, Kaufman S. Hyperphenylalaninemia: phenylalanine hydroxylase deficiency. In: Scriver CR, Beaudet AL, Sly WS, Valle D (editors). The Metabolic and Molecular Basis of Inherited Disease, 8th ed. New York: McGraw-Hill, 2001:1667–724.

6.   Blau N, Thony B, Cotton RG, Hyland K. Disorders of tetrahydrobiopterin and related biogenic amines. In: Scriver CR, Beaudet AL, Sly WS, Valle D (editors). The Metabolic and Molecular Basis of Inherited Disease, 8th ed. New York: McGraw-Hill, 2001:1725–76.

7.   Medical Research Council Working Party on Phenylketonuria. Recommendations on the dietary management of phenylketonuria. Arch Dis Child 1993;68:426–7.

8.   Waisbren SE, Zaff J. Personality disorder in young women with treated phenylketonuria. J Inherit Metab Dis 1994;17:584–92.

9.   Beasley MG, Costello PM, Smith I. Outcome of treatment in young adults with phenylketonuria detected by routine neonatal screening between 1964 and 1971. Q J Med 1994;87:155–60.

10. Lou HC, Toft PB, Andresen J et al. An occipito-temporal syndrome in adolescents with optimally controlled hyperphenylalaninaemia. J Inherit Metab Dis 1992;15:687–95.

11. Pennington BF, van Doorninck WJ, McCabe LL et al. Neuropsychological deficits in early treated phenylketonuric children. Am J Ment Defic 1985;89:467–74.

12. Medical Research Council Working Party on Phenylketonuria. Phenylketonuria due to phenylalanine hydroxylase deficiency: an unfolding story. BMJ 1993;306:115–9.

13. Smith I, Beasley MG, Ades AE. Intelligence and quality of dietary treatment in phenylketonuria. Arch Dis Child 1990;65:472–8.

14. Shortland D, Smith I, Francis DE et al. Amino acid and protein requirements in a preterm infant with classic phenylketonuria. Arch Dis Child 1985;60:263–5.

15. Monch E, Herrmann ME, Brosicke H et al. Utilisation of amino acid mixtures in adolescents with phenylketonuria. Eur J Pediatr 1996;155(Suppl. 1):S115–20.

16. Acosta PB, Wenz E, Williamson M. Nutrient intake of treated infants with phenylketonuria. Am J Clin Nutr 1977;30:198–208.

17. Hillman L, Schlotzhauer C, Lee D et al. Decreased bone mineralization in children with phenylketonuria under treatment. Eur J Pediatr 1996;155(Suppl. 1):S148–52.

18. Fisberg RM, Da Silva-Femandes ME, Fisberg M et al. Plasma zinc, copper and erythrocyte superoxide dismutase in children with phenylketonuria. Nutrition 1999;15:449–52.

19. Acosta PB. Nutrition studies in treated infants and children with phenylketonuria: vitamins, minerals, trace elements. Eur J Pediatr 1996;155(Suppl. 1):S136–9.

20. Hanley WB, Feigenbaum AS, Clarke JT et al. Vitamin B12 deficiency in adolescents and young adults with phenylketonuria. Eur J Pediatr 1996;155(Suppl. 1):S145–7.

21. Lombeck I, Jochum F, Terwolbeck K. Selenium status in infants and children with phenylketonuria and in maternal phenylketonuria. Eur J Pediatr 1996;155(Suppl. 1):S140–4.

22. Jochum F, Terwolbeck K, Meinhold H et al. Effects of a low selenium state in patients with phenylketonuria. Acta Paediatr 1997;86:775–7.

23. Sierra C, Vilaseca MA, Moyano D et al. Antioxidant status in hyperphenylalaninemia. Clin Chim Acta 1998;276:1–9.

24. Schoeffer A, Herrmann ME, Brosicke HG et al. Influence of single dose amino acid mixtures on the nitrogen retention in patients with phenylketonuria. J Nutr Med 1994;4:415–8.

25. Thompson AJ, Smith I, Brenton D et al. Neurological deterioration in young adults with phenylketonuria. Lancet 1990;336:602–5.

26. Rey F, Abadie V, Plainguet F et al. Long-term follow up of patients with classical phenylketonuria after diet relaxation at 5 years of age. The Paris study. Eur J Pediatr 1996;155(Suppl.1):S39–44.

27. Azen C, Koch R, Friedman E et al. Summary of findings from the United States collaborative study of children treated for phenylketonuria. Eur J Pediatr 1996;155(Suppl. 1):S29–32.

28. Smith I, Beasley MG, Ades AE. Effect on intelligence of relaxing the low phenylalanine diet in phenylketonuria. Arch Dis Child 1991;66:311–6.

29. Brenton DP, Tarn AC, Cabrera-Abreu JC et al. Phenylketonuria: treatment in adolescence and adult life. Eur J Pediatr 1996;155(Suppl. 1):S93–6.

30. Bickel H. Phenylketonuria: past, present, future. J Inherit Metab Dis 1980;3:123–32.

31. Hanley WB, Koch R, Levy HL et al. The North American maternal phenylketonuria collaborative study, developmental assessment of the offspring: preliminary report. Eur J Pediatr 1996;155(Suppl. 1):S169–72.

32. Cipcic-Schmidt S, Trefz FK, Funders B et al. German maternal phenylketonuria study. Eur J Pediatr 1996;155(Suppl. 1):S173–6.

33. Brenton DP, Lilburn M. Maternal phenylketonuria. A study from the United Kingdom. Eur J Pediatr 1996;115(Suppl.1):S177–80.

34. Waisbren SE, Chang P, Levy HL et al. Neonatal neurological assessment of offspring in maternal phenylketonuria. J Inherit Metab Dis 1998;21:39–48.

35. Dhondt JL. Tetrahydrobiopterin deficiencies: preliminary analysis from an international survey. J Pediatr 1984;104:501–8.

36. Brusilow SW, Maestri NE. Urea cycle disorders: diagnosis, pathophysiology and therapy. Adv Pediatr 1996;43:127–70.

37. Burton BK. Inborn errors of metabolism in infancy: a guide to diagnosis. Pediatrics 1998;102:E69.

38. Bachmann C, Colombo JP. Increased tryptophan uptake into the brain in hyperammonemia. Life Sci 1983;33:2417–24.

39. Brusilow SW, Horwich AL. Urea cycle enzymes. In: Scriver CR, Beaudet AL, Sly WS, Valle D (editors). The Metabolic and Molecular Basis of Inherited Disease, 8th ed. New York: McGraw-Hill, 2001:1909–63.

40. Brusilow SW. Phenylacetylglutamine may replace urea as a vehicle for waste nitrogen excretion. Pediatr Res 1991;29:147–50.

41. Maestri NE, McGowan KD, Brusilow SW. Plasma glutamine concentration: a guide in the management of urea cycle disorders. J Pediatr 1992;121:259–61.

42. Whitington PF, Alonso EM, Boyle JT et al. Liver transplantation for the treatment of urea cycle disorders. J Inherit Metab Dis 1998;21(Suppl.1):112–8.

43. Dewey KG, Beaton G, Fjeld C et al. Protein requirements of infants and children. Eur J Clin Nutr 1996;50(Suppl. 1):S119–47.

44. Sweetman L, Williams JC. Branched chain organic acidurias. In: Scriver CR, Beaudet AL, Sly WS, Valle D (editors). The Metabolic and Molecular Basis of Inherited Disease, 8th ed. New York: McGraw-Hill, 2001:2125–63.

45. Fenton WA, Gravel RA, Rosenblatt DS. Disorders of propionate and methylmalonate metabolism. In: Scriver CR, Beaudet AL, Sly WS, Valle, D (editors). The Metabolic and Molecular Basis of Inherited Disease, 8th ed. New York: McGraw-Hill, 2001:2165–93.

46. Goodman SI, Frerman FE. Organic acidemias due to defects in lysine oxidation: 2-ketoadipicacidemia and glutaric acidemia. In: Scriver CR, Beaudet AL, Sly WS, Valle D (editors). The Metabolic and Molecular Basis of Inherited Disease, 8th ed. New York: McGraw-Hill, 2001:2195–204.

47. Saudubray JM, Ogier H, Charpentier C. Diagnostic procedures: function tests and postmortem protocol. In: Saudubray JM, Fernandes J, van den Berghe G (editors). Inborn Metabolic Diseases. Berlin: Springer, 1995:3–40.

48. Fernades J, Saudubray JM. Clinical approach to metabolic disease. In: Fernandes J, Saudubray JM, van den Berghe G (editors). Inborn Metabolic Diseases. Berlin: Springer, 1995:41–6.

49. Ogier de Baulny H, Saudubray JM. Emergency treatments. In: Fernandes J, Saudubray JM, van den Berghe G (editors). Inborn Metabolic Diseases: Diagnosis and Treatment, 2nd ed. Berlin: Springer, 1995:47–55.

50. Leonard JV. The management and outcome of propionic and methylmalonic acidaemia. J Inherit Metab Dis 1995;18:430–4.

51. van't Hoff WG, Dixon M, Taylor J et al. Combined liver-kidney transplant in methylmalonic acidemia. J Pediatr 1998;132:1043–4.

52. Mahoney MJ, Bick D. Recent advances in the inherited methylmalonic acidemias. Acta Paediatr Scand 1987;76:689–96.

53. Hoffman GF. Glutaric aciduria type I and related cerebral organic acid disorders. In: Fernandes J, Saudubray JM, van den Berghe G (editors). Inborn Metabolic Disease. Berlin: Springer, 1995:229–36.

54. Leonard JV, Daish P, Naughten ER et al. The management and long-term outcome of organic acidaemias. J Inherit Metab Dis 1984;7:13–7.

55. Sanjurjo P, Ruiz JI, Montejo M. Inborn errors of metabolism with a protein-restricted diet: effect on polyunsaturated fatty acids. J Inherit Metab Dis 1997;20:783–89.

56. Kyllerman M, Skjeldal OH, Lundberg M et al. Dystonia and dyskinesia in glutaric aciduria type I: clinical heterogeneity and therapeutic considerations. Mov Disord 1994;9:22–30.

57. Holton JB, Walter JH, Tyfield LA. Galactosemia. In: Scriver CR, Beaudet AL, Sly WS, Valle D (editors). The Metabolic and Molecular Basis of Inherited Disease, 8th ed. New York: McGraw-Hill, 2001:1553–87.

58. Gitzelmann R, Steinmann B, van den Berghe G. Disorders of fructose metabolism. In: Scriver CR, Beaudet AL, Sly WS, Valle D (editors). The Metabolic and Molecular Basis of Inherited Disease, 8th ed. New York: McGraw-Hill, 2001:1489–520.

59. Chen Y-T. Glycogen storage diseases. In: Scriver CR, Beaudet AL, Sly WS, Valle D (editors). The Metabolic and Molecular Basis of Inherited Disease, 8th ed. New York: McGraw-Hill, 2001:1521–51.

60. Ng WG, Xu YK, Kaufman FR et al. Biochemical and molecular studies of 132 patients with galactosemia. Hum Genet 1994;94:359–63.

61. Walter JH, Collins JE, Leonard JV. Recommendations for the management of galactosaemia. Arch Dis Child 1999;80:93–6.

62. Kaufman FR, McBride-Chang C, Manis FR et al. Cognitive functioning, neurologic status and brain imaging in classical galactosemia. Eur J Pediatr 1995;154:S2–5.

63. Schweitzer S, Shin Y, Jakobs C et al. Long-term outcome in 134 patients with galactosaemia. Eur J Pediatr 1993;152:36–43.

64. Lee P. Glycogen storage diseases. Curr Pediatr 1997;7:108–13.

65. Goldberg T, Slonim AE. Nutrition therapy for hepatic glycogen storage disease. J Am Diet Assoc 1993;93:1423–30.

66. Lee PJ, Dixon MA, Leonard JV. Uncooked cornstarch – efficacy in type I glycogenosis. Arch Dis Child 1996;74:546–7.

67. McCallion N, Irranca M, Naughten E et al. Uncooked cornflour compared to high protein diet in the treatment of glycogen storage disease type III. J Inherit Metab Dis 1998;21(Suppl. 2):93.

68. Davies ML. Morphology and natural history of atherosclerotic lesions in the human artery tree. In: Davies MJ, Woolf N (editors). Atheroma: Atherosclerosis in Ischaemic Heart Disease. Volume 1: The Mechanisms. London: Science Press, 1990:2.1–2.52.

69. Hegsted DM, Ausman LM, Johnson JA et al. Dietary fat and serum lipids: an evaluation of the experimental data. Am J Clin Nutr 1993;57:875–83.

70. Shekelle RB, Stamler J. Dietary cholesterol and ischaemic heart disease. Lancet 1989;1:1177–9.

71. Judd JT, Clevidence BA, Muesing RA et al. Dietary trans fatty acids: effects on plasma lipids and lipoproteins of healthy men and women. Am J Clin Nutr 1994;59:861–8.

72. Van Horn L. Fiber, lipids and coronary heart disease. Circulation 1997;95:2701–4.

73. Gidding SS, Leibel RL, Daniels S et al. Understanding obesity in youth. Circulation 1996;94:3383–7.

74. Rocchini AP. Adolescent obesity and hypertension. Pediatr Clin North Am 1993;40:81–92.

75. Connor WE, DeFrancesco CA, Connor SL. N-3 fatty acids from fish oil. Effects on plasma lipoproteins and hypertriglyceridemic patients. Ann NY Acad Sci 1993;683:16–34.

76. Nordoy A, Rodset JM. The influences of dietary fats on platelets in man. Acta Med Scand 1971;190:27–34.

77. Malinow MR, Bostom AG, Krauss RM. Homocysteine, diet and cardiovascular diseases. Circulation 1999;99:178–82.

78. Howard BV, Kritchevsky D. Phytochemicals and cardiovascular disease. Circulation 1997;95:2591–3.

79. Tribble DL. Antioxidant consumption and risk of coronary heart disease: emphasis on vitamin C, vitamin E and b carotene. Circulation 1999;99:591–5.

80. Elliott P, Dyer A, Stamler R et al. Correcting for regression dilution in INTERSALT. Lancet 1993;342:1123.

81. Simons-Morton DG, Obarzanek O. Diet and blood pressure in children and adolescents. Pediatr Nephrol 1997;11:244–9.

82. Aggett PJ, Haschke F, Heine W et al. Committee Report: childhood diet and prevention of coronary heart disease. J Pediatr Gastroenterol Nutr 1994;19:261–9.

83. Pesonen E, Norio R, Sarna S. Thickenings in the coronary arteries in infancy as an indication of genetic factors in coronary heart disease. Circulation 1975;51:218–25.

84. Akerblom HK, Viikari J, Raitakari OT et al. Cardiovascular risk in young Finns study: general outline and recent developments. Ann Med 1999;31(Suppl. 1):45–54.

85. Feinstein JA, Quivers ES. Pediatric preventive cardiology: healthy habits now, healthy hearts later. Curr Opin Cardiol 1997;12:70–7.

86. Williams CL, Bollella M. Guidelines for screening, evaluating and treating children with hypercholesterolemia. J Pediatr Health Care 1995;9:153–61.

87. American Academy of Pediatrics. National Cholesterol Education Program. Report of the expert panel on blood cholesterol levels in children and adolescents. Pediatrics 1992;89(3 Pt 2):525–84.

88. Wray R, Neil H, Rees J. Screening for hyperlipidaemia in childhood. Recommendations of the British Hyperlipidaemia Association. J R Coll Physicians Lond 1996;30:115–8.

89. DHSS. Nutritional aspects of cardiovascular disease. Department of Health Report on Health and Social Subjects No. 46. London: HMSO, 1994.

90. Golding J, Emmett PM, Rogers IS. Does breastfeeding have any impact on non-infectious, non-allergic disorders? Early Hum Dev 1997;49:S131–42.

91. Fredrickson DS, Levy RI, Lees RS. Fat Transport in lipoproteins – an integrated approach to mechanisms and Disorders. N Engl J Med 1967;276(1):34–42.

92. Tonstad S, Knudtzon J, Sivertsen M et al. Efficacy and safety of cholestyramine therapy in peripubertal and prepubertal children with familial hypercholesterolemia. J Pediatr 1996;129:42–9.

93. Couture P, Brun LD, Szots F et al. Association of specific LDL receptor gene mutations with different plasma lipoprotein response to simvastatin in young French Canadians with heterozygous familial hypercholesterolemia. Arterioscler Thromb Vasc Biol 1998;18:1007–12.

94. Ose L, Tonstad S. The detection and management of dyslipidaemia in children and adolescents. Acta Paediatr 1995;84:1213–5.

95. Assman G, von Eckardstein A, Cullen P. Dyslipidaemias. In: Fernandes J, Saudubray JM, van den Berghe G, editors. Inborn Metabolic Disease. Berlin: Springer, 1995:261–85.

96. Seddon HR, Green A, Gray RG et al. Regional variations in medium-chain acyl-CoA dehydrogenase deficiency. Lancet 1995;345:135–6.

97. Roe CR, Ding J. Mitochondrial fatty acid oxidation disorders. In: Scriver CR, Beaudet AL, Sly WS, Valle D (editors). The Metabolic and Molecular Basis of Inherited Disease, 8th ed. New York: McGraw-Hill, 2001:2297–326.

98. Strauss AW, Bennett MJ, Rinaldo P et al. Inherited long-chain 3-hydroxyacyl-CoA dehydrogenase deficiency and a fetal-maternal interaction cause maternal liver disease and other pregnancy complications. Semin Perinatol 1999;23:100–12.

99. Saudubray JM, Martin D, de Lonlay P et al. Recognition and management of fatty acid oxidation defects: a series of 107 patients. J Inherit Metab Dis 1999;22:488–502.

100. Rinaldo P. Mitochondrial fatty acid oxidation disorders and cyclic vomiting syndrome. Dig Dis Sci 1999;44(Suppl. 8):97S–102S.

101. Stanley CA. Disorders of fatty acid oxidation. In: Fernandes J, Saudubray JM, van den Berghe G (editors). Inborn Metabolic Disease. Berlin: Springer, 1995:133–43.

chapter 5

Carbohydrate Malabsorption

To a degree, carbohydrate malabsorption is physiologic. Impaired carbohydrate absorption found in lactating infants may be due to the oligosaccharides present in breast milk and also, in part, to lactose malabsorption. In other infants, sugar malabsorption can be the result of an imbalance between the amount of dietary carbohydrate ingested and the functional capacity for digestion and absorption, particularly in those infants who are overfed. Such malabsorption may also result from the combined presence of fructose and sorbitol in the proportions found in certain fruit juices (e.g. apple and pear), which makes them less absorbable than if they were administered separately. The absorption of fructose is facilitated by the presence of glucose. Carbohydrate malabsorption can be demonstrated by the presence of sugar in the stools, fecal pH below 5.5 and elevated hydrogen gas in the breath (see p. 166).

Physiologic carbohydrate malabsorption produces no symptoms other than flatulence. The causes for pathologic carbohydrate malabsorption, which leads to excessive flatulence, abdominal pain and/or diarrhea, can be congenital or acquired (Table 5.1).

The main carbohydrate ingested by infants is the disaccharide lactose; in contrast, in older children and adults sucrose and starches represent the main sources.

BASIC CHEMISTRY OF SUGARS

D-glucose is a hexose sugar, i.e. it contains six carbon atoms (Fig. 5.1). Glucose molecules can be linked to form a disaccharide or a polysaccharide such as starch, which is made up of amylopectin and, to a lesser extent, amylose (Figs 5.2 and 5.3). Amylose is formed by a straight chain of 200–2000 glucose units linked via α-1,4 oxygen bonds (the α designation means the OH at C-1 is below the plane of the ring). Salivary and pancreatic α-amylases can attack the interior α-1,4 junctions but not the outermost links – therefore maltose (two glucose units) and maltotriose (three glucose units) are the final products.

Amylopectin is highly branched, containing 250–5000 glucose units. The main linkage is α-1,4, but, at the branch site, a third unit of glucose is joined in the 6 position (see Fig. 5.3). Salivary and pancreatic amylases attack the interior α-1,4 glucose–glucose links, but cannot hydrolyze the exterior bonds or those at the branching points. Therefore, the end products of starch digestion are maltose, maltotriose and α-dextrins (see Fig. 5.2). Alpha-dextrins are hydrolyzed to glucose by mucosal α-dextrinase (isomaltase).

Congenital	Acquired
Lactase deficiency (rare)	Acute diarrhea
Sucrase–isomaltase deficiency	Chronic diarrhea
Fructose malabsorption	Enteropathy due to dietary protein intolerance
Glucose–galactose malabsorption	Small-bowel bacterial overgrowth
Cystic fibrosis	Giardiasis in patients with secretory IgA deficiency
	Short-bowel syndrome
	Celiac disease (mild and transient lactose malabsorption)

Table 5.1 Causes of carbohydrate malabsorption.

Diet (percentage of carbohydrate intake)	Luminal enzymes	Oligosaccharides and disaccharides presented to mucosa	Mucosal enzymes	End products
Starch (60%)		Maltose Maltotriose (α-1,4 linkage) ⟶	Maltase	Glucose
	Amylopectin ⟶ Salivary and pancreatic α-amylases	α-Dextrins (α-1,6 linkage) ⟶	α-Dextrinase (isomaltase)	Glucose
	Amylose ⟶ Salivary and pancreatic α-amylases	Maltose Maltotriose (α-1,4 linkage) ⟶	Maltase	Glucose
Sucrose (30%)	⟶	Sucrose ⟶	Sucrase	Glucose and fructose
Lactose (10%)	⟶	Lactose ⟶	Lactase	Glucose and galactose

Table 5.2 Carbohydrate digestion. Modified from Gray GM. Carbohydrate digestion and absorption. Gastroenterology 1970;58:100.

The major catalytic enzymes responsible for carbohydrate hydrolysis are (Table 5.2):

- Maltase (maltose and maltotriose to glucose)
- Lactase (lactose to glucose and galactose; Fig. 5.4a)
- Sucrase (sucrose to glucose and fructose; Fig. 5.4b)

Lactase reaches its peak level in the term neonate: the enzyme's activity is suboptimal in preterm infants, which explains the lactose malabsorption seen in very immature babies. The epithelial cells in the proximal jejunum have the highest concentration of brush-border enzymes. There is least activity in the terminal ileum.

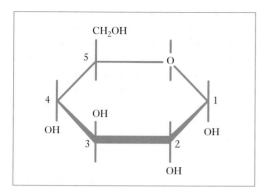

Figure 5.1 Haworth projection formula of sugars. For clarity, all carbon atoms have been omitted except the sixth.

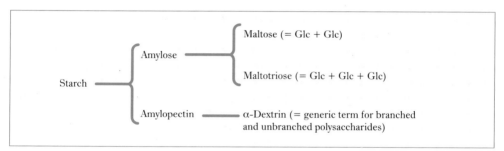

Figure 5.2 The composition of starch. Glc = glucose.

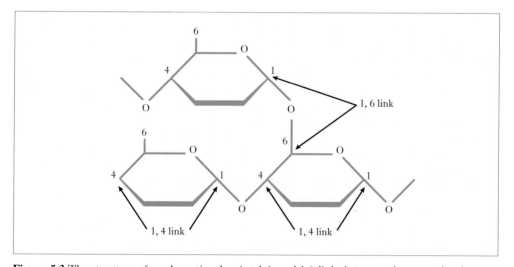

Figure 5.3 The structure of amylopectin, showing 1,4- and 1,6-links between glucose molecules.

MONOSACCHARIDE MALABSORPTION

Glucose–galactose malabsorption

Glucose–galactose malabsorption is a rare autosomal recessive defect leading to impaired absorption of the two separate monosaccharides transported by a common mechanism [1]. Glucose and galactose are the monosaccharides derived from the hydrolysis of lactose by

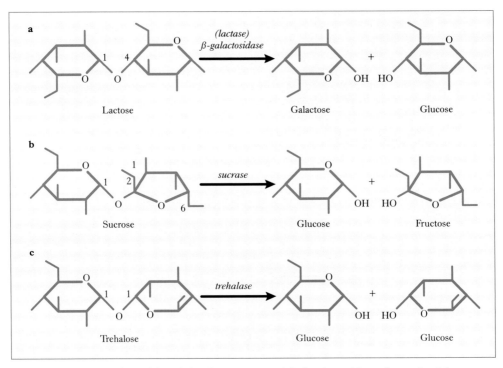

Figure 5.4 The action of brush-border enzymes: **(a)** β-galactosidase (lactase); **(b)** sucrase; **(c)** trehalase.

lactase, the brush-border enzyme predominantly distributed in the outermost part of the small-bowel villi. In glucose–galactose malabsorption, lactase activity is intact. The problem resides in the absence of the transmembrane glucose carrier [2].

Presentation
Diarrhea is seen when the baby is given a glucose solution such as a water–electrolyte preparation or a feed containing either lactose or a glucose polymer. Stools are explosive and watery. Presenting features are similar to those seen in disaccharidase deficiencies (see p. 165). Symptoms become less severe in the second or third year of life as the child develops a greater capacity to ferment the malabsorbed carbohydrates in the colon.

Diagnosis
Diagnosis is based on the following:

- pH of stool supernatant is below 5.5

- Presence of reducing substances or glucose in feces – in normal neonates, however, this finding may be physiologic

- Symptoms resolve when the patient is fasted

- Hydrogen breath test (see p. 166), using lactose as the loading sugar

- Jejunal biopsy – both small-bowel architecture and disaccharidase activity level are normal; this test is not necessary if the diagnosis can be made by the hydrogen breath test (see p. 166)

Management

Glucose, galactose and lactose must all be excluded from the diet. The alternative milk substitute is a preparation containing fructose (e.g. Galactomin in the UK; Appendix IV.1) or a feeding regimen using a protein and fat module that is free of lactose, to which fructose can be added (e.g. Ross Carbohydrate Free in the USA; Appendix IV.2).

Fructose malabsorption

Fructose, a ketohexose, is absorbed by facilitated diffusion. Absorption is maximal when the monosaccharide is given in a solution that contains a similar amount of glucose. When fructose is combined with sorbitol, carbohydrate malabsorption occurs. Excessive intake of fruit juices that contain fructose and sorbitol, such as pear and apple, can result in diarrhea and/or abdominal pain.

Diagnosis

Diagnosis is based on the following:

- A thorough dietary history

- Hydrogen breath test (see p. 166)

- Complete disappearance of the symptoms upon withdrawal of fructose from the diet

Acquired fructose malabsorption

Damage to the villi can cause malabsorption of this monosaccharide. The clinical features are similar to those seen in other sugar intolerances.

DISACCHARIDE MALABSORPTION

Sucrase–isomaltase deficiency [3]

Isolated deficiency of the brush-border enzyme complex sucrase/isomaltase (= sucrase/α-dextrinase) is the result of an inherited autosomal recessive disorder (see Fig. 5.4b). The incidence in most populations is between 1:500 and 1:30,000, but in the Eskimos of Greenland it is as high as 10%. The defect of the two enzymes, sucrase and isomaltase, always coexists. Isomaltase activity (measured as palatinase) concerns the α-1,6 glucosidic linkage. Secondary deficiency of sucrase–isomaltase will be seen as a result of severe mucosal damage (e.g. post enteritis), in which case the disaccharidase lactase will also be decreased (see below).

Presentation

Clinical manifestations of sucrose intolerance arise from incomplete hydrolysis of this disaccharide and starch. Undigested sucrose in the jejunum will increase the osmotic load of the intraluminal contents, thus causing watery diarrhea. Abdominal distension and cramps will occur when the malabsorbed carbohydrate is fermented in the colon.

Diagnosis

Diagnosis is based on the following:

- Presence of carbohydrate in stools (Clinitest reaction; see below) – because sucrose is a non-reducing sugar two volumes of 1 N hydrochloric acid should be added to one volume of liquid stool, then boiled for 30 seconds *before* carrying out the Clinitest reaction (see below)

- Fecal pH below 5.5 if there is carbohydrate malabsorption

- Hydrogen breath test (see p. 166)

- Jejunal biopsy – although enzyme assay in a small-bowel biopsy sample demonstrating low activity, in the presence of normal histology, is the definitive diagnostic test, this is rarely necessary

- Complete disappearance of the symptoms upon withdrawal of sucrose and starches from the diet

Clinitest reaction

This is a test for reducing substances in the fluid portion of the stool (not with Clinistix, which is specific for glucose). A small volume of liquid stool should be placed in a test tube and twice its volume of water added. One Clinitest tablet should be added to 15 drops of suspension.

Results

- 0.25% = negative (normal)

- 0.25%–0.5% = suspect

- >0.5% = abnormal

Management

Removal of concentrated sources of sucrose from the diet is the most important aspect of management. In infants this means ensuring that the normal milk formula used is sucrose-free. In the primary condition, where there is an isolated enzyme deficiency, the ability to hydrolyze glucose polymers, cornstarch and dextrins should be normal. Sweetened fruit drinks and syrups should be eliminated from the diet and care needs to be taken to ensure that any medicines do not have a sucrose base. When infant solid foods are introduced, they should be free of sucrose and starch. A list of suitable items is given in Appendix IV.28.

In the older child without severe symptoms the diet need not be so restrictive. Although the 1,6-linkage of starch cannot be hydrolyzed owing to lack of isomaltase, these α-limit dextrins constitute only about 30% of the hydrolyzed starch molecule, and do not impose a high osmotic load in the gut lumen. In practice, foods containing starch can be given in limited quantities. Tolerance to starch improves with age because of the increased capacity of the colonic flora to ferment malabsorbed carbohydrate. Foods such as fruit with natural sucrose complexed with fiber tend to be better tolerated than processed foods containing added sucrose. Parents and children tend to construct a diet that suits the individual, perhaps limiting their intake to one normal-sized serving of starch-containing foods and one small serving of natural sucrose per meal. Soy flour can be used in place of wheat flour where the child wishes to eat more baked foods than can be tolerated. Soy flour has a relatively low starch content (15 g per 100 g) when compared with wheat flour (80 g per 100 g). Because it does not contain gluten, it will not rise and does not give a light, aerated product.

Where only small amounts of fruit and potato are tolerated and green vegetables are not taken, a supplement of ascorbic acid and folate should be given.

Congenital and genetically acquired lactase deficiency

Lactase-phlorizin hydrolase (LPH) is a membrane-bound brush-border enzyme that hydrolyzes lactose to its two monosaccharide components, glucose and galactose (see Fig. 5.4a). The protein is synthesized by enterocytes as a 220-kilodalton precursor, which is then processed to the mature 150-kilodalton protein. In contrast to the situation in non-human mammals, LPH remains active during the adult life of some humans. Unlike the other intestinal disaccharidases, lactase develops early in the fetus, from the second trimester, to reach a peak of activity in the perinatal period. Thus, it is not unusual for an immature neonate to demonstrate a transient developmental intolerance to lactose. There is no evidence that lactase is an inducible enzyme, i.e. that offering a baby the substrate lactose promotes enzymal activity. Most of the lactase is localized in the outermost part of the intestinal villi, making it very vulnerable to mucosal damage.

Congenital lactase deficiency

The existence of this very rare congenital disorder of lactose malabsorption is disputed by some. Symptoms arise immediately after birth when breast milk or a lactose-containing formula is offered.

Genetically acquired lactase deficiency

This form of hypolactasia, also known as adult-type hypolactasia, is the most common disaccharidase deficiency, affecting one-third to almost one-half of the population worldwide. It was reported for the first time in 1959 [4]. Several factors have been implicated in the decline of LPH in human hypolactasia, such as reduction of (pre) pro-LPH synthesis, slow processing of the protein and the fact that only some enterocytes continue to produce LPH.

Symptoms

As with other cases of disaccharidase deficiency, flatulence, abdominal pain and/or diarrhea follow the ingestion of milk. Many individuals may not be aware of the relationship between milk intake and the symptoms described [5,6]. Lactase deficiency needs to be considered among the causes of abdominal pain, particularly in the older pediatric population and especially if they are not of north European descent (see Chapter 9).

Secondary lactase deficiency

Acquired, secondary or transient lactase deficiency is frequently the result of an intestinal infection. The following conditions can cause transient lactase deficiency:

- Enteritis (viral, parasitic, bacterial, fungal)

- Dietary protein intolerance

- Celiac disease

Lactose intolerance is a common complication of gastroenteritis in infants and young children living in the developed world. The incidence of severe lactose intolerance in the post-enteritis syndrome has decreased substantially in the last 15 years, in association with the use of oral (rather than intravenous) rehydration and early reintroduction to feeding or both.

Presentation

Diarrhea is the major feature seen in malabsorption of lactose, irrespective of the basic pathology. Explosive diarrhea and the presence of watery, acidic stools become evident after milk ingestion. Non-hydrolyzed disaccharides cause considerable movement of electrolytes and water into the gut lumen and this provokes osmotic diarrhea (Fig. 5.5). Excoriation of the perianal area is common because of the acidic stools. Incompletely absorbed lactose is passed from the small bowel to the colon, where it is fermented by bacteria to acids and gas. Abdominal distension, with or without vomiting, may appear, and the infant will not thrive. In some situations, blood (macroscopic or microscopic) may be found in the stools. In the developing world, infection with more than one pathogen (e.g. *Salmonella* and *Entamoeba histolytica*) can involve the colon, and the stools may contain mucus.

The differential diagnosis includes secretory diarrheas. Secretory diarrhea is characterized by a fecal sodium concentration of more than 90 mmol/l, and a volume greater than 200 ml/day. Fecal osmolarity is less than plasma osmolarity (= <300 mOsm/kg) and there is a persistence of fecal losses despite fasting. Characteristically, diarrhea caused by carbohydrate malabsorption improves when the patient is fasted.

Cow milk protein intolerance can produce an enteropathy in the upper gastrointestinal tract with lactose malabsorption and, uncommonly, colitis (milk-sensitive) in the large bowel.

Diagnosis

Diagnosis is based on the following:

- Clinitest reaction (see p. 166) – this is only valid if lactose is still being ingested

- Stool pH – if <5.5, sugar is present

- Hydrogen breath test, using lactose as the loading sugar (see p. 166) – stools should be examined for pH and the Clinitest reaction during and following the test period

- Jejunal biopsy – this may be helpful in patients with post-enteritis syndrome who are not responding to dietary manipulations

Management

The dietary treatment of adverse reactions to lactose relates to the severity of the symptoms. Weight loss in a small infant necessitates the removal of virtually all lactose from the diet, while a less intense reaction may respond to a temporary reduction in lactose intake. Although most pill-type medicines contain lactose as a filler, it is rarely necessary to remove lactose entirely from the diet of an infant or young child; a reduction in the lactose concentration of the diet may be sufficient to alleviate symptoms.

A minimal lactose regimen means that no milk from any species can be used, because lactose is the carbohydrate in human, cow, goat and sheep milk. A milk without lactose should be

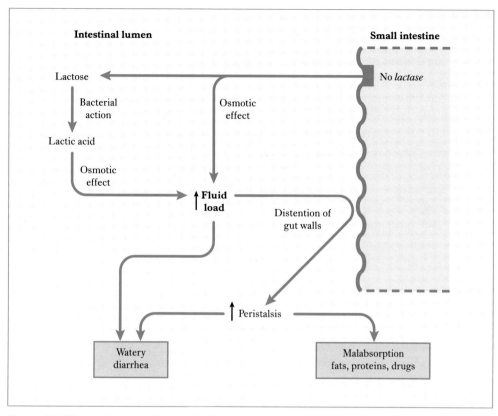

Figure 5.5 The mechanism of congenital lactase deficiency. (Courtesy of WF Balistreri.)

used (Appendix IV.2). Because it is sometimes difficult to differentiate between adverse reactions to lactose and to other components of cow milk, particularly protein, it may be prudent to use a preparation that does not include intact cow milk protein. This type of formula (Appendices IV.2 and IV.3) is always free of lactose. A normal infant formula which contains glucose polymers rather than lactose would be the most suitable if protein intolerance is not suspected; milks with this type of composition are discussed in the section on normal milks (Appendix II.7). For older children who are receiving unmodified cow milk, preparations of the enzyme lactase can be added to the milk to remove approximately 70% of the lactose [7]. No advantage in terms of growth or improved nutrient retention has been shown in children with primary lactose intolerance from whom milk is withheld.

Small infants who are taking solid foods and have shown a severe reaction to lactose should be offered a lactose-free weaning diet (Appendix IV.29). The duration of the diet is a matter of clinical judgement. It is important that the infant should be tolerating the feed and gaining weight before any attempt is made to reintroduce lactose. Although lactase levels are not influenced by substrate concentrations, there should be a slow reintroduction of this sugar into the diet to prevent the reappearance of symptoms. Approximately 10% of the lactose-free formula should be replaced by a normal infant formula or breast milk for the first 24 h. This 10% should not be given in one feed but be divided and combined with the lactose-free formula. The quantity of lactose-containing milk can be increased over a period of 4–5 days until full-lactose milk is consumed.

Lactose and sucrose intolerance – management

Where there is severe trauma to the small-bowel mucosa, both lactase and sucrase–isomaltase enzymes may be depleted, leading to malabsorption of all disaccharides and starch (see Table 5.2). Digestion of glucose polymer, hydrolyzed cornstarch and dextrins may also be affected because the hydrolysis of short-chain oligosaccharides requires α-glucosidase, which is a brush-border enzyme. For the young infant, treatment is identical to that of lactose intolerance alone, with the proviso that the lactose-free formula selected contains only glucose, or glucose with fructose, as the carbohydrate. If symptoms persist, solids free of lactose and sucrose should be given. Care should be taken when introducing starch, as only small quantities may be tolerated. Until normal gut function returns, gluten should be omitted from the diet because there may be a transient and secondary gluten intolerance. A list of suitable foods is shown in Appendix IV.35.

Complete carbohydrate intolerance – management

In addition to reduced disaccharidase activity, where there is severe damage to the mucosa of the small intestine, the absorptive mechanism for monosaccharides may also fail. Small infants, particularly those who are malnourished, do not have large glycogen stores and are inefficient converters of glucogenic amino acids to glucose by gluconeogenesis. Consequently, it is vital that a parenteral source of glucose is given. If total parenteral nutrition is not possible, provided that glucose is given parenterally, a carbohydrate-free oral feed may be tolerated. Examples of preparations containing protein and fat, either singly or in combination, are described in the section on modular feeding in Appendices IV.14–IV.19. If solid foods are administered, it needs to be remembered that protein foods that are free of carbohydrate are meat, poultry, fish and eggs.

When the infant appears to be tolerating a carbohydrate-free regimen and is maintaining weight (weight gain is unlikely), small quantities of a monosaccharide can be introduced. A mixture of glucose and fructose is likely to be better tolerated than a higher concentration of either sugar alone. Initially, 1 g glucose per 100 ml feed can be added in the first 24 h. If the sugar does not appear in the feces and the stool frequency does not increase, then 1 g fructose per 100 ml feed can also be added. When a total of 6 g mixed carbohydrate per 100 ml feed is tolerated, the procedure and feeding regimen is as for lactose/sucrose intolerance.

Trehalase deficiency

This is a very rare disorder due to the absence (or deficiency) of the intestinal enzyme trehalase (Fig. 5.4c). The major source of trehalose, a non-reducing sugar, is the young mushroom; it is converted to glucose in the older mushroom. This sugar intolerance is characterized by watery diarrhea soon after young mushrooms are ingested. This can be treated by eliminating the offending source of the carbohydrate from the diet.

REFERENCES

1.   Lindquist B, Meeuwisse GW, Melin, K. Glucose-galactose malabsorption. Lancet 1962;ii:666.

2.   Wright EM. The intestinal Na^+/glucose cotransporter. Annu Rev Physiol 1993;55:575–89.

3.   Auricchio S. Genetically determined disaccharidase deficiencies. In: Walker WA, Durie PR, Hamilton JR et al. editors. Pediatric Gastrointestinal Disease: Pathophysiology, Diagnosis, Management. Volume 1. Philadelphia: BC Decker, 1991:647–67.

4.   Holzel A, Schwarz V, Sutcliffe, KW. Defective lactose absorption causing malnutrition in infancy. Lancet 1959;i:1126–8

5.   Bedine MS, Bayless TM. Intolerance of small amounts of lactose by individuals with low lactase level. Gastroenterology 1973;65:735–43.

6.   Caspary WF. Diarrhea associated with carbohydrate malabsorption. Clin Gastroenterol 1986;15:631–55.

7.   Biller JA, King S, Rosenthal A et al. Efficacy of lactase-treated milk for lactose intolerant pediatric patients. J Pediatr 1987;111:91–4.

chapter 6

Malabsorption Syndromes

In addition to the entities described in detail below, malabsorption can be seen in a variety of situations such as:

- Chronic diarrhea (see Chapter 7)

- Protein-sensitive enteropathy (see Chapter 8)

- Giardiasis, particularly in patients with IgA deficiency

- Crohn's disease (see Chapter 11)

- Cystic fibrosis (see Chapter 15)

- Short-bowel syndrome (see Chapter 12)

CELIAC DISEASE (GLUTEN-SENSITIVE ENTEROPATHY)

Celiac disease is a life-long disorder caused by an intolerance to gluten, the germ protein present in wheat and other cereals [1,2]. A temporary gluten intolerance can arise as a secondary phenomenon. The prevalence of celiac disease varies widely within Europe, ranging from 1:3000 in England, through 1:1850 in Scotland, 1:890 in Switzerland and 1:496 in eastern Austria, to a peak of 1:300 in the Galway region of western Ireland and 1:184 in Italy. One American community study in Minnesota revealed a prevalence of less than 1:5000 [3]. There is a high frequency (1.6%) in Down syndrome [4,5]. In an Italian study of 63 children (mean age of 11 years) with Williams syndrome there was a prevalence in the series of 9.6%. This was comparable to the level seen in both the chromosomal disorders Down and Turner syndromes, and higher than that in the general population in Italy (0.54%) [6]. The difference in prevalence between Europe and America has been attributed to the difference in the structure of their grains. The decreasing incidence of celiac disease in some countries over the last two decades has been linked to an increase in breastfeeding, a reduction in the protein content and osmolality of infant milk, and later introduction of weaning in Western countries [7]. In Sweden, the incidence has decreased as a result of a national policy to reduce gluten intake in infants. In The Netherlands, in contrast with many other countries, the incidence has increased in the last 15 years [8].

Celiac disease was originally described in the first century AD by Aretaeus of Cappadocia. A vivid and classic clinical description of this alimentary tract disease was written by Samuel Gee in the St Bartholomew's Hospital Report of 1888: "Faeces, being loose, ... bulky, ... pale, ... stinking." In more contemporary times, Dicke in Holland noted the link between wheat and steatorrhea [9].

CLINICAL FEATURES

Commonly, celiac disease presents before the age of 2 years and usually within 6 months of starting cereals, but may be diagnosed only in late childhood or even adulthood. Frequently, these children are referred to pediatricians because of irritability, apathy, a delay or regression of motor development, hypotonia, malaise, anorexia, failure to thrive, the passage of foul, bulky stools and vomiting. They may have dental enamel defects [10]. Edema may arise secondary to a protein-losing enteropathy that has caused hypoproteinemia. Muscle wasting is a useful sign and is usually most evident around the shoulders, hips or buttocks. The classic presentation with abdominal distension is less common nowadays as physicians are more aware of the disease [11]. However, the gastrointestinal symptoms sometimes can be subtle with a variable expression (Fig. 6.1), and the child's main feature might be small stature [12]. Monosymptomatic forms of celiac disease have been reported, such as severe constipation, anemia, dental enamel hypoplasia [10,13], delayed puberty and sterility in women [14]. The commonest type of anemia in celiac disease is due to iron deficiency; megaloblastic anemia is rare. Serum iron, serum folate and red cell folate are all usually reduced in patients older than 1 year. The infant should be examined for digital clubbing and clinical evidence of anemia.

There is a highly significant increase in the incidence of histocompatibility antigens HLA-B8, HLA-DR3 and HLA-DR7 in patients with celiac disease when compared with controls [15]. HLA-B8 has a very high frequency within the Galway population mentioned above. Furthermore, a lymphocyte antigen independent of the HLA system has been identified in many cases of celiac disease [16].

The precise mechanism of the toxic effect of gluten is unknown. Gluten is a large complex molecule that consists of gliadin, glutenin and globulins. Electrophoresis shows gliadin to be composed of about 40 different compounds – the α-gliadin fraction is the most toxic.

DIAGNOSIS

In regions where celiac disease is prevalent, or when the index of suspicion is high – such as when the patient has juvenile chronic arthritis [17] or insulin-dependent diabetes [18], or has a close relative with the disease [19] – most pediatric gastroenterologists will perform a small-bowel biopsy (see below) without requesting any preliminary tests. This is justified because, if the prevalence of the disease is high, in the presence of compatible symptomatology, the patient is more likely than not to have celiac disease. On the other hand, in regions where celiac disease is not very prevalent, most specialists may want to perform some preliminary tests that will justify the small-bowel biopsy. If the only symptom is failure to thrive and the index of suspicion is not high, nutritional supplementation for a limited time, with a diet not excluding gluten, may be the best approach. Exclusion of gluten will confuse the diagnosis.

Laboratory investigations

The following investigations are available to the clinician.

Serum antigliadin antibodies

This test has a relatively good sensitivity and very good specificity for the suspicion of celiac disease [12,20]. The IgA immunofluorescent test is more specific but less sensitive than the

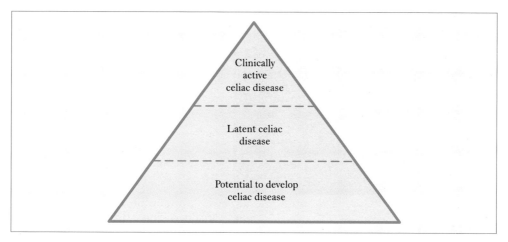

Figure 6.1 Iceberg model of celiac disease.

IgG one. False positivity increases with age, with a relatively high number of false positives in asymptomatic prepubertal children.

Serum antiendomysial antibodies

This test is more sensitive than antigliadin antibodies [21,22]. It measures antibodies of the IgA subclass. It should be remembered that false-negative results may be seen in those with IgA deficiency, the frequency of which is relatively high among patients with celiac disease. According to a study conducted in Italy [23], of 2098 patients with celiac disease, 54 (2.6%) had IgA deficiency, more than 10 times the rate observed in the general population. Consequently, it may be necessary to request quantitative serum immunoglobulins to rule out IgA deficiency or antigliadin.

Tissue transglutaminase (tTG) is the predominant autoantigen recognized by endomysial antibodies. Thus, the tTG-based enzyme-linked immunosorbent assay is the preferred serologic test [24,25]. However, false negative antibody results can occur in a mild enteropathy, as well as in those less than two years of age and especially in the presence of IgA deficiency [26].

Fecal smear for fat globules

This is a simple test which is considered to be abnormal if more than 100 globules per high-power field are seen. It is not specific.

Fecal fat collection for 72 h

This is used for the quantification of fat excretion using colorant markers to time the collection together with calculation of the total fat intake during the study. It is a cumbersome and non-specific test. Although steatorrhea occurs in 80% of cases of celiac disease, it may only be evident later in the disease, and, indeed, in some infants there is no increase in the stool fat content. An abnormal fat collection result is greater than 10% excretion; exceeding 5 g/24 h in infants and 3.5 g/24 h in children.

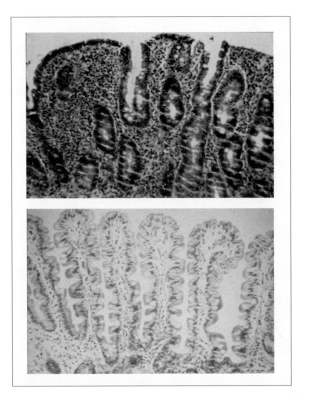

Figure 6.2 (a) Histologic appearance showing flattened villi of the proximal small intestine in celiac disease. **(b)** Normal appearance for comparison – tall fingerlike villi.

Intestinal permeability test

This test determines the ratio of the urinary excretion of two partially absorbable sugars of different molecular weight administered by mouth [27]. As the test is not very sensitive it will be abnormal only in cases where the mucosa is at least moderately affected. It is not used in routine clinical practice.

Xylose absorption

This test is of limited value and has almost been abandoned. Although there is a high degree of correlation between a severely abnormal biopsy and a low 1-h blood xylose after a load of 5 g (14.2 g/m^2) as a 10% solution, the test is less sensitive when the mucosal lesion is not that severe.

Biopsy

Diagnosis is made histologically from a duodenal or jejunal biopsy [28]. Biopsies can be obtained through an endoscope or by a thin tube-like device that is swallowed and allowed to advance to the angle of Treitz (duodenojejunal junction). On histology, there is a diffuse lesion of the proximal small intestine with atrophy of villi (Figs 6.2 and 6.3), lymphocyte infiltration and deepening of the crypts [29]. However, these findings are not pathognomonic of celiac disease or of transient gluten intolerance. In addition to loss of villi and crypt hyperplasia, there is inflammatory cell infiltration of the lamina propria and an increase in the number of

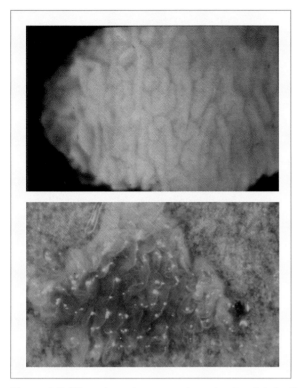

Figure 6.3 Dissecting microscope views showing **(a)** the flat mucosa seen in celiac disease; **(b)** normal mucosa for comparison. (Courtesy of Dr M Brueton.)

intraepithelial lymphocytes. Severe villous atrophy is likely to be accompanied by a deficiency of one or both of the brush-border disaccharidases – lactase and sucrase. There are some other causes of villus damage, such as post-enteritis syndrome and dietary protein intolerance.

The original recommendations to make a diagnosis of celiac disease required three small-bowel biopsies over an unspecified period:

- Initial biopsy revealing damaged or flattened villi
- Normal biopsy findings on a gluten-free diet
- Histologic relapse following a gluten-containing diet or after challenge with 20 g daily of gluten powder

These so-called Interlaken criteria were formerly agreed upon at a meeting of the European Society for Paediatric Gastroenterology in 1969 [30]. Although there is still no universal agreement, most authors consider that these criteria do not always need to be met in order to make the diagnosis.

There may be difficulties in distinguishing celiac disease from a transient gluten intolerance. If challenge with gluten causes no histologic or clinical deterioration and if gluten were responsible originally, then, following a normal biopsy, the problem is a temporary and not a permanent intolerance.

Condition	Difference/Diagnosis
Cystic fibrosis	Sweat test
Cow milk and/or soy protein intolerance	Generally more eosinophils in biopsy
Tropical sprue	Bacteria can be seen attached to mucosa
Giardiasis, particularly in patients deficient in secretory IgA	*Giardia* antigen in stools; *Giardia* attached to mucosa (seen by electron microscopy)
Lymphoma of small intestine (mainly in adults)	Characterize cells
Immunodeficiency, congenital or acquired	Quantitative serum immunoglobulins, skin tests, HIV tests
Bacterial overgrowth of the small bowel	Breath hydrogen test; culture of small-bowel contents
Crohn's disease	Rarely villus damage; other manifestations such as perianal signs and extraintestinal features (e.g. arthritis, uveitis and erythema nodosum) and positive serology (anti-*Saccharomyces cerevisiae* antibody)
Autoimmune enteropathy	+ antienterocyte antibodies

Table 6.1 Differential diagnosis of celiac disease.

Gluten challenge

Various methods of gluten administration and times of post-challenge biopsy have been proposed. Some favor the use of up to 20 g/day of commercially prepared gluten powder; this has the disadvantage that the gluten ingested is not in the same form as cooked gluten in food, and its toxicity may be altered. If natural foods are used, it is important to ensure that an adequate amount is taken: 10 g of wheat protein daily (equivalent to 130 g [approximately 2 slices] of bread or 90 g of flour) for 3–4 months appears to be sufficient in many – but not in all – with celiac disease. In a few, even the so-called 2-year rule is insufficient time to induce a relapse.

DIFFERENTIAL DIAGNOSIS

Other disorders that may produce symptoms of celiac disease are listed in Table 6.1.

DIETARY MANAGEMENT OF CELIAC DISEASE

The treatment for celiac disease and gluten-induced enteropathies is a gluten-free diet (see Appendix IV.35). Whether the enteropathy is thought to be true celiac disease – requiring life-long adherence to the diet – or a transient gluten intolerance, the principles of management are the same. There is general agreement that wheat and rye should be completely excluded from the diet. The position is less clear when oats and possibly barley are considered, although there is clinical evidence that they are toxic [31]. In England, it has been demonstrated that only 12% of children with celiac disease are adversely affected by the inclusion of oats in their diet. A recent study in children has indicated that intake of oats may

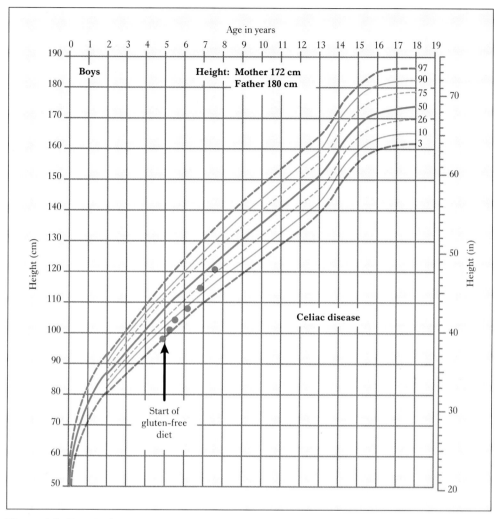

Figure 6.4 Growth chart of a child with celiac disease, showing improvement after the introduction of a gluten-free diet.

be safe in children with newly diagnosed celiac disease [32]. All four cereals, along with beer and malt, continue to be excluded in most centers in the UK and USA until further long-term evidence is available to support the inclusion of oats or barley. Following the introduction of a strict gluten-free diet, an impressive growth spurt is seen; however, it might take 2–3 years before the peak velocity of growth height is achieved (Fig. 6.4). If there is evidence of lactose intolerance, temporary limitation of lactose may be necessary.

Compliance with the restrictive diet is likely to be poor, particularly among adolescents. Failure to comply with the diet during childhood is associated with short stature and depressed brush-border enzyme activity, particularly lactase. Poor contractility of the gallbladder – worsening fat absorption – has been documented in patients with untreated celiac disease.

Foods allowed and forbidden

All wheat, rye, barley and products derived from these cereals should be excluded from the regimen. It is controversial whether oats should be excluded as well (see above).

Processed foods

With the enormous variety of manufactured food products available in Western countries, it is impossible to give comprehensive instructions for the avoidance of gluten in processed foods (see Appendix IV.35). Unless the ingredients are included on the packaging, it is wise to omit them. Careful scrutiny of labels each time a food is purchased is important, as the composition of complex products can change. In the UK, owing to the efforts of the Coeliac Society, some major food retailers whose products are guaranteed free of wheat products put a gluten-free symbol on their packaging. The UK Coeliac Society also publishes a list, regularly updated, of foodstuffs that are gluten-free (http://www.coeliac.co.uk), as does the American Society (http://www.celiac.com/). In all countries where stringent food regulations exist and information is available, dieticians should be able to compile a list of gluten-free manufactured products.

Special gluten-free foods

In countries where wheat is the staple cereal, it is advantageous to include specially prepared gluten-free equivalents of bread, bagels, biscuits, cookies and pasta in the diet. Without these products, the diet can prove to be expensive, unless substantial amounts of pulses, lentils and nuts are taken, as large quantities of animal protein foods will be needed to provide an adequate energy intake for a growing child. Special foods are generally prepared from purified wheat starch. This has given rise to some controversy recently as to whether the small portion of cereal protein left over after treatment of the wheat starch is harmful. There is no evidence to suggest that this small residue causes adverse effects in celiac disease, and biopsies demonstrate that the mucosa returns to normal when these products are included in the diet. There are standards laid down for gluten-free foods by the Committee on Foods for Special Dietary Use of the Codex Alimentarius Commission of the World Health Organization. These standards state that a residual cereal nitrogen content of 0.05% is acceptable, providing that the residual material contains no gliadin. Bagels contain a large amount of glutenous flour and therefore should be avoided.

In the UK and USA, a number of proprietary breads, bread mixes, biscuits, cookies, crackers, flours and pasta are available for use in celiac disease, for purchase or on prescription. A full list of these foods is available from dieticians and from the Celiac Societies.

Research has been carried out recently on the use of strains of wheat thought to be naturally lacking in a fraction of the gliadin molecule, but to date they have not proved to be of any practical use.

Vitamin and mineral supplements

Various deficiency states have been described in celiacs prior to treatment. Because of the generalized malabsorption, it is advisable to give a multivitamin supplement, including a water-miscible form of the fat-soluble vitamins (see Appendix II.14). If there is a prolonged prothrombin time, parenteral vitamin K is indicated initially, especially prior to any small-bowel biopsy. A trace element preparation, administered either orally or parenterally, may be useful in children with long-standing malabsorption or failure to thrive (see Appendix II.14).

Supplements should not be considered a permanent part of a gluten-free regimen. A varied diet will provide an adequate intake, and vitamins and minerals are absorbed normally after improvement of the small-bowel histology and may thus be discontinued when the child has shown a good response to the diet [33].

COMPLICATIONS

Failure to thrive

Where diagnosis has been delayed, infants or children may present with severe failure to thrive, resembling frank protein–energy malnutrition (PEM). These patients will achieve catch-up growth and show an earlier response to dietary treatment if they are given a generous protein and energy intake, as well as supplemental vitamins, minerals and trace elements. Steatorrhea is the consequence of defects in absorption, lipolysis, micelle formation and the enterohepatic circulation, as well as suspected exocrine pancreatic insufficiency [34]. Because fat is malabsorbed, a milk containing medium-chain triglycerides may be better tolerated than one with long-chain fatty acids. Precautions should be taken to ensure that this is not introduced too rapidly (Appendix IV.13). Alternatively, a high-protein, high-energy formula based on skimmed milk can be used (Appendix III.8).

Celiac crisis

This is a rare life-threatening complication in which dehydration provoked by diarrhea accompanies malabsorption. Although this was not an uncommon mode of presentation in Western countries previously, it is rarely seen now, probably owing to increased awareness and earlier referral. However, children in less-developed countries may still present in this dramatic manner, particularly where a hot climate or intercurrent infection exacerbates dehydration. Acidosis, hypokalemia and hypoglycemia, along with low serum levels of calcium and magnesium, may be encountered. Correction of the fluid, electrolyte and mineral status is of first importance. When the infant is able to take oral feeds, he or she should be treated with a multiple malabsorption regimen – excluding not only gluten but also milk and soy protein and disaccharides – until the diagnosis has been established.

PROBLEMS ARISING FROM A GLUTEN-FREE DIET

Dental problems

There is no evidence to suggest that a gluten-free diet has a deleterious effect on tooth development, and the incidence of caries appears not to be increased in children with celiac disease. However, parents should be warned that caries will result if they ply children with sweets in order to compensate for dietary restrictions. Delay in diagnosis and subsequent poor nutrition can lead to enamel hypoplasia, which may be severe [10].

Constipation

A gluten-free diet is necessarily low in cereal fiber, the main source of this in Western diets being wholemeal wheat products. Constipation can be a problem in those children who do

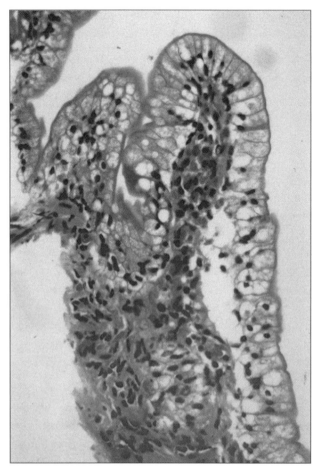

Figure 6.5 Small-bowel biopsy in abetalipoproteinemia. Note the epithelial cells are vacuolated by lipids which cannot be transported. (Courtesy of Dr N Croft and Dr S Naik.)

not care for vegetables and fruit. Even when reasonable quantities of these items are eaten, difficulty can still be encountered. The inclusion of pulses, beans (including gluten-free varieties of baked beans), nuts and lentils should be encouraged, as they can be helpful. Gluten-free bread enriched with soy bran compares favorably with wheat bran in its properties and should prove useful where constipation is a problem (Appendix IV.35).

ABETALIPOPROTEINEMIA (BASSEN–KORNZWEIG SYNDROME)

Abetalipoproteinemia is a rare disorder of lipid metabolism inherited in an autosomal recessive manner and characterized by the following: failure to thrive and steatorrhea early in infancy, and progressive ataxia (degeneration of spinocerebellar tracts) and retinitis pigmentosa later in childhood [35]. Although acanthocytes (thorny red cells) in the peripheral blood smear are pathognomonic, it can be difficult to distinguish these malformed erythrocytes from burr cells. The primary defect is the deficiency of apoprotein

B and low-density lipoprotein (LDL), a β-lipoprotein. LDL is needed to form chylomicrons; in its absence, dietary fat accumulates within the engorged enterocyte as it cannot be transported away. Beta-lipoproteins transport more than 50% of the cholesterol of human plasma, and their deficiency leads to abnormally low levels of lipids in the plasma. Dietary triglycerides are normally re-esterified in the intestinal mucosa and then transported through the lymphatic system as chylomicrons. However, without β-lipoproteins, chylomicrons cannot be formed. Coagulation abnormalities in patients presenting with hemorrhages have been described in abetalipoproteinemia. A jejunal biopsy will show distended small-intestinal epithelial cells full of triglyceride (Fig. 6.5).

INVESTIGATIONS

Typical findings include the following:

- Blood film shows acanthocytosis of erythrocytes (crenated red cells with spiny/thorny excrescences)
- Low plasma cholesterol (<2.0 mmol/1)
- Low plasma triglyceride (<0.25 mmol/1)
- Only high-density lipoprotein (α-lipoprotein) band present on lipid electrophoresis
- Jejunal biopsy shows normal villi morphologically but distended with lipid drops (see Fig. 6.5)

MANAGEMENT

Early treatment in infancy prevents retinal and neurological complications.

DIETARY TREATMENT

Some of the clinical manifestations of abetalipoproteinemia resemble those of deficiencies of the fat-soluble vitamins A, D, E and K. Thus, it is essential that these vitamins are given in a water-miscible form as soon as the diagnosis is made. If an oral supplement such as Ketovite liquid (UK) or Liquid Adeks (USA; Scandipharm) (Appendix II.14) is not absorbed, it may be necessary to use a parenteral source of these vitamins. Initially, a minimal fat regimen is recommended, as described on p. 153 for intestinal lymphangiectasia. After weaning, the fat content of the diet should remain as low as is practical. It is important to note that the energy content of the diet may be low and careful attention must be paid to providing calories from suitable non-fat sources.

REFERENCES

1. Littlewood JM. Coeliac disease in childhood. Baillieres Clin Gastroenterol 1995;9:295–327.

2. Troncone R, Greco L, Auricchio S. Gluten-sensitive enteropathy. Pediatr Clin North Am 1996;43:355–73.

3. Talley NJ, Valdovinos M, Petterson TM et al. Epidemiology of celiac sprue: A community-based study. Am J Gastroenterol 1994;89:843–6.

4. George EK, Mearin ML, Bouquet J et al. High frequency of celiac disease in Down syndrome. J Pediatr 1996;128:555–7.

5. Bonamico M, Rasore-Quartino A, Mariani P et al. Down syndrome and coeliac disease: Usefulness of antigliadin and antiendomysium antibodies. Acta Paediatr 1996 85:1503–5.

6. Gianotti A, Tiberio G, Castro M. Coeliac disease in Williams syndrome. J Med Genet 2001;38:767–8.

7. George EK, Mearin ML, van der Velde EA et al. Low incidence of childhood celiac disease in The Netherlands. Pediatr Res 1995;37:213–8.

8. George EK, Mearin ML, Franken HC et al. Twenty years of childhood coeliac disease in The Netherlands: A rapidly increasing incidence? Gut 1997;40:61–6.

9. Dicke WK. Coeliakie [MD thesis]. Utrecht: University of Utrecht, 1950.

10. Martelossi S, Zanatta E, Del Santo E et al. Dental enamel defects and screening for coeliac disease. Acta Paediatr Suppl 1996;412:47–8.

11. Cucchiara S, Bassotti G, Castellucci G et al. Upper gastrointestinal motor abnormalities in children with active celiac disease. J Pediatr Gastroenterol Nutr 1995;21:435–42.

12. de Lecea A, Ribes-Koninckx C, Polanco I et al. Serological screening (antigliadin and antiendomysium antibodies) for non-overt coeliac disease in children of short stature. Acta Paediatr Suppl 1996;412:54–5.

13. Aine L. Coeliac-type permanent-tooth enamel defects. Ann Med 1996;28:9–12.

14. Sher KS, Mayberry JF. Female fertility, obstetric and gynaecological history in coeliac disease: A case control study. Acta Paediatr Suppl 1996;412:76–7.

15. Mäki M, Collins P. Coeliac disease. Lancet 1997;349:1755–9.

16. Spencer J, Isaacson PG, MacDonald TT et al. Gamma/delta T cells and the diagnosis of coeliac disease. Clin Exp Immunol 1991;85:109–13.

17. Lepore L, Martelossi S, Pennesi M et al. Prevalence of celiac disease in patients with juvenile chronic arthritis. J Pediatr 1996;129:311–3.

18. Thain ME, Hamilton JR, Ehrlich RM. Coexistence of diabetes mellitus and celiac disease. J Pediatr 1974;85:527–9.

19. Bonamico M, Mariani P, Mazzilli MC, et al. Frequency and clinical pattern of celiac disease among siblings of celiac children. J Pediatr Gastroenterol Nutr 1996;23:159–63.

20. Bonamico M, Ballati G, Mariani P et al. Screening for coeliac disease: The meaning of low titres of anti-gliadin antibodies (AGA) in non-coeliac children. Eur J Epidemiol 1997;13:55–9.

21. Grodzinsky E, Jansson G, Skogh T et al. Anti-endomysium and anti-gliadin antibodies as serological markers for coeliac disease in childhood: A clinical study to develop a practical routine. Acta Paediatr 1995;84:294–8.

22. Korponay-Szabo IR, Kovacs JB, Lorincz M et al. Prospective significance of antiendomysium antibody positivity in subsequently verified celiac disease. J Pediatr Gastroenterol Nutr 1997;25:56–63.

23. Cataldo F, Marino V, Ventura A et al. Prevalence and clinical features of selective immunoglobulin A deficiency in coeliac disease: an Italian multicentre study. Gut 1998;42:362–5.

24. Troncone R, Maurano F, Rossi M et al. IgA antibodies to tissue transglutaminase: An effective diagnostic test for celiac disease. J Pediatr 1999;134:166–71.

25. Feighery C. Coeliac disease. BMJ 1999;319:236–9.

26. Farrell RJ, Kelly CP. Celiac Sprue. N Eng J Med 2002;346:180–188.

27. van Elburg RM, Uil JJ, Kokke FT et al. Repeatability of the sugar-absorption test, using lactulose and mannitol, for measuring intestinal permeability for sugars. J Pediatr Gastroenterol Nutr 1995;20:184–8.

28. McClean P, Dodge JA, Nunn S et al. Surface features of small-intestinal mucosa in childhood diarrheal disorders. J Pediatr Gastroenterol Nutr 1996;23:538–46.

29. Weizman Z, Ben-Zion YZ, Binsztok M et al. Correlation of clinical characteristics and small bowel histopathology in celiac disease. J Pediatr Gastroenterol Nutr 1997;24:555–8.

30. Meeuwisse GW. European Society for Paediatric Gastroenterology Meeting in Interlaken September 18, 1969. Diagnostic criteria in coeliac disease. Acta Paediatr Scand 1970;59:461–4.

31. Schmidt J. Lack of oats' toxicity in coeliac disease. BMJ 1997;314:159–60.

32. Hoffenberg EJ, Haas J, Drescher A, Barnhurst R et al. A trial of oats in children with newly diagnosed celiac disease. J Pediatr 2000;137:361–6.

33. Rea F, Polito C, Marotta A et al. Restoration of body composition in celiac children after one year of gluten-free diet. J Pediatr Gastroenterol Nutr 1996;23:408–12.

34. Schmitz J. Maldigestion and malabsorption. In: Walker WA, Durie PR, Hamilton JR et al. editors. Pediatric Gastrointestinal Disease. Pathophysiology, Diagnosis, Management, 3rd ed. Hamilton, Ontario: BC Decker, 2000:46–58.

35. Desjeux JF, Taminiau JAJM, Abely M. Congenital intestinal transport defects. In: Walker WA, Durie PR, Hamilton JR et al. editors. Pediatric Gastrointestinal Disease. Pathophysiology, Diagnosis, Management, 3rd ed. Hamilton, Ontario: BC Decker, 2000:701–26.

chapter 7

Acute and Chronic Diarrhea

'Too much stress can be put on poverty as a prime cause of diseases and malnutrition, but poverty of knowledge and initiative is, in nearly every case, as important as poverty of material possessions.'

Williams and Jelliffe, 1972

ACUTE DIARRHEA

At the end of the 19th century, the mortality caused by dehydration from diarrhea among hospitalized infants worldwide was in the order of 80%. Now, in the USA, within the population under the age of 3 years, the overall incidence of acute diarrhea is about 1.3 episodes per child per year, but among children who attend daycare the rate is almost double. Diarrhea accounts for approximately 9% of all hospitalizations of children under the age of 5 years, and almost 300 children die each year as a consequence of dehydration from diarrhea. Principally affected are premature infants, children of adolescent mothers, children of mothers who have received inadequate prenatal care and children of mothers who are poor and/or belong to minority groups. The combined cost of inpatient and outpatient care for pediatric diarrhea is greater than US$2 billion per year.

Most of the acute diarrheal episodes in children are caused by rotavirus and are malabsorptive (impaired dietary carbohydrate absorption) and characterized by the following:

- Diarrhea stops when enteral nutrition is discontinued

- Stools may demonstrate presence of carbohydrate (positive response to reducing substances or presence of glucose)

- Fecal pH is ≤ 5.5

- Stool sodium concentration is <60 mmol/l

- Stool volume is <20 ml/kg per day

In cases of severe carbohydrate malabsorption, continuation of feedings with high amounts of carbohydrate can lead to hypertonic diarrhea.

MANAGEMENT
Historical perspective

In 1935, Darrow and Yannet [1] demonstrated that hypotonicity and cell swelling are the result of a deficit in sodium chloride, which creates a relative excess of water, while the converse produces hypertonicity and a loss of cell water. In the following years, determination of serum sodium levels became more readily available and hyponatremia and hypernatremia were noted as frequent complications of diarrheal dehydration. One factor in clinical practice that contributed to the occurrence of hyponatremia was the low concentration of the sodium solutions used in the replacement therapy for dehydration from diarrhea. To correct hyponatremia, oral solutions containing an excess of salt and/or sugar were developed, but the use of these resulted in an increase in the incidence of hypernatremia, which is associated with brain injury. Excessively rapid correction of hypernatremia causes convulsions. The recommended treatment, using the deficit therapy model, was to infuse a hypotonic solution calculated to correct the hypernatremia over 48–72 h. These calculations for correction of hyponatremia and hypernatremia added complexity to the deficit therapy regimen.

The first report of success using oral rehydration therapy (ORT) to treat dehydration in infants with diarrhea came from Hirschhorn and colleagues in 1973 [2]. By 1980, the experience was that 90% of infants with dehydration successfully recovered with ORT without the need for intravenous therapy [3]. In 1996, a meta-analysis of data from published randomized, controlled trials in which the safety and efficacy of glucose-based ORT were compared with those of intravenous therapy and/or oral rehydration solutions of varying sodium content found that the combined overall rate of ORT failure was less than 4% [4]. It has been demonstrated in ambulatory children in the USA that oral rehydration solutions containing 90, 50 or 30 mmol/l of sodium can be used safely for the treatment of mild acute diarrhea [5].

The success of ORT suggests that calculating rehydration volumes based on estimated fluid deficit may not be necessary. Today, the recommendation is the aggressive use of ORT, only preceded by intravenous saline when needed.

Current recommendations
The treatment of choice to replace fluid and electrolyte losses is ORT, as it can successfully rehydrate most infants and children at a lower cost and with fewer complications than intravenous therapy. A certain amount of emesis is not a contraindication for attempting to use ORT (information on oral rehydration solutions is provided in appendices II.9 and II.10).

Administration of small volumes (5 ml) on a frequent basis (every 1–2 min) may be successful. The use of a nasogastric tube, including the possibility of a continuous infusion, is another option. The stool number and total volume, duration of diarrhea and rate of weight gain are similar with both oral and intravenous therapies. Children who are dehydrated rarely refuse ORT, despite its salty flavor (sodium concentration ranges from 45 to 50 mmol/l in the solutions used in developed countries).

Recommended treatment guidelines for dehydrated children who are between 1 month and 5 years of age, live in developed areas, are well nourished and have no serious underlying illnesses are listed in Table 7.1.

All kinds of beverages with a high carbohydrate content and electrolytes at non-physiologic concentrations have been used inappropriately to treat children with diarrhea. The use of

> **Mild dehydration (3–5%)**
> 50 ml/kg oral rehydration solution + ongoing losses replaced at 10 ml/kg
>
> **Moderate dehydration (6–9%)**
> 100 ml/kg oral rehydration solution + ongoing losses replaced over a 40-h period
>
> **Severe dehydration (>10%)**
> 20–60 ml/kg Ringer's lactate solution (or normal saline) intravenously over a 15- to 60-min period until circulation, extracellular fluid volume and renal perfusion are restored, followed by oral rehydration therapy and early refeeding

Table 7.1 Guidelines for rehydration therapy for children 1 month to 5 years of age. These guidelines apply to children who are well nourished and have no serious underlying illnesses.

such drinks can exacerbate the problem, as they have very low electrolyte concentrations and are hypertonic due to their high carbohydrate content.

Laboratory analysis

There is no need to perform quantification of serum electrolytes as a routine, as most diarrheal episodes in well-nourished infants lead to isotonic dehydration. These laboratory tests, however, may be helpful in moderately dehydrated children, particularly those whose histories or physical findings are inconsistent with a pure diarrheal episode, and in all severely dehydrated children [6].

Feeding the child who has diarrhea

The old concept of bowel rest has been completely abandoned for children with uncomplicated acute diarrhea. Many studies have now demonstrated that, once rehydrated, children with diarrhea should receive their usual diet. It has been shown that unrestricted, age-appropriate diets not only do not worsen mild diarrhea, but also can result in a lower stool output compared to treatment with ORT or intravenous therapy alone [7]. A multicenter study has demonstrated that, when treating well-nourished infants, there is no need to delay the reintroduction of nutrients [8]. Early refeeding during diarrhea has been found to shorten the duration of symptoms by 0.43 days, which, although small, is relevant when one considers the benefit of improved nutrition [9]. At present, in well-nourished infants in the developed world, carbohydrate malabsorption rarely follows rotavirus illness [10].

Brown et al. [11] performed a meta-analysis to compare the effects of continued feeding of lactose-containing versus lactose-free regimens to young children during acute diarrhea. The results suggested that children with mild or no dehydration, and those who are managed according to appropriate treatment protocols, such as that promoted by the WHO, can be treated as successfully with lactose-containing diets as with those lacking lactose. The conclusion of this and many other published studies is that the majority of young children with acute diarrhea can be successfully managed with continued feeding of undiluted non-human milks. Routine dilution of milk and use of a lactose-free milk formula are therefore not necessary, especially when ORT and early feeding (in addition to milk) form the basic approach to the clinical management of diarrhea in infants and children. Early introduction of age-appropriate foods is also recommended [12,13].

Vaccine and medications

After exhaustive international trials, RotaShield, an oral tetravalent rotavirus vaccine, was introduced in 1998. The Advisory Committee on Immunization Practices (ACIP) recommended infants in the USA routinely receive three doses, at 2, 4, and 6 months, respectively. However, almost 1 year after the vaccine was licensed and 1.5 million doses had been administered, the CDC postponed the program because of an association with intussusception, and the product was withdrawn. Notwithstanding, it is estimated that in Africa, Asia and South America, three million children die annually because of diarrhea, 600,000 to 800,000 of which cases are caused by rotavirus. The vaccine would have prevented 80% of these deaths. Hence, if a new vaccine takes 3–5 years to develop, the wait will have caused 1.4 to 3.2 million preventable deaths in these territories [14,15].

Although some studies have demonstrated beneficial effects of certain medications for the management of acute diarrhea in children, the American Academy of Pediatrics – in common with other academic bodies – does not recommend the routine use of antiemetics, antiperistaltics or antisecretories. One of the drugs found to be beneficial in the treatment of acute diarrhea, when used in conjunction with ORT, is loperamide [16]. However, many studies have reported a high incidence of side effects associated with this agent, such as ileus, lethargy, respiratory depression, coma and even death, especially in infants [17]. Use of bismuth subsalicylate in children, every 4 h for 5 days, has been associated with a (modest) decrease in the duration of diarrhea and frequency of loose stools [18]. It should be remembered, however, that salicylate can be absorbed and result in toxicity. The supplementation of infant formula with *Bifidobacterium bifidum* and *Streptococcus thermophilus* has been shown to reduce the incidence of acute diarrhea and rotavirus shedding, a factor of relevance in hospitalized infants. Several studies in young children have demonstrated that administration of *lactobacillus rhamnosus GG* can reduce the duration of diarrhea caused by rotavirus [19,20].

CHRONIC DIARRHEA

Diarrhea lasting more than 14 days is considered to be chronic. Awareness of the causes for chronic diarrhea has resulted in earlier diagnosis and a lower number of consultations. In developed countries, severe, protracted diarrhea has become far less common. Another frequent cause for consultation used to be chronic, non-specific (or toddler) diarrhea, but physicians who treat children have become more familiar with its benign course. Most chronic diarrheas are due to nutrient malabsorption and/or excessive fluid intake rather than secretory (Table 7.2). Most common causes need to be ruled out before performing any complicated investigations. Malabsorptive diarrheas improve dramatically when the child is fasted or given oral rehydration solution alone. Secretory diarrheas persist even when the patient is fasted. In children, the majority of the secretory diarrheas are infectious; neuroendocrine tumor is a rare cause.

The etiology of chronic diarrhea varies according to age. Table 7.3 lists the causes of chronic diarrhea seen in various age groups.

> **Common causes**
> Excessive intake of formula or other fluid (water, fruit juice, high-carbohydrate beverages)
> Chronic non-specific diarrhea of the toddler
> Irritable bowel syndrome
> Encopresis (overflow diarrhea)
>
> **Less common causes**
> Parasitosis (*Giardia lamblia*, *Cryptosporidium*)
> Celiac disease
> Post-enteritis syndrome

Table 7.2 Causes of chronic diarrhea.

0–6 months	7–23 months	24 months and older
Carbohydrate malabsorption: acquired congenital	Chronic non-specific diarrhea ('toddler diarrhea') (usually 11 months or older)	Irritable bowel syndrome
Protein hypersensitivity	Small-bowel bacterial overgrowth	Adult-type hypolactasia
Excessive intake of formula, water or fruit juice	Celiac disease	Encopresis
Post-enteritis syndrome and intractable diarrhea	Immunodeficiency	Inflammatory bowel disease
Infections	Munchausen syndrome by proxy	Excessive intake of laxatives
Cystic fibrosis and other causes of fat malabsorption	Graft-versus-host enteropathy	Excessive intake of fruit juice/high-carbohydrate drinks
Immunodeficiency	Autoimmune enteropathy	Infections
Lymphangiectasia	Carbohydrate malabsorption	Small-bowel bacterial overgrowth
Neuroblastoma	Protein hypersensitivity	Celiac disease
Congenital chloridorrhea	Excessive intake of fruit juice/high-carbohydrate drinks	Munchausen syndrome by proxy
Intestinal villi inclusion disease	Post-enteritis syndrome	Graft-versus-host enteropathy
Congenital defective jejunal Na$^+$/H$^+$ exchange	Cystic fibrosis	Carbohydrate malabsorption
	Infections	
	Fat malabsorption	
	Neuroblastoma	

Table 7.3 Causes of chronic diarrhea in various age groups.

DIAGNOSTIC TESTS

Feces

Stools should be examined for the following:

- pH and presence of reducing substances to characterize carbohydrate malabsorption (normally stool pH is >5.5 and carbohydrate is negative, but the latter may be minimally present in the neonate)

- Presence of fat globules (seen under the microscope); prolonged (72-h) fecal collection for quantitation of fat is rarely necessary

- Occult blood – this may be present in protein-hypersensitive colitis, but a severe diaper rash with skin excoriation can also result in a positive test

- Parasites – the yield is increased if samples from three bowel movements are collected; however, assay of *Giardia* antigen is much more sensitive than observation under the microscope and one sample is sufficient

- Macroscopic evidence of non-digested food – this is not necessarily indicative of malabsorption but is frequently seen in toddler diarrhea.

- Electrolytes, for the diagnosis of secretory diarrhea – care should be taken to ensure that urine does not contaminate the sample

Blood

Blood tests are not very useful in the work-up of chronic diarrhea except as an aid to determine electrolyte balance and specific nutrient deficiencies.

Peripheral eosinophilia may be seen in cases of protein-hypersensitive enteritis or colitis.

Urine

Urinary tract infection can be associated with diarrhea in young infants.

Radiologic

Flocculation of barium in the small bowel may be indicative of malabsorption (flocculation caused by excessive amounts of luminal fluid). This phenomenon, however, may be a normal finding in the first year of life.

Contrasted studies for the investigation of chronic diarrhea are rarely helpful in infants and children, unless a stricture or inflammatory bowel disease is suspected.

Breath hydrogen test

This is difficult to interpret in infants for the following reasons:

- Carbohydrate (lactose) malabsorption is normal in the first 6 months of life

- Mouth-to-cecum transit time is shorter than in adults, making it difficult to reach conclusions regarding small-bowel bacterial overgrowth

- Crying children hyperventilate and dilute the hydrogen in the sample, which can result in a falsely negative test

1 g/kg of the carbohydrate to be tested should be used in a 20% solution.

CARBOHYDRATE MALABSORPTION

Acquired

Up to 10% of well-nourished infants may suffer transient lactose intolerance which can last 10 to 15 days following an episode of acute gastroenteritis [21]. Malnourished infants, those who have experienced an episode of diarrhea in the recent past and those with a history of severe gastroenteritis are more likely to suffer from lactose malabsorption [22]. Lactose malabsorption can also be seen when the intestinal mucosa is damaged by protein hypersensitivity [23]. Prolonged lactose intolerance can complicate acute gastroenteritis in malnourished infants [24]. In cases of lactose malabsorption, other carbohydrates need to be used. Glucose polymers are digested by glucoamylase and maltase, enzymes that are quite resistant to damage of the intestinal mucosa [25]. However, in cases of severe damage to the integrity of the intestinal villi, malabsorption of glucose polymers can also occur.

Diagnosis

Characteristically, diarrhea occurs after feeding with formula, mainly if it contains lactose, and improves when the child is kept hydrated with oral rehydrating solution or intravenous fluids. Stools are watery, with an acid pH (<5.0), and reducing substances or glucose are present.

The breath hydrogen test is difficult to interpret in infants and may have false negatives in acute diarrhea [26]. However, it may help in confirming carbohydrate malabsorption after recovery from diarrhea.

Treatment

As a general rule, 'no bowel rest'. A formula containing glucose polymers should be used in place of lactose (information on specialized formulas is provided in Appendix IV). If the infant has intolerance to glucose polymers the following should be considered:

(a) protein hypersensitivity – try a formula with hydrolyzed protein

(b) administering the formula as a constant intragastric infusion.

Care must be taken not to administer an insufficient amount of calories (100 kcal/kg body weight in the first 6 to 9 months of life) for more than 2 or 3 days. If an infant is unable to tolerate formula by constant infusion, parenteral nutrition should be initiated.

The duration of lactose intolerance in chronic diarrhea is difficult to predict, and can extend from 10 days to several months [27,28]. Gradual reintroduction of lactose and monitoring of stools is the best way to determine tolerance. Feeding lactose to a lactose-intolerant child with chronic diarrhea can have adverse effects on nutritional recovery [22].

Congenital

Sucrase–isomaltase deficiency

This congenital disaccharidase deficiency, inherited as an autosomal recessive trait, is caused by a complete or almost total lack of sucrase activity, a decrease of maltase to about one-third of normal and a very marked reduction of isomaltase. Molecular studies have revealed at least three phenotypes:

• One in which sucrase–isomaltase protein accumulates intracellularly, probably in the endoplasmic reticulum, as a membrane-associated high-mannose precursor

• One in which the intracellular transport of the enzyme may be blocked in the Golgi apparatus

• One where the catalytically altered enzyme is transported to the cell surface [29]

It is probable that small mutations in the sucrase–isomaltase gene lead to the synthesis of transport-incompetent or functionally altered enzymes, which result in congenital sucrose intolerance. Symptoms develop following the introduction of cereals or table sugar to the diet, or when an infant formula has been changed to one containing sucrose or glucose polymers.

Diagnosis

Diagnosis can be made by a breath hydrogen test following the ingestion of a sucrose solution. Confirmation requires a small-bowel biopsy and assay for disaccharidases. Histologic features will be normal.

Treatment

Starches, sucrose and glucose polymers should be excluded from the diet until the child is older: colonic fermentation of malabsorbed carbohydrate may result in gas and short-chain fatty acid formation but less diarrhea than in an infant. Appendix IV.28 gives information on foods containing sucrose and starch. The diet must be planned according to individual tolerance, ensuring nutritional adequacy for growth. Recently, an enzyme preparation (sacrosidase) has been marketed to produce sucrose hydrolysis *in vivo* for patients with sucrase–isomaltase deficiency [30].

Glucose–galactose malabsorption

This rare autosomal recessive disease results from a specific defect in the intestinal Na$^+$/glucose co-transporter (SGLT1). The SGLT1 gene – located on chromosome 22q13.1 – encodes the primary carrier protein responsible for the uptake of dietary glucose and galactose from the intestinal lumen. The 75-kD glycoprotein is localized in the brush border of the intestinal epithelium and is predicted to comprise 12 membrane spanning regions. In two patients with glucose–galactose malabsorption, the underlying cause was found to be a missense mutation in SGLT1, and the Asp28→Asn change was demonstrated *in vitro* to eliminate SGLT1 transport activity [31].

Following the first feeding, infants have profuse diarrhea with evidence of carbohydrate malabsorption (carbohydrate in stools). Initially, fecal pH is not below 5.0 because the fecal flora has not yet developed; thus, there is no colonic fermentation of malabsorbed carbohydrate. Diarrhea rapidly resolves when the infant is fasted and receives intravenous fluids, but recurs after feeding. Fructose is well tolerated.

Treatment

Substitution of fructose in place of glucose-yielding carbohydrates including glucose, galactose, lactose, sucrose, glucose polymers and starches is the only effective treatment [32]. Fructose can be added to an infant formula that does not contain any carbohydrate (RCF, Ross Carbohydrate-Free, Ross Laboratories) or a fructose formula can be used (Galactomin 19, Fructose Formula, SHS). The diet is initially very limited (Appendix IV.26); however, in the second or third year of life, as the colonic capacity to ferment carbohydrates is better developed, children can ingest limited amounts of a greater variety of carbohydrates, resulting in formation of gas, but generally not diarrhea. Careful dietary planning by a specialized pediatric dietician is required to ensure a nutritionally adequate diet.

Congenital lactase deficiency

The existence of this is questioned by some authors. If real, it is an extremely rare condition, characterized by watery acidic stools and the presence of carbohydrate following the ingestion of lactose-containing milk. Symptoms resolve if the infant is fed a lactose-free milk.

PROTEIN HYPERSENSITIVITY

Diarrhea caused by hypersensitivity to dietary protein may occur primarily in the first month of life, and secondarily in the first 6 months of life or at any time after an episode of severe gastroenteritis (see Chapter 17). As a consequence of mucosal damage, there can be blood in the stools and/or carbohydrate malabsorption.

EXCESSIVE FORMULA, WATER OR FRUIT JUICE INTAKE

The capacity of the small bowel to digest carbohydrate, as well as that of both the small and large bowel to absorb water, can be overwhelmed by excessive formula intake and this can result in diarrhea. Excessive fluid intake can also cause diarrhea [33]. Unfortunately, it is not unusual to see children with all-day access to a bottle or a 'sippy-cup' of juice and achieving daily fluid intakes as high as 2 l. Infants and children have difficulty absorbing volumes larger than 200 ml/kg per day; an excess results in diarrhea. In fact, diarrhea can occur at much lower volumes with certain fruit juices, particularly those which contain a mixture of carbohydrates in a proportion that impairs absorption, such as apple juice [34].

Diagnosis

Detailed questions about dietary intake should be part of the routine history-taking in patients with diarrhea. Stools may have the presence of carbohydrate and an acidic pH, but these may also be normal. Sometimes parents continue to offer the child (excess) fluids to prevent dehydration after an episode of acute diarrhea.

Treatment

Fluids should be reduced, allowing a milk intake of up to 600–800 ml a day in those aged 18–24 months and 500 ml in older children. Total fluid intake should be no more than 200 ml/kg per day during the first 2 years of life. Juice intake should also be limited [35].

Parents of infants who have diarrhea due to an excessive intake of formula need advice on appropriate feeding practices.

POST-ENTERITIS SYNDROME AND INTRACTABLE DIARRHEA

Post-enteritis syndrome is the persistence of diarrhea following an episode of acute gastroenteritis. This is characterized by carbohydrate malabsorption, and there may be a component of protein hypersensitivity [36]. The typical history is that of a previously healthy infant, formula-fed or (less commonly) breastfed, who develops an episode of acute gastroenteritis and, instead of improving over the following 3–7 days, continues with loose, watery, explosive stools, with evidence of carbohydrate malabsorption. Although oral hydration and small amounts of diluted formula may be tolerated, the infant is unable to ingest an appropriate amount of calories and therefore loses weight.

Intractable diarrhea or idiopathic prolonged diarrhea, also known as acquired monosaccharide intolerance [37], is a syndrome whereby the patient has persistent malabsorptive diarrhea with severe villus atrophy and acquired disaccharidase deficiency with complete intolerance to oral or enteral nutrition. It is possible that this is the extreme of post-enteritis syndrome [38,39]. In the developing world, this syndrome is still seen in large numbers, and affects infants after weaning (6–18 months of age). In developed countries, intractable diarrhea was more common among formula-fed than breastfed infants, and occurred predominantly in the first 3 months of life. Nowadays, intractable diarrhea is rarely seen in developed countries, probably as a consequence of one or more of the following therapeutic modalities for acute gastroenteritis:

- Oral rehydration

- Elimination of the 'bowel rest' policy (prolonged fasting) recommended in former times for treatment of acute diarrhea

- Elimination of lactose in cases of persistent diarrhea

- Use of protein hydrolysates when there is suspicion of protein intolerance

The two major groups of intractable diarrhea are due to (1) primary epithelial abnormalities (which usually present within the first few days of life) and (2) immunologically mediated abnormalities (which generally present after the first few weeks of life).

Diagnosis

There are no specific tests for the diagnosis of post-enteritis syndrome or intractable diarrhea. Suggestive features include:

- History of acute diarrhea with partial recovery and relapse

- Diarrhea with evidence of carbohydrate intolerance and inability to feed the infant a sufficient amount of calories to gain weight

In intractable diarrhea, a flat intestinal mucosa can be seen in the biopsy.

Treatment

Early identification of the problem, and change to a formula that can be tolerated, is the only effective approach in the treatment of post-enteritis syndrome. In cases where diarrhea becomes chronic and does not respond to replacement of carbohydrate by a more digestible preparation, temporary formula dilution or small, frequent volumes, then protein hypersensitivity should be suspected. Elimination of sensitizing dietary proteins (casein and soy) will be necessary to prevent further inflammation of the small-bowel mucosa and consequent villous damage. For more details, see information above regarding the treatment of carbohydrate malabsorption and protein hypersensitivity. Total intravenous nutrition and complete bowel rest may be necessary in cases of intractable diarrhea.

INFECTIONS

A urinary tract infection can cause chronic diarrhea in young infants.

Viruses

Although viruses do not produce chronic diarrhea, they may be the cause of the initial illness which may subsequently lead to post-enteritis syndrome, or predispose to protein-hypersensitive enteropathy or even intractable diarrhea. Rotavirus is the most common pathogen associated with gastroenteritis [40]. Enteric adenovirus and Norwalk agent may also lead to chronic diarrhea.

Bacteria

The most common organisms that produce diarrhea are [41]:

- *Campylobacter jejuni*
- *Escherichia coli*
- *Salmonella enteritidis*
- *Shigella*
- *Clostridium difficile*

E. coli

In addition to the enterotoxigenic, enteroinvasive and enterohemorrhagic *E. coli*, there is an enteroadhesive or pathogenic organism that does not invade the mucosa, but adheres to the brush border and affects its integrity. Children may present with an acute episode of secretory diarrhea from which they do not completely recover, followed by diarrhea with malabsorptive characteristics, and then possibly present with another episode of secretory diarrhea. Progressive malnutrition occurs until an appropriate diagnosis is made and suitable antibiotic treatment instituted.

Salmonella

This causes a colitis with bloody, mucusy stools. Antibiotic treatment of diarrhea caused by *S. typhi* is only indicated for immunocompromised hosts, including the neonate, children with sickle cell disease and those in a toxic state.

Shigella

The diarrhea is bloody and mucusy. Infections by *Shigella* may lower the tone of the anal sphincter, and rectal prolapse can occur. Shigellosis involves the colon and is a self-limiting disease.

Clostridium difficile

This may be present in the bowel of normal neonates, and between 10% and 50% of asymptomatic infants and young children have *C. difficile* toxin. By the end of the first year of life, fewer than 5% of these infants excrete the organism and an even smaller number the toxin. The absence of toxin receptors may explain why infants can be asymptomatic.

Parasites

Giardia lamblia (a protozoon) and *Cryptosporidium* species are among the most common parasites affecting children. In a study performed in Canada [42], it was found that the prevalence of enteric parasites in hospitalized children was 4% (35 of 829) compared with rates of 10% and 13% for children attending the emergency room or other outpatient clinics and the gastroenterology clinic, respectively. *G. lamblia* was found most often (31%), followed by *Dientamoeba fragilis* (23%), *Entamoeba coli* (16%), *Blastocystis hominis* (13%), *Cryptosporidium* (8%), *Endolimax nana* (4%), *Enterobius vermicularis* (2%), *Hymenolepis nana* (2%) and *Iodamoeba buetschlii* (1%). Most children (85%) were colonized/infected with a single parasite. Both *Giardia* and *Cryptosporidium* parasites can be found in asymptomatic children, particularly those attending daycare centers. Chronic diarrhea is the commonest symptom caused by these parasites. Excessive burping and/or intestinal gas can be produced by small-bowel bacterial overgrowth associated with the parasite.

Diagnosis

A number of stool samples need to be cultured and analyzed for parasites and *Giardia* antigen before any invasive tests are performed in children with chronic diarrhea, unless the history or other symptoms indicate another problem such as inflammatory bowel disease.

Treatment options

These include:

- *C. jejuni* – erythromycin

- *E. coli* – trimethoprim–sulfamethoxazole

- *Salmonella* – trimethoprim–sulfamethoxazole, ampicillin, chloramphenicol

- *Shigella* – trimethoprim–sulfamethoxazole

- *Giardia* – metronidazole, 30 mg/kg/day for 3 days; tinidizole, 30 mg/kg as a single dose; mepacrine, 2 mg/kg three times a day for 7 days; furazolidone, 1.25 mg/kg four times a day for 7 days

- *Cryptosporidium* – parasite numbers and stool volume can be lowered with antibiotics such as erythromycin, spiramycin and clindamycin

CYSTIC FIBROSIS AND OTHER CAUSES OF FAT MALABSORPTION

Stools are pale-white, malodorous and shiny. When fat malabsorption is significant, infants have failure to thrive and diarrhea, and may present with clinical evidence of fat-soluble vitamin and essential fatty acid deficiency. Fat malabsorption may be associated with any of the following:

- Post-enteritis syndrome

- Cystic fibrosis (see Chapter 15)

- Celiac disease (see Chapter 6)

- Giardiasis in a patient with immunodeficiency (e.g. selective IgA)

- Intrahepatic or extrahepatic cholestasis

- Shwachman syndrome (neutropenia, metaphyseal chondrodysplasia and other features – see Chapter 15)

- Impaired bile acid synthesis

- Congenital malabsorption of bile acids

- Congenital enterokinase deficiency

- Congenital trypsinogen deficiency

Cystic fibrosis (see Chapter 15) must be considered as a cause of chronic diarrhea, particularly in the presence of any of the following:

- History of meconium ileus, peritonitis or plug

- Poor weight gain

- Hyperinflation of lungs, pneumonia

- Recurrent pulmonary infections

Breast milk or standard infant formula is recommended for the majority of infants with CF. In a small number of infants who have required gut resection or have increased fat malabsorption, a formula with medium chain tryglycerides may be indicated and in some instances protein absorption may be enhanced by using a formula containing hydrolyzed protein. Pancreatic enzymes should be given with all milks and formulas.

In the older child a normal diet is recommended, with additional calorie and protein supplements being required by many. Pancreatic enzymes are required with all meals and snacks. Additional vitamins are recommended for all infants and children with CF.

Pancreatic enzymes contain lipase, protease and amylase. Dosage is generally based on lipase content. The recommended starting dose for infants is 2000–4000 units of lipase per 120 ml formula or breast feed. For children under 4 years of age, 1000 units of lipase/kg body weight/meal and for children over 4 years of age 500 units of lipase/kg body weight/meal can be used as a guide. Very high doses of lipase have been associated with fibrosing colonopathy in CF patients (see Chapter 15).

Diagnosis (see Chapter 15)
Fat malabsorption can be documented by the presence of fat globules in stools. Confirmation of diagnosis is by sweat test. Sodium values above 70 mmol/l (or mEq/l) are abnormal.

Treatment
Use a formula with medium-chain triglycerides. Protein absorption may be enhanced by use of a formula with hydrolyzed protein. Breastfed infants and those fed a soy-based formula may develop hypoproteinemia.

Pancreatic enzymes are frequently required to optimize lipolysis of dietary fats. The usual dosage of pH-sensitive microspheres is as follows:

- Infants – 8000 U lipase per 120 ml formula
- Children – 24,000 U lipase per meal

IMMUNODEFICIENCY STATES

Acquired immunodeficiency (AIDS)

Perinatal transmission of HIV infection can present as failure to thrive with or without diarrhea. The long-term effects are demonstrated in results from a study that showed that a decline in weight occurred in the first 4 months of life, followed by decreased linear growth [43]. In older children, weight and height seem to fall in parallel, but loss of lean body mass may occur prior to a decline in weight [44]. Adequate caloric intake can improve weight gain, but has little effect on height velocity and lean body mass [45]. Long-term survivors with HIV infection are shorter than anticipated, and these changes cannot be explained solely by inadequate nutrition or by endocrine abnormalities [46]. Diffuse lymphoadenopathy, oral candidiasis resistant to therapy and hepatosplenomegaly are frequently present. Recurrent or intractable diarrhea with malabsorption is common and difficult to manage. Organisms known to produce disease of the gastrointestinal tract are similar to those affecting adult patients with AIDS [47]. Children diagnosed in the first few months of life have worse outcome than those who present with symptoms later.

Treatment

Children with AIDS suffering from chronic diarrhea may benefit from nutritional supplements orally or delivered by nasogastric tube as a constant infusion. The use of formulas that are lactose-free and contain hydrolyzed protein and medium-chain triglycerides may result in better dietary tolerance.

Congenital immunodeficiency

Congenital immunodeficiency usually becomes symptomatic in infants older than 6 months of age, particularly if they are breastfed, because maternal immunoglobulins will protect them during the first few months of life. The most common immunodeficiencies associated with chronic diarrhea are listed below.

X-linked agammaglobulinemia

Typically, the patient is a male, 6 to 9 months of age, with severe respiratory infection or meningitis and diarrhea that may or may not be associated with pathogens or bacterial overgrowth.

Selective IgA deficiency

IgA deficiency is the commonest form of primary immune deficiency. Diarrhea and malabsorption due to giardiasis may be present. A number of disorders are associated with reduced or absent IgA, including celiac disease and inflammatory bowel disease.

Severe combined immunodeficiency

The infant presents with major infections, chronic persistent diarrhea, malabsorption and failure to thrive. The diarrhea may become bloody or mucopurulent.

LYMPHANGIECTASIA

Intestinal lymphangiectasia is a rare disorder of the small bowel that impairs lymphatic flow from the intestine. It can be due to a congenital malformation, or secondary to cardiovascular anomalies such as constrictive pericarditis or operations (e.g. the Fontan procedure for hypoplastic left heart syndrome), infection, inflammatory bowel disease or drugs. Primary intestinal lymphangiectasia is associated with hypoalbuminemia, hypogammaglobulinemia (particularly IgG), hypolipidemia and lymphopenia, with an increased vulnerability to infections. Diarrhea and edema are found frequently. Many of the clinical features are similar to those seen in celiac disease. Lymphangiectasia has been associated with other syndromes. In a study of eight patients, the presenting features were diarrhea (n=6), vomiting (n=4) and growth deficit (n=7) [48]. Additional conditions in these patients included asthma, urinary tract infection, esophageal atresia, hydrops fetalis, inflammatory bowel disease, malabsorption syndrome and thymic hypoplasia. Hypoalbuminemia and edema (n=4) were more prominent in patients under 5 years of age. The patients responded variably to hyperalimentation and dietary supplements, depending on the extent of their lymphangiectasia and the age at onset of symptoms. Dilated lymphatics were seen in the small-intestinal mucosa under the surface epithelium. Lesions were often focal, requiring several biopsies or serial sections for detection (see Fig. 8.1). Other common findings were lymphoplasmocytic inflammation and mild-to-moderate villous injury with blunting and edema. Mild inflammation without lymphangiectasia was also present in esophageal, gastric or colonic biopsies. Thus, diagnosis should be made on the basis of endoscopic findings or in small-intestinal inflammatory conditions, even in the absence of a classic clinical picture. Histologic confirmation may require more than one serially sectioned biopsy.

NEUROBLASTOMA

Rarely, neuroblastoma is associated with diarrhea, which is of a secretory nature as a result of the vasoactive intestinal peptide produced by tumor cells. Approximately 77% of neuroblastomas occur in children under 5 years of age and 90% under the age of 7. Peak age is between 1 and 3 years. Increased amounts of urinary homovanillic acid and vanillylmandelic acid derived from catecholamine metabolism are found in 75% of patients.

CONGENITAL CHLORIDORRHEA

This is a rare autosomal recessive disorder of the chloride transport mechanism which results in secretory diarrhea and alkalosis [49]. The condition begins *in utero* and is lifelong. Treatment has not been successful. Fluid replacement is the mainstay approach, although proton-pump inhibitors have been used [50].

INTESTINAL VILLI INCLUSION DISEASE

This congenital abnormality of the structure of the intestinal mucosa results in chronic secretory and malabsorptive diarrhea [51].

CONGENITAL DEFECTIVE JEJUNAL NA⁺/H⁺ EXCHANGE

This rare disorder results in secretory diarrhea. It is seen in those between 7 and 23 months of age.

CHRONIC NON-SPECIFIC DIARRHEA ('TODDLER DIARRHEA') (see Chapter 9)

The exact cause of this diarrhea is not known, but it may be the result of an inability of the colon to handle the fluid load [52]. Typically, the patient is a healthy 11- to 24-month-old whose only problem is the presence of watery and runny stools. By definition, if no dietary restrictions are imposed in an attempt to control the diarrhea, the child continues to gain weight normally. Unfortunately, parents or physicians often discontinue milk, dairy products and other foods; so, eventually, the child may experience failure to thrive or actual weight loss. In many cases, excessive fluid intake can be identified as a possible cause (see below). In an attempt to prevent dehydration, carers provide even more fluids, creating overhydration diarrhea, which perpetuates the problem. The child's sleep is not interrupted by the diarrhea, and dehydration does not arise.

Diagnosis

The diagnosis is suspected by a combination of the following:

- Age between 11 and 24 months

- Healthy-looking, well-hydrated child (unless dietary restrictions have been imposed)

- Up to 10 loose bowel movements a day, containing undigested and recognizable items of food (e.g. corn, peas and carrots).

- Feces contain no blood but often mucus

The common dietary transgressions observed are:

- Low-fat milk and a low fat, often very high fiber, diet

- Excess milk, water, juices and/or fruit

Tests

The feces should be tested for:

- Electrolytes – sodium should be less than 40 mmol/l (mEq/l)

- Evidence of carbohydrate – negative test for reducing substances

- pH – >5.5

- Parasites – screen for *G. lamblia* antigen (a test that is not as yet universally available) and *C. difficile* toxin

Treatment

If dietary transgressions are identified, correction to a normal healthy balanced diet with adequate fat intake can improve or resolve the problem completely. In some cases, fiber supplementation may help by giving bulk to the stools.

SMALL-BOWEL BACTERIAL OVERGROWTH

The causes of small-bowel bacterial overgrowth in children are the same as in adults. It may occur after infection with *Giardia* or prolonged diarrhea, and could be a component of post-enteritis syndrome. Bacterial overgrowth can also be associated with cystic fibrosis, previous abdominal surgery (e.g. for intestinal atresia), intestinal pseudo-obstruction, short-bowel syndrome, Crohn's disease and tropical enteropathy.

The main symptoms are excessive burping and passage of gas, abdominal distension, abdominal pain and diarrhea, which can be malabsorptive and/or secretory.

Diagnosis

The diagnosis is mainly clinical. The breath hydrogen test can be helpful if the baseline is elevated or if a peak is obtained 10 or 20 min after ingestion of lactulose (0.5 g/kg). Peaks appearing later than this could correspond to colonic fermentation, because transit time, particularly in young children, may be short compared with that in adults [53].

Treatment

Patients may respond to metronidazole (30 mg/kg/day divided into three doses a day, for 7 to 10 days). Co-trimoxazole (trimethoprim–sulfamethoxazole; 8 mg/kg/day divided into two doses a day, for 7 to 10 days) can also be used.

CELIAC DISEASE

Celiac disease has a prevalence of 1:2000–1:6000 in parts of Europe, but is less common in the USA and Canada. There is a peak estimated prevalence of 1:300 in the west of Ireland. Therefore, if both of the child's parents have Irish ancestry, the index of suspicion should be increased. Onset of diarrhea can be identified by history: it develops some weeks to months after the introduction of wheat to the diet and, depending on weaning practices, can occur from age 6 to 18 months (or in adulthood). Children may have abdominal distension and foul-smelling, pale and frothy stools, appear moody and experience weight loss or inadequate weight gain (see Chapter 6).

Diagnosis

Diagnosis is based on the following:

- Fat globules in stool

- Presence of serum antiendomysial and/or antigliadin antibodies and tissue transglutaminase antibodies

- Small-bowel biopsy

MUNCHAUSEN SYNDROME BY PROXY

This syndrome involves falsification of the child's medical history, usually by the mother. Pediatricians as well as neonatologists are becoming increasingly aware of its existence. Gastrointestinal bleeding, diarrhea and vomiting are common complaints, resulting in extensive and unnecessary investigation and treatment of fabricated illnesses. Symptoms can at times be confused with intestinal pseudo-obstruction [54].

Symptoms are generally absent when the involved carer is not in attendance. He or she presents as concerned, usually refusing to leave the hospital. Intravenous lines may be tampered with or become contaminated; medications reportedly are vomited. Frequently, the carer has had some medical or nursing training.

Diagnosis

Suspect Munchausen syndrome by proxy whenever there are inconsistent symptoms, signs and/or features that only the main carer reports, and there is an absence of associated symptoms, etc. The carer may be noted to eavesdrop when doctors and nurses are privately discussing the child. Filming the carer with infant using a hidden camera, entering the room without warning and observation when urine samples are collected, as well as searching the room for laxatives or other drugs, may be helpful in making the diagnosis. Phenolphthalein is a commonly used laxative in these cases. Its presence can be identified by the development of a pink color when stools are alkalinized to pH 8.5. Fecal sulfate and magnesium can also be determined to establish the illicit use of laxatives. Screen urine from both the patient (for poisons) and the carer (for evidence of drug abuse). In a long-term follow up of 54 victims of this syndrome in Leeds, England, 13 had been exposed to repetitive poisoning [55].

GRAFT-VERSUS-HOST ENTEROPATHY

Following bone marrow transplantation, graft-versus-host disease can affect the intestine, causing protein-losing enteropathy. Weisdorf et al. [56] measured fecal protein losses before and after transplantation in 25 consecutive patients. The mean α_1-antitrypsin concentration and serum clearance before transplantation were below 2.6 mg/g stool and 13.0 ml/day, respectively (upper limits for normals). Values for all patients increased moderately after pretransplant conditioning. Levels for patients who did not develop graft-versus-host disease of the intestine returned to baseline; however, those for patients with graft-versus-host disease of the intestine became markedly and persistently elevated (concentration ranged from 16.6 to 51.1 mg/g, clearance from 66.6 to 384.5 ml/day). Usually this problem improves with corticosteroid therapy.

AUTOIMMUNE ENTEROPATHY

This is a rare small-bowel disorder characterized by damaged intestinal mucosa secondary to an autoimmune mechanism. Infants have chronic diarrhea and, characteristically, crypt hyperplasia, villous atrophy with enterocyte autoantibodies in the blood, activation of mucosal lymphocytes and increased epithelial HLA-DR. There is no cure and the prognosis is poor. Treatment includes high doses of corticosteroids and immunosuppressants [57].

IRRITABLE BOWEL SYNDROME (see Chapter 9)

In children, episodes of diarrhea alternate with those of constipation and/or abdominal pain, particularly under stressful conditions [58]. Many preadolescent and adolescent patients use this as a pretext to miss school or to pay frequent visits to the nurse's station when they ought to be in the classroom. Characteristically, constipation and pain is worse during daytime, and improves on weekends and in vacation time. Some parents who are separated or divorced report diarrhea when the child returns from visiting the former partner and may use this against the other party for the manipulation of their preferred visitation rights.

ADULT-TYPE HYPOLACTASIA

Genetically determined hypolactasia can become symptomatic at 10 or 11 years of age, and cause chronic diarrhea and/or abdominal pain. The incidence is higher in non-whites. Diagnosis can be made by elimination of lactose from the diet and confirmed by a lactose breath hydrogen test.

ENCOPRESIS

Encopresis is defined as the act of defecation in socially non-acceptable places, and the initial complaint may be of chronic diarrhea (see Chapter 9). The liquid stool is by overflow.

INFLAMMATORY BOWEL DISEASE

Crohn's disease and ulcerative colitis can occur at almost any age, but primarily affect preadolescents and adolescents. One of the common forms of presentation is chronic diarrhea (see Chapter 11).

EXCESSIVE INTAKE OF LAXATIVES

In children, excessive use of laxatives can be seen in Munchausen syndrome by proxy and in anorexia nervosa and bulimia nervosa.

Purgatives to consider include:

- Diphenolic laxatives (phenolphthalein)

- Anthraquinones (senna, cascara, rhubarb aloe, frangula and dantheron)

- Osmotic laxatives such as lactulose, sodium sulfate, sodium phosphate, magnesium sulfate and magnesium citrate

Ricinoleic acid should be included when screening the stool for laxatives and electrolytes.

REFERENCES

1.   Darrow DC, Yannet H. The changes in the distribution of body water accompanying increase and decrease in extracellular electrolyte. J Clin Invest 1935;14:266–75.

2.   Hirschhorn N, McCarthy BJ, Ranney B et al. Ad libitum oral glucose-electrolyte therapy for acute diarrhea in Apache children. J Pediatr 1973;83:562–71.

3. Hirschhorn N. The treatment of acute diarrhea in children: An historical and physiological perspective. Am J Clin Nutr 1980;33:637–63.

4. Gavin N, Merrick N, Davidson B. Efficacy of glucose-based oral rehydration therapy. Pediatrics 1996;98:45–51.

5. Santosham M, Burns B, Nadkarni V et al. Oral rehydration therapy for acute diarrhea in ambulatory children in the United States: A double-blind comparison of four different solutions. Pediatrics 1985;76:159–66.

6. Holliday M. The evolution of therapy for dehydration: Should deficit therapy still be taught? Pediatrics 1996;98:171–7.

7. Ulshen MH. Refeeding during recovery from acute diarrhea. J Pediatr 1988;112:239–40.

8. Sandhu BK, Isolauri E, Walker-Smith JA et al. A multicentre study on behalf of the European Society of Paediatric Gastroenterology and Nutrition Working Group on Acute Diarrhoea. Early feeding in childhood gastroenteritis. J Pediatr Gastroenterol Nutr 1997;24:522–7.

9. Brown KH, Gastanaduy AS, Saavedra JM et al. Effect of continued oral feeding on clinical and nutritional outcomes of acute diarrhea in children. J Pediatr 1988;112:191–200.

10. Beattie RM, Vieira MC, Phillips AD et al. Carbohydrate intolerance after rotavirus gastroenteritis: A rare problem in the 1990s. Arch Dis Child 1995;72:466.

11. Brown KH, Peerson JM, Fontaine O. Use of nonhuman milks in the dietary management of young children with acute diarrhea: A meta-analysis of clinical trials. Pediatrics 1994;93:17–27.

12. Brown KH. Dietary management of acute childhood diarrhea: Optimal timing of feeding and appropriate use of milks and mixed diets. J Pediatr 1991;118:S92–8.

13. Lifschitz CH, Torun B, Chew F et al. Absorption of carbon 13-labeled C-rice in milk by infants during acute gastroenteritis. J Pediatr 1991;118:526–30.

14. Melton L. Lifesaving vaccine caught in an ethical minefield. Lancet 2000;356:318.

15. Weijer C. The future of research into rotavirus vaccine. BMJ 2000;321:525–6.

16. Diarrhoeal Diseases Study Group (UK). Loperamide in acute diarrhoea in childhood: Results of a double-blind, placebo controlled multicentre clinical trial. BMJ (Clin Res Ed) 1984;289:1263–7.

17. Bowie MD, Hill ID, Mann MD. Loperamide for treatment of acute diarrhoea in infants and young children. A double-blind placebo-controlled trial. S Afr Med J 1995;85:885–7.

18. Soriano-Brucher H, Avendano P, O'Ryan M et al. Bismuth subsalicylate in the treatment of acute diarrhea in children: A clinical study. Pediatrics 1991;87:18–27.

19. Isolauri E, Juntunen M, Rautanen T et al. A human Lactobacillus strain (Lactobacillus casei sp strain GG) promotes recovery from acute diarrhea in children. Pediatrics 1991;88:90–7.

20. Pant AR, Graham SM, Allen SJ et al. Lactobacillus GG and acute diarrhoea in young children in the tropics. J Trop Pediatr 1996;42:162–5.

21. Hyams JS, Krause PJ, Gleason PA. Lactose malabsorption following rotavirus infection in young children. J Pediatr 1981;99:916–8.

22. Penny ME, Paredes P, Brown KH. Clinical and nutritional consequences of lactose feeding during persistent postenteritis diarrhea. Pediatrics 1989;84:835–44.

23. Walker-Smith JA. Cow's milk intolerance as a cause of post-enteritis diarrhoea. J Pediatr Gastroenterol Nutr 1982;1:163–73.

24. Penny ME, Brown KH. Lactose feeding during persistent diarrhoea. Acta Paediatr Suppl 1992;381:133–8.

25. Lebenthal E, Lee PC. Glucoamylase and disaccharidase activities in normal subjects and in patients with mucosal injury of the small intestine. J Pediatr 1980;97:389–93.

26. Solomons NW, Garcia R, Schneider R et al. H2 breath tests during diarrhea. Acta Paediatr Scand 1979;68:171–2.

27. Davidson GP, Goodwin D, Robb TA. Incidence and duration of lactose malabsorption in children hospitalized with acute enteritis: Study in a well-nourished urban population. J Pediatr 1984;105:587–90.

28. Lifschitz CH, Bautista A, Gopalakrishna GS et al. Absorption and tolerance of lactose in infants recovering from severe diarrhea. J Pediatr Gastroenterol Nutr 1985;4:942–8.

29. Naim HY, Roth J, Sterchi EE et al. Sucrase-isomaltase deficiency in humans. Different mutations disrupt intracellular transport, processing, and function of an intestinal brush border enzyme. J Clin Invest 1988;82:667–79.

30. Treem WR, McAdams L, Stanford L et al. Sacrosidase therapy for congenital sucrase-isomaltase deficiency. J Pediatr Gastroenterol Nutr 1999;28:137–42.

31. Turk E, Klisak I, Bacallao R et al. Assignment of the human Na^+/glucose cotransporter gene SGLT1 to chromosome 22q13.1. Genomics 1993;17:752–4.

32. Abad-Sinden A, Borowitz S, Meyers R et al. Nutrition management of congenital glucose-galactose malabsorption: A case study. J Am Diet Assoc 1997;97:1417–21.

33. Greene HL, Ghishan FK. Excessive fluid intake as a cause of chronic diarrhea in young children. J Pediatr 1983;102:836–40.

34. Kneepkens CM, Hoekstra JH. Fruit juice and chronic nonspecific diarrhea. J Pediatr 1993;122:499.

35. Lifschitz CH. Carbohydrate absorption from fruit juices in infants. Pediatrics 2000;105:e4.

36. Sullivan PB, Marsh MN, Mirakian R et al. Chronic diarrhea and malnutrition – histology of the small intestinal lesion. J Pediatr Gastroenterol Nutr 1991;12:195–203.

37. Gryboski JD. The role of allergy in diarrhea: Cow's milk protein allergy. Pediatr Ann 1985;14:31–2, 33–4, 36.

38. Nichols VN, Fraley JK, Evans KD et al. Acquired monosaccharide intolerance in infants. J Pediatr Gastroenterol Nutr 1989;8:51–7.

39. Murch SH. The molecular basis of intractable diarrhoea of infancy. Baillieres Clin Gastroenterol 1997;11:413–40.

40. Greenberg HB, Clark HF, Offit PA. Rotavirus pathology and pathophysiology. Curr Top Microbiol Immunol 1994;185:255–83.

41. Kotloff KL. Bacterial diarrheal pathogens. Adv Pediatr Infect Dis 1999;14:219–67.

42. Kabani A, Cadrain G, Trevenen C et al. Practice guidelines for ordering stool ova and parasite testing in a pediatric population. The Alberta Children's Hospital. Am J Clin Pathol 1995;104:272–8.

43. McKinney RE, Robertson JW. Effect of human immunodeficiency virus infection on the growth of young children. Duke Pediatric AIDS Clinical Trials Unit. J Pediatr 1993;123:579–82.

44. Miller TL, Evans SJ, Orav EJ et al. Growth and body composition in children infected with the human immunodeficiency virus-1. Am J Clin Nutr 1993;57:588–92.

45. Henderson RA, Saavedra JM, Perman JA et al. Effect of enteral tube feeding on growth of children with symptomatic human immunodeficiency virus infection. J Pediatr Gastroenterol Nutr 1994;18:429–34.

46. Winter H. Gastrointestinal tract function and malnutrition in HIV-infected children. J Nutr 1996;126(10 Suppl.):2620S–2622S.

47. Benkov KJ. Gastrointestinal aspects of acquired immunodeficiency syndrome in children. In: Wyllie R, Hyams JS, editors. Pediatric Gastrointestinal Disease. Pathophysiology, Diagnosis, Management. Philadelphia: WB Saunders,1993:712–23.

48. Abramowsky C, Hupertz V, Kilbridge P et al. Intestinal lymphangiectasia in children: A study of upper gastrointestinal endoscopic biopsies. Pediatr Pathol 1989;9:289–97.

49. McReynolds EW, Roy S, Etteldorf JN. Congenital chloride diarrhea. Am J Dis Child 1974;127:566–70.

50. Aichbichler BW, Zerr CH, Santa Ana CA et al. Proton-pump inhibition of gastric chloride secretion in congenital chloridorrhea. N Engl J Med 1997;336:106–9.

51. Desjeux J-F. Congenital transport defects. In: Walker WA, Durie PR, Hamilton JR, Walker-Smith JA, Watkins JB, editors. Pediatric Gastrointestinal Disease, Volume 1. Philadelphia: BC Decker, 1991:668–88.

52. Treem WR. Chronic nonspecific diarrhea of childhood. Clin Pediatr (Phila) 1992;31:413–20.

53. Perman JA, Modler S, Barr RG et al. Fasting breath hydrogen concentration: Normal values and clinical application. Gastroenterology 1984;87:1358–63.

54. Baron HI, Beck DC, Vargas JH et al. Overinterpretation of gastroduodenal motility studies: Two cases involving Munchausen syndrome by proxy. J Pediatr 1995;126:397–400.

55. Bools CN, Neale BA, Meadow SR. Follow up of victims of fabricated illness (Munchausen syndrome by proxy). Arch Dis Child 1993;69:625–30.

56. Weisdorf SA, Salati LM, Longsdorf JA et al. Graft-versus-host disease of the intestine: A protein losing enteropathy characterized by fecal alpha 1-antitrypsin. Gastroenterology 1983;85:1076–81.

57. Bousvaros A, Leichtner AM, Book L et al. Treatment of pediatric autoimmune enteropathy with tacrolimus (FK506). Gastroenterology 1996;111:237–43.

58. Schuster MM. Irritable bowel syndrome. In: Sleisenger MH, Fordtran JS, editors. Gastrointestinal Diseases: Pathophysiology, Diagnosis, Management, 4th ed. Philadelphia: WB Saunders, 1989:21–52.

chapter 8

Protein-Losing Enteropathies

Many disorders cause protein loss from the mucosal surface of the gastrointestinal tract [1,2], including burns [3]. Altered gut permeability may be seen in ulcerative colitis, enteritis [4], celiac disease, kwashiorkor, cystic fibrosis and nephrosis. Protein loss will also occur if there is lymphatic stasis [5], as in primary intestinal lymphangiectasia, congestive heart failure, constrictive pericarditis and lymphoma [6,7]. A small protein loss can be more severe in the presence of malnutrition or malabsorption. The basis of therapy is to treat the primary cause whenever possible [8,9].

PATHOGENESIS

Serum albumin will fall if hepatic synthesis cannot compensate for the enteric loss of protein (Table 8.1). Proteins that have the longest half-life (albumin and γ-globulin) are more depressed than proteins with a short half-life (e.g. prealbumin, fibrinogen, fibronectin and retinol-binding protein).

QUANTIFICATION OF THE ENTERIC PROTEIN LOSS

In clinical practice, the only acceptable way to assess intestinal protein loss is to measure α_1-antitrypsin in a random fecal sample. α_1-antitrypsin is a glycoprotein protease inhibitor that is resistant to degradation by intestinal bacteria. This method has the advantage of being non-radioactive and is easy to perform.

DIETARY TREATMENT

Dietary treatment is only a partial remedy, as the underlying cause must be managed [10]. In cases of intestinal lymphangiectasia (see below), in addition to a high-protein source of nutrition, the quantity of dietary fat should be reduced and the composition modified to provide mostly medium-chain triglycerides (MCTs) rather than long-chain triglycerides (LCTs). Because MCTs are transported by the portal vein, they (unlike LCTs) do not increase lymph flow; however, they do provide an important source of energy, albeit in the absence of essential fatty acids. A low-LCT, high-protein diet for infants and children with lymphangiectasia is described on p. 154.

In contrast, where protein loss is due to altered gut permeability, there is no need to restrict fat unless there is steatorrhea. Where fat does not need to be restricted, a high-protein, high-energy regimen, as described in the section on enteral feeding (p. 37), can be followed.

Subjects	Serum albumin level (g/100 ml)	Albumin synthesis (mg/kg/24 h)	Albumin degradation (percentage plasma albumin pool/24 h)	Exchangeable albumin pool (g/kg)	Intravascular albumin (%)
13 days–14 months	3.3–4.3	180–300	10–11	6.0–8.0	33–43
Over 36 months	4.2–5.0	130–170	6–9	3.0–4.0	46–51

Table 8.1 Normal albumin data (data only available for 13 days–14 months and over 36 months).

It is important to monitor the vitamin, mineral and trace element status in all cases of enteropathy causing malabsorption, and to supplement these accordingly.

INTESTINAL LYMPHANGIECTASIA

This disease is characterized by congenital abnormalities of the small-bowel lymphatic system. Hypoplasia of the lymphatic channels may also be seen in the limbs. Obstruction to the lymphatic drainage of the intestine results in rupture of the lacteals, with leakage of lymph into the lumen of the bowel. There is marked protein loss from the bowel mucosa; there may also be fat loss. Chronic loss of lymphocytes and immunoglobulins from the gastrointestinal tract increases susceptibility to infection. An acquired form of the disease is caused by constrictive pericarditis, congestive heart failure or obstruction of other lymphatic channels.

Clinical features

Intestinal lymphangiectasia may present with failure to thrive, steatorrhea, edematous limbs, repeated infections and tetany. The gastrointestinal symptoms include diarrhea, abdominal distension and pain [11]. The disorder may be associated with autoimmune polyglandular disease type 1 and celiac disease [12].

Pathology

The lymphatics of the lamina propria and/or submucosa and/or serosa and mesentery are dilated, and macrophages may be present. Enterocytes at the tip of the villi contain lipid droplets (Fig. 8.1).

Investigations

The following findings are characteristic of intestinal lymphangiectasia:

- Low total proteins (3.4–5.5 g per 100 ml)

- Low serum albumin (1.1–2.7 g per 100 ml)

- Low immunoglobulin

- Lymphopenia

- ± Anemia (low serum iron and folate)

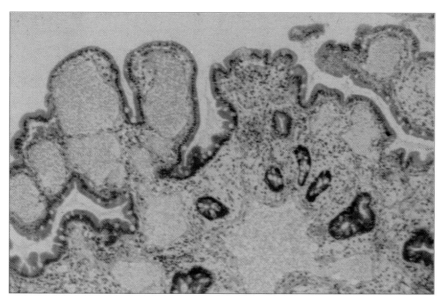

Figure 8.1 Small-bowel biopsy showing dilated lymphatics and presence of lipids in intestinal lymphangiectasia. (Courtesy of Dr P Domizzo and Dr N Meadows.)

- Hypocalcemia

- Steatorrhea

- Increased stool protein loss (measured by α_1-antitrypsin)

- Many lymphocytes seen on stool smear

- Dilated lacteals demonstrated on small-bowel biopsy

- Increased intestinal and mucosal folds, spiculation, jejunization of ileum and dilatation of lumen seen on barium studies of the small bowel

- Obstruction demonstrated by lymphangiography

Treatment

Localized disease might be remedied with resection at the site of obstruction or the creation of an anastomosis. Complete remissions have been described. However, fundamentally, the aim of treatment must be to provide nutrients in a form in which they can be readily absorbed. The presence of LCTs increases the intralymphatic pressure; this may result in rupture of the channels, leading to an increased loss of lymphocytes and protein from the lacteals [13].

Early removal of most of the LCTs is essential. MCTs are absorbed directly into the portal venous system, thus bypassing the lymphatics (Fig. 8.2), and can be offered to replace the energy that is normally derived from dietary LCT. It is important to introduce MCTs very slowly; so, initially, a low-fat feed based on skimmed milk powder is advisable. This feed can also be used in situations where MCT formulas are not available. To prevent deficiency of

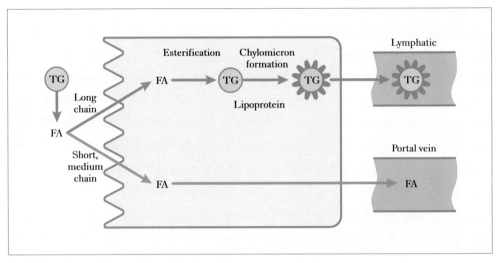

Figure 8.2 Lipid transport in the mucosa. FA = fatty acids; TG = triglycerides.

essential fatty acids, approximately 1.0 g LCT per 100 ml feed or per 60–70 kcal (250–290 kJ) should be consumed. Once the infant is tolerating this, the energy intake can be improved by the gradual introduction of either an MCT formula (e.g. Portagen – see Appendix IV.7), or a formula with hydrolyzed protein and MCT (Pregestimil, Alfare or Alimentum). The protein intake needed in intestinal lymphangiectasia depends upon the quantity being lost from the gut. This loss should decrease once the LCT content of the feed is reduced. Generally, the requirement is 5–10 g of protein per kilogram of actual weight daily, although serum protein and blood urea levels must be monitored to ensure that the correct intake has been achieved. Infant formulas incorporating MCT will not provide sufficient protein unless large quantities are consumed, and a modular regimen might be needed. Alternatively, a protein module (Appendix IV.15) can be used to supplement an MCT formula.

Fat-soluble vitamins are poorly absorbed; hence, up to double the recommended dosage in a water-miscible form is suggested. If the feed is based on skimmed milk or a specially designed modular regimen, water-soluble vitamins may be indicated. Since anemia is a feature of this condition, iron will be required at least until intestinal protein losses are minimal.

When weaning foods are introduced, they should contain no LCTs. Foods such as potato, rice, fruit and vegetables should form the basis of the diet. In older children, the LCT intake ought to be less than 10 g daily, and only foods with a very low fat content (Appendix IV.30) should be included. Additional energy in the form of glucose polymer and MCT will be necessary to achieve sufficient growth. A high-protein, high-energy, low-fat drink, such as that described in Appendix III.8, could be a useful source of nutrients. Furthermore, MCTs can be used in cooking, as described in Appendix IV.9.

REFERENCES

1. Molina JF, Brown RF, Gedalia A et al. Protein losing enteropathy as the initial manifestation of childhood systemic lupus erythematosus. J Rheumatol 1996;23:1269–71.

2. Sullivan PB, Lunn PG, Northrop-Clewes CA et al. Parasitic infection of the gut and protein-losing enteropathy. J Pediatr Gastroenterol Nutr 1992;15:404–7.

3. Matoth I, Granot E, Gorenstein A et al. Gastrointestinal protein loss in children recovering from burns. J Pediatr Surg 1991;26:1175–8.

4. Dansinger ML, Johnson S, Jansen PC et al. Protein-losing enteropathy is associated with Clostridium difficile diarrhea but not with asymptomatic colonization: a prospective, case-control study. Clin Infect Dis 1996;22:932–7.

5. Hardikar W, Smith AL, Chow CW. Neonatal protein-losing enteropathy caused by intestinal lymphatic hypoplasia in siblings. J Pediatr Gastroenterol Nutr 1997;25:217–21.

6. Kaulitz R, Luhmer I, Bergmann F et al. Sequelae after modified Fontan operation: postoperative haemodynamic data and organ function. Heart 1997;78:154–9.

7. Davis CA, Driscoll DJ, Perrault J et al. Enteric protein loss after the Fontan operation. Mayo Clin Proc 1994;69:112–4.

8. Zellers TM, Brown K. Protein-losing enteropathy after the modified Fontan operation: oral prednisone treatment with biopsy and laboratory proved improvement. Pediatr Cardiol 1996;17:115–7.

9. Yamada M, Sumazaki R, Adachi H et al. Resolution of protein-losing hypertrophic gastropathy by eradication of Helicobacter pylori. Eur J Pediatr 1997;156:182–5.

10. Stanley AJ, Gilmour HM, Ghosh S et al. Transjugular intrahepatic portosystemic shunt as a treatment for protein-losing enteropathy caused by portal hypertension. Gastroenterology 1996;111:1679–82.

11. Van der Meer SB, Forget PP, Willebrand D. Intestinal lymphangiectasia without protein loss in a child with abdominal pain. J Pediatr Gastroenterol Nutr 1990;10:246–8.

12. Perisic VN, Kokai G. Coeliac disease and lymphangiectasia. Arch Dis Child 1992;67:134–6.

13. Vardy PA, Lebenthal E, Shwachman H. Intestinal lymphangiectasia: a reappraisal. Pediatrics 1975;55:842–51.

chapter 9

Chronic and Recurrent Abdominal Pain

Peine in the belly is a common disease of childre.

Thomas Phaire, *The Boke of Chyldren* (1553)

Chronic abdominal pain is one of the most common reasons for a family practitioner to refer a child to a general pediatrician. Various field studies in the UK have determined that between 10% and 15% of school-aged children experience recurrent abdominal pain (RAP) [1]. A commonly agreed definition for RAP is that of at least three discrete episodes over a minimum period of 3 months. The pain must be serious enough to interfere with school attendance and other usual activities [2].

Regardless of the fact that there are between 60 and 80 known disorders characterized by RAP, clinicians more often than not determine that the cause of this chronic symptom, in those older than 2 years, is not secondary to serious disease [3]: for example, in a well-known English epidemiological study of 1000 Bristol school children, psychogenic factors were deemed to be responsible for RAP in 90% of cases [4]. A clinician might feel taxed and dissatisfied when challenged with such a long-suffering child and family. There will be a suspicion that the young 'bellyacher' will become an adult one and be at an increased risk of a future psychiatric disorder [5].

However, many now believe that this approach is not valid. It takes little skill to unjustly invoke, on negative grounds, a psychogenic causation. The frequent bias of the clinician toward making an instant diagnosis of RAP secondary to stress is unfair to the patient and family. Such a 'blinkered' approach could lead to an organic and treatable disorder, such as peptic ulceration, going unrecognized.

Diagnosis is dependent upon taking an extensive history before conducting the physical examination. An in-depth record of the previous, present, family and social history is the hallmark of the more determined pediatrician. The history has to be exceptionally comprehensive and include questions relating to a family history of atopy, food intolerance, migraine equivalent syndrome, abdominal pain, irritable bowel syndrome (IBS), peptic ulceration, inflammatory bowel disease, fruit juice intake and, especially in African and African-American families, Asians and those of Jewish ancestry, lactose intolerance. When taking a personal history from carers, note must be taken of earlier colic and the impact, where relevant, when lactation ceased and whether the switch to formula was associated with adverse symptoms or a suggestion of milk-sensitive or food-sensitive colitis. A full psychosocial history of both the child and carers is essential, combined with details of the school attendance record.

The site of the abdominal pain is important because it is well known that the greater the distance from the umbilicus the more likely it is to be linked to a serious ailment (Fig. 9.1). Furthermore, the clinician must determine if there is blood in the stool and whether RAP is associated with an urge to defecate as in proctitis. Abdominal fullness or distension is common in those with IBS and lactose intolerance. In adolescents and adults, certain criteria can be used to establish a diagnosis (Manning or Rome criteria) [6].

During the history taking it is essential to observe the emotional and physical interactions between the child and the parents or other carers. Also, if other siblings are present, the clinician will be able to obtain key clues as to the nature of all the 'subunits', and which members of the family couple or group together for mutual support during the consultation. Where causation is due to personality and emotional issues, it is often apparent to the perceptive physician before the child is even examined. An interviewer needs to be cognizant of the relationship between emotional, physical and sexual abuse and chronic abdominal pain. Although the clinical examination is frequently non-contributory, it must be thorough both for diagnostic reasons and to establish credibility with the carers. Relevant investigations are listed in Table 9.1.

In our experience the most common disorders responsible for chronic and recurrent abdominal pain are (Fig. 9.2):

- IBS

- Psychogenic pain

- Constipation

- Food intolerance (migraine equivalent syndrome)

- Esophagitis

- Lactose intolerance and fruit juice malabsorption

- *Helicobacter pylori* infection

- Inflammatory bowel disease (see Chapter 11)

- A combination of any of the above

Management of the common causes is outlined in Fig. 9.3.

IRRITABLE BOWEL SYNDROME

(chronic non-specific diarrhea, toddler diarrhea, irritable colon syndrome of infancy)

This benign and self-limiting condition, known by a number of descriptive terms, is a syndrome of abnormal intestinal motility seen in children between 6 months and 5 years of age. IBS is the most common disorder to be characterized by chronic diarrhea in a child who

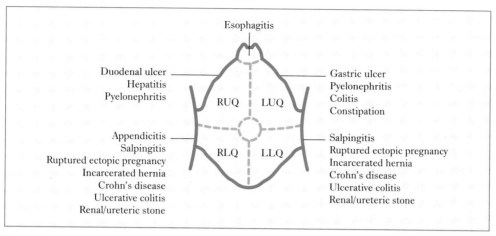

Figure 9.1 Causes of non-central abdominal pain. RUQ = right upper quadrant; LUQ = left upper quadrant; RLQ = right lower quadrant; LLQ = left lower quadrant.

General
- White cell count and differential
- ESR or CRP
- Liver function and amylase
- Urea and creatinine
- Mid-stream urine for microscopy, culture and sensitivity
- IgE (useful in absence of atopy – if ↑, suggests parasitic infestation)

Stomach and small intestine
(i) To exclude lactose intolerance: hydrogen breath test post lactose load (see p. 107)
(ii) To identify *Helicobacter pylori*: ¹³C breath test – if not available, offer Rapid Office screening blood test or *H. pylori* antibody test
(iii) To identify *H. pylori* or small-bowel enteropathy: endoscopy + biopsy + duodenal fluid aspirate for *Giardia lamblia* and parasite identification
(iv) Radiology: barium ± follow-through studies (e.g. if Crohn's disease is suspected)

Colon
(i) Stools: microscopy, culture and sensitivity (×7 before excluding pathogen)
(ii) Nuclear: white cell scanning with indium or selenium
(iii) Endoscopy, biopsy and stool culture: for mycobacteria, amebae and other pathogens; also to exclude IBD

ESR = erythrocyte sedimentation rate; CRP = C-reactive protein.

Table 9.1 Chronic and recurrent abdominal pain: investigations.

does not have a state of malabsorption or failure to thrive. Indeed, IBS is one of the most frequent gastrointestinal syndromes seen in infants and toddlers.

The features often include colicky intestinal pains, increased flatus [7] and distension of the abdomen. One study of American senior- and middle-school students revealed 17% of the former and 8% of the latter had IBS-type symptoms [8]. Moreover, the scores for anxiety and depression among those affected were significantly higher than the scores for students lacking such symptoms. Not surprisingly, there is commonly a strong family history of so-called functional bowel disorders. Carers are concerned because of the presence of

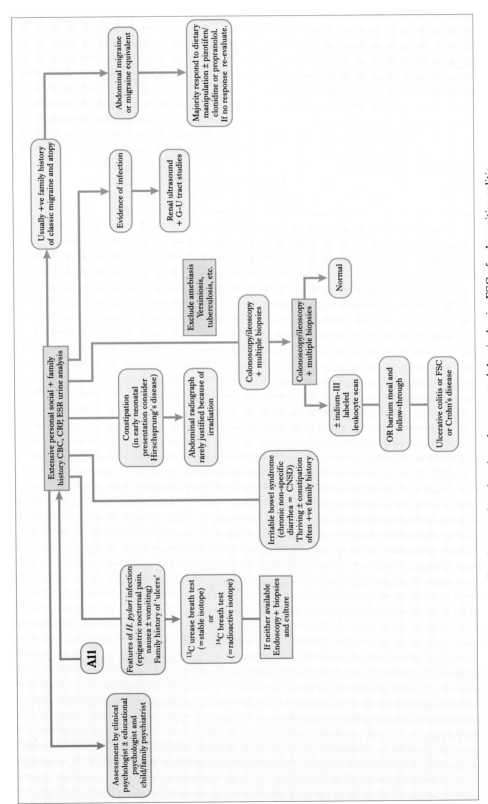

Figure 9.2 Evaluation options of the major disorders causing chronic and recurrent abdominal pain. FSC=food sensitive colitis.

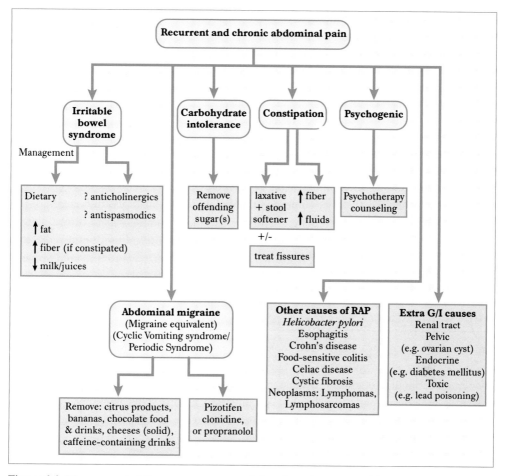

Figure 9.3 Management of the common causes of chronic and recurrent abdominal pain.

undigested items of food such as peas, corn and carrots in the loose, foul-smelling stools. These unaltered vegetables reflect the reduced intestinal transit time. Paradoxically, the same child will often be troubled at times by constipation. Usually, no stools are passed at night. Nonetheless, families reassuringly report that the child is thriving in terms of height and weight gain as well as development. However, the state of nutrition might be unsatisfactory when attempts are made to control the symptoms by reducing the caloric intake.

PATHOPHYSIOLOGY

There is morphologically normal small-bowel mucosa. Both congenital and acquired disease processes may be associated with this disorder [9].

Studies of upper small intestinal motility in IBS have provided evidence of an abnormality of the migrating motor complexes (MMCs). This is present not when fasting but upon initiation of feeding and during postprandial activity. It has been proposed that this anomalous pattern of MMCs results in reduced gut transit time. Rapid emptying of the contents of the small bowel into the colon, with partially digested food and incomplete reabsorption of bile salts, promotes colonic secretion. Degeneration by colonic bacteria, with the presence of excess bile salts, will produce hydroxy fatty acids that act as secretagogues.

TREATMENT

This is based upon clinical findings. However, it is essential to reassure the carers that, despite the presence of foul-smelling and loose stools, the child is well. Usually, simple measures are effective – such as increasing the fat content of the diet if the child is eating a low-fat diet, normalizing the fiber content of the diet, reducing an excess milk intake or the volume of fruit juice to no more than 200 ml per day and excluding sugary drinks. Rarely, loperamide (0.1 mg/kg/day) can be resorted to for short and intermittent periods of time. Psyllium may have a role [10]. Also, naloxone, an opioid antagonist, appears to hold promise in patients with IBS [11].

PSYCHOGENIC ABDOMINAL PAIN

Unfortunately, too many children and adolescents with RAP are readily – and often falsely – labeled as being ill secondary to psychogenic disorders. In recent years, there has been greater understanding of gastrointestinal infections due to *H. pylori* and of the pervasiveness of lactose intolerance, particularly within certain ethnic groups. This heightened awareness has facilitated better diagnoses and so reduced the risk of incorrect use of the label 'emotional disorders'.

Psychogenic disease in childhood is diffuse, complex and one of the most labor-intensive in terms of history taking and the need for time to be set aside for periods of observation with counseling. Parents with little insight often resent the absence of an organic disorder. A number of lengthy family meetings may be necessary to elicit the true picture. Adequate history taking is essential in an endeavor to identify triggering factors that provoked the pain, particularly when the child comes from a so-called dysfunctional family. Invariably, such pain is unaltered by antacids, H_2 blockers, anticholinergics or analgesics. In addition, it is associated with times of stress, such as returning to school on a Monday morning, following a school vacation or witnessing a family quarrel.

A number of studies have revealed mutual themes of depression between mother and child where RAP is present. Precipitating factors or a so-called significant life event, at home or school, must be sought. If the onset of pain coincided with a tragic event involving a relative, friend, schoolteacher or perhaps a pet, or the anniversary of such, that might be the explanation.

Initially, the clinician will need to exclude organic disease by performing a comprehensive battery of investigations. While it is true that a clinical psychologist or a child and family psychiatrist might be more positive in making a diagnosis based upon an emotional etiology, this approach can sometimes be inappropriate. We have all seen patients who are suffering from gastrointestinal disease but who are also emotionally ill, either in response to their ailment or in an unlinked manner. It is a sobering exercise to note the considerable number of children who have been referred to psychiatrists because of anorexia, weight loss and depression, but who suffer from undiagnosed Crohn's disease. Hence, the pediatrician is obliged to investigate fully before negating organic bowel disease and transferring the patient to the psychologist or psychiatrist. It is essential that a finite stage is promptly reached, and flagged within the family, after which no further clinical investigations are undertaken. Only then will the patient and family accept that the pain, although genuine, is related to psychogenic factors.

In the presence of features suggesting psychosocial ailments, such as a tic, phobias, night terrors, depression in the child, family members or peers or conflict between any persons attending the sessions, it is evident that an emotional disorder might be responsible for the pain [12]. Furthermore, a positive response to any intervention from the psychologist or psychiatrist reinforces the likelihood of non-organic disease being present. Rarely does a child present as an overt malingerer, lacking any genuine pain but nonetheless announcing, if not broadcasting, his or her need for skilled professional help.

ABDOMINAL MIGRAINE (migraine equivalent syndrome)

There is nothing that is so coueniet for the meygrym as tranquillietie and rest.

The Regiment of Life (1544)

It was in 1765 that Whyatt observed how 'gastralgia' alternated with migraine: more than two centuries later, we can still affirm that association. The term abdominal migraine was suggested by Brams in 1922 [13]. However, it has since become evident that this expression is etymologically inappropriate and it has been suggested that 'migraine equivalent' might be a better alternative.

Abdominal migraine is a well-recognized condition in childhood and is responsible for many with RAP [14]. Despite its high prevalence, it is often underdiagnosed by primary care physicians, and at times by pediatricians. Characteristically, the central abdominal pain is accompanied by marked pallor, headache, anorexia, nausea and/or vomiting, and there is a strong family history of migraine [15]. In at least 25% of cases, there is a personal history of travel sickness. In our experience, the mean age at onset is 8.2 ± 1.9 years, with the abdominal pain resolving at 10.6 ± 2.4 years.

In 1933, Wyllie and Schlesinger described 'the periodic group of disorders in childhood' [16] and, in 1963, Cullen and MacDonald equated the 'periodic syndrome' with 'juvenile migraine' [17]. However, there is still confusion and disagreement regarding what constitutes and distinguishes abdominal migraine, the periodic syndrome and cyclic vomiting syndrome (CVS) [18]. Many regard CVS as being part of the syndrome of abdominal migraine, while others see it as a separate entity but one having a close interrelationship [19,20]. In CVS, the dominant feature is recurrent and explosive vomiting lasting hours or even days [21].

DIET AND BIOCHEMICAL THEORIES

The study of abdominal migraine has been hindered by an absence of distinct diagnostic laboratory markers. For centuries it has been known that certain foodstuffs, particularly those containing vasoactive amines, can trigger cephalgic migraine. There are many common provoking dietary agents: namely, citrus fruits and drinks, chocolate and its derivatives, coffee, tea, nuts and solid cheeses. Some adult migraineurs cannot oxidize tyramine or phenylethylamine. The former is contained in a number of cheeses (Appendix IV.41), and the latter in chocolates as well as some red wines.

Food allergens and RAST (radioallergosorbent test)

It has been claimed that food intolerance can provoke or accentuate migraine. Katchburian et al. [22] reported a normal IgE level and negative RAST results in non-atopic children with abdominal migraine. This suggests that if the pathogenesis is in part immunologic, it is not reaginic. Michie [23] demonstrated that when his group of patients improved, the bowel mucosal permeability decreased. Enterocytes are capable of expressing MHC class 2 antigen and secreting chemokines, and so might initiate immune responses in the epithelial lymphocyte population under the influence of dietary antigens.

MANAGEMENT

The key component of therapy is dietary manipulation, with the removal of citrus fruits and drinks, solid cheeses, chocolate and its derivatives and caffeine-containing drinks (e.g. tea, coffee, cocoa and cola drinks). Where a diet fails to achieve a prompt and impressive improvement, and there has been proper dietary compliance under the surveillance of a pediatric dietitian, the diagnosis must be reconsidered. Usually, an oligoantigenic (or 'few foods') diet is not indicated. In those not responding to dietary exclusions, we have resorted to pizotifen, ketotifen or clonidine.

ESOPHAGITIS (*see also* Chapter 13)

The majority of infants and children with gastroesophageal reflux experience some degree of esophagitis. The intensity of pain, epigastric discomfort, 'heartburn', colic and, in babies, restlessness, will relate to the degree of reflux and its perseverance. A crying and sleepless baby might be in pain or persistent discomfort from esophagitis. Symptoms will be much influenced by the presence of prematurity (with an immature gastroesophageal junction), the feeding and weaning regimen, as well as physical posture when sleeping. Older children might have substernal chest pain or swallowing difficulties.

SELECTED DISORDERS OF CARBOHYDRATE ABSORPTION

LACTOSE MALDIGESTION (*see also* Chapter 5)

Despite the abundance of available literature on lactose intolerance, in terms of pathogenesis and geographic distribution, there is little agreement in respect of its classification. Globally,

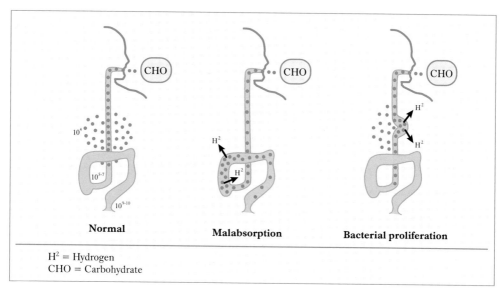

Normal **Malabsorption** **Bacterial proliferation**

H^2 = Hydrogen
CHO = Carbohydrate

Figure 9.4 Situation leading to the production of hydrogen in man. The powers of 10 shown in the left-hand diagram indicate the number of bacteria per milliliter of intestinal fluid.

lactose-intolerant individuals outnumber those with tolerance to this carbohydrate. The term lactose intolerance is appropriate where it is the result of a damaged intestinal mucosa causing secondary lactase deficiency. Moreover, in the rare instances of congenital primary alactasia, it is acceptable. In the case of the genetically determined decrease of lactase activity during childhood, however, low lactase levels suggest that most of the world's population is 'abnormal', whereas those of Caucasian ancestry with high levels of the enzyme within the brush-border villi are then considered 'normal'. Rings et al. [24] suggest it would be better to ascribe racial and ethnic lactose malabsorption as the result of a genetically determined reduction of lactase activity, rather than implying an 'abnormality' by use of the term deficiency.

Lactose intolerance is common in children from southeast Asia and the Pacific (e.g. Chinese, Japanese, Koreans, Thais, Fijians, Filipinos and Australian Aborigines). Although there is a high prevalence in Africans and African-Americans, those originating from areas of cattle-raising nomads, as would be anticipated, are not lactose intolerant.

The condition is uncommon in west Europeans and those from the Middle East. In Europe, the frequency increases in the southern and eastern directions, reaching levels of 70% in southern Italy and Turkey. The lowest prevalence is in Scandinavia and northwest Europe (3–8%), which contrasts with almost 100% in parts of southeast Asia [25]. For an interesting and concise review, in terms of the biology and an anthropological appraisal of this disaccharide see [26].

SECONDARY LACTOSE INTOLERANCE

This transient problem, which results from damage to the mucosa of the small-bowel wall, can be attributed to a considerable number of diseases. It is by far the commonest cause of lactose malabsorption [27].

The following conditions are an example of some that may be associated with temporary lactose intolerance:

- Enteritis (viral, bacterial or fungal)
- Dietary milk protein intolerance
- Parasitic infestation (e.g. *Giardia lamblia*)
- Celiac disease or a transient gluten enteropathy
- Cystic fibrosis (seen in 25%)
- Protein–energy malnutrition
- Drugs (e.g. neomycin, methotrexate)
- Immunodeficiency syndrome (e.g. HIV [28])

Diagnosis

Diagnosis is based on the following:

- Stool Clinitest reaction (see p. 108)
- Stool pH – if below 5.5, a sugar is present
- Hydrogen breath test (see below)
- Small-bowel biopsy with disaccharidase assay (see below)

Hydrogen breath test

This test depends upon the presence of bacteria in the colon fermenting non-absorbed carbohydrates (Fig. 9.4). In normal circumstances, only a trace of (or zero) hydrogen is present in expired breath. However, given the presence of abnormal quantities of sugar and adequate bacteria, there is a semi-quantitative relationship between the expired hydrogen and the malabsorption of the carbohydrate. The end expiratory air should be sampled in duplicate, using nasal prongs or an airtight facemask attached to a 20 ml syringe with a stopcock or bag.

The patient should be fasted for 4–6 h (infants) or for 12 h (older children), the baseline breath hydrogen measured and then a load of 1–2 g/kg (max. 50 g) in a 20% solution (10% in infants less than 6 months of age) of the carbohydrate in question (lactose, sucrose etc.) given. The end-expiratory air should be sampled in duplicate at 15, 30, 60, 90, 120 and 180 min. If the expired breath hydrogen exceeds 20 parts per million above the baseline (= pre-carbohydrate load), sugar malabsorption is present. An elevated baseline result suggests small-bowel bacterial overgrowth [40].

With the greater availability of user-friendly, handheld, bedside hydrogen breath analyzers (e.g. Bedfont Scientific Gastrolyzer, UK), this test will become easier to perform.

Duodenojejunal biopsy

Given the absence of the few contraindications, such as significant hypoprothrombinemia or a disorder of blood clotting, a small-bowel biopsy is indicated if an enteropathy is to be excluded. Increasingly, in tertiary centers, a biopsy is taken during endoscopy as opposed to blind duodenal intubation with a Crosby or Watson capsule.

Management

The dietary treatment of recurrent and chronic abdominal pain secondary to lactose intolerance relates to the severity of the symptoms. Most pill-type medicines contain lactose as a filler. A reduction in the lactose content of the diet may be sufficient to alleviate the pain and other features. In older children who are receiving unmodified cow milk, preparations of the enzyme lactase (e.g. Lactaid) can be added to the milk to remove much of the lactose. In the presence of severe villous atrophy, sucrose will also need to be removed until the mucosa has healed.

FRUIT-JUICE CARBOHYDRATE MALABSORPTION

Excessive intake of fruit juices, particularly those in which the carbohydrate composition may lead to carbohydrate malabsorption, has been identified as another cause of abdominal pain. The mixture of a low glucose concentration relative to that of fructose and the presence of sorbitol, such as found in apple and pear juice, results in impaired absorption of carbohydrate which, when fermented in the colon, will produce gas and abdominal pain [29].

HELICOBACTER PYLORI INFECTION

Few microorganisms have achieved such a meteoric rise in attention within so relatively short a time as has *H. pylori*. The significance of *H. pylori* infection in children is controversial, but it is acknowledged to cause gastritis and RAP.

MICROBIOLOGY

Helicobacter-like organisms were first observed by veterinary pathologists in the 1800s. Interest was subsequently rekindled in 1983, when Warren and Marshall wrote in *The Lancet* of the little-known "unidentified curved bacilli on gastric epithelium in active chronic gastritis" [30]. Only 14 years later, the complete genome sequence of this high-profile microbe was identified and published in *Nature* [31].

Originally, the organism was named *Campylobacter pyloridis* because of its similarity to the species, and later became known as *C. pylori*. However, this microorganism is quite distinct from other *Campylobacter* species that can cause acute enteritis with diarrhea. In 1989, *C. pylori* acquired recognition as a new genus, in part due to its enzymatic properties, and so was named *H. pylori* [32]. There are 40 epidemiologically unrelated strains of *H. pylori*.

Genetic studies suggest that *H. pylori* strains are very diverse and that this reflects the bacteria's ancient ancestry and the readiness with which it exchanges genes with other *H. pylori* strains [33]. Moreover, this diversity has clinical relevance in that different genetic loci have been identified and those with particular alleles have associated types of duodenogastric disease.

INCIDENCE AND TRANSMISSION

The organism's prevalence is associated with the child's homeland, socioeconomic standard and density of living, as well as age. In the West, it is relatively uncommon, especially among the affluent and in those under 5 years of age; yet, beyond 50 years, there is serologic evidence to show that 50% have had an infection. *H. pylori* infection is present in 15% of 12-year-old Americans. In France, 3.5% of children are infected within the first decade of life, which contrasts with 45–90% in that same period in Algeria and Gambia.

H. pylori can pass from person to person and there is a high rate of cross-infection among those in institutions. Mothers chewing food before feeding it to their infants (premastication) or using a community feeding bowl are means of spreading the disease. Mouth-to-mouth resuscitation and inadequate endoscope cleansing techniques have been identified as other avenues of cross-infection.

The fecal–oral route of transmission has been substantiated by the isolation of *H. pylori* from the feces of 48% of subjects colonised with the microbe. Clustering within families is a well-described phenomenon.

CLINICAL FEATURES

Chronic abdominal pain has been the principal clinical finding in children who, upon endoscopy, have evidence of *H. pylori* [34]. However, there have been conflicting reports as to the evidence for a link between *H. pylori* gastritis and abdominal pain in children. In one small Finnish study of 82 children with RAP, 22% were infected with *H. pylori* [35]; yet, in a Belfast-based investigation, which revealed a high prevalence of *H. pylori* seropositivity, there was no association with recurrent and chronic abdominal pain [36]. The latter group of researchers did not carry out endoscopy and biopsy. When the organism is causing antral nodular gastritis in children, as diagnosed by tissue biopsy, there is a relationship with RAP [37].

PATHOGENESIS

This microbe, in common with other bacteria, can induce inflammatory responses in tissues by a number of mechanisms. At endoscopy, a nodular appearance due to lymphoid hyperplasia within the antrum is commonly seen in *H. pylori* gastritis.

Mediators of inflammation include chemotaxin for neutrophils, proteins that induce the expression of interleukin (IL)-2 receptors, IL-1, tumor necrosis factor, leukotriene B_4, leukocyte migration inhibition factor and platelet-activating factor. These mediators are present in increased amounts in tissue infected with *H. pylori*. In addition, the increased levels of gastrin associated with this microorganism will also explain the tissue injury. In pediatrics, there is a close relationship between *H. pylori* and primary gastritis. Approximately 90% of children with proven duodenal ulcers have an associated *H. pylori* gastritis, but it is not a significant cause of gastric ulcers within the pediatric population.

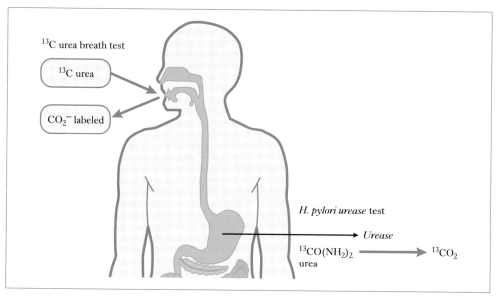

Figure 9.5 ^{13}C urea breath test and *H. Pylori* urease test.

DIAGNOSIS

An important feature of this organism is the presence of the enzyme urease, which is responsible for the conversion of urea into ammonium and bicarbonate, then carbon dioxide. Urease is a convenient diagnostic tool for the clinician. Its activity can be identified from biopsied tissue samples obtained at endoscopy, or by the ^{13}C or ^{14}C urea breath test.

Urea breath test

This test is carried out using urea labeled with either non-radioactive ^{13}C or, in adults, radioactive ^{14}C. A test meal of labeled urea (together with pure orange juice to delay gastric emptying) is given, and the expired breath CO_2 then measured (Fig. 9.5). ^{13}C is a naturally occurring substance, normally present in small quantities in expired breath. However, when *H. pylori* is present, following a meal of ^{13}C-labeled urea, the amount of the stable isotope in expired breath will be higher than normal. The urea test is both highly specific (93%) and highly sensitive (96%). Neither this test nor the one using ^{14}C should be carried out within at least a month of receiving antibiotics. Other explanations for false-negative findings include the use of bismuth salts or omeprazole.

Other tests

There are a number of alternatives now available using direct and indirect techniques to establish a diagnosis and to monitor eradication. One such option is an enzyme immunoassay that detects *H. pylori* antigen in feces [38,39]. This low-cost non-invasive test has been described as both reliable and accurate [40].

Screening young dyspeptic patients for *H. pylori* and avoiding endoscopy in those who are seronegative can reduce the endoscopy workload by 30% [41]. However, endoscopy and histology of the antral mucosa enables a definitive diagnosis to be made [42]. Furthermore, there is the opportunity with biopsied tissue to carry out a rapid urea test on the sample. This is performed using a pellet or solution of urea and a pH indicator: if present, *H. pylori* will hydrolyze the urea and thus create a change in the color indicator and pH reading. This option is both rapid and – apart from the cost of endoscopy and biopsy procedure – inexpensive. Multiple biopsies should be obtained and the tissue stained with Giemsa, Gram, acridine or silver. Specimens can be cultured, but if a polymerase chain reaction (PCR) technique is used, the organism can be directly identified without the need to have cultured the microbe.

A less sophisticated and non-invasive screening method, and one not requiring access to a central laboratory with a gas isotope ratio mass spectrometer, involves the measurement of specific *H. pylori* antibodies. This enzyme-linked immunosorbent assay (ELISA) technique is reliable and highly sensitive as well as specific [32].

The 'Rapid Office Test' is a commercial kit that allows the use not only of serum but also possibly saliva or gingival secretions. The disadvantage is the high rate of false-positive results: those who are positive require further investigation, namely the costly ^{13}C urea breath test.

The Helisal Rapid whole-blood test is a recently introduced diagnostic tool. In a group of adults it has been found to be 88% sensitive and 91% specific. When coupled with a gold-standard battery of tests it could dramatically reduce the number of endoscopies [43].

TREATMENT

There is still much controversy regarding the optimal therapeutic regimen for children, but similar disagreements prevail among adult gastroenterologists [44]. Despite the appearance of over 700 publications on eradication therapy in the past decade, the guidelines are ever changing, as is the sensitivity of this ubiquitous microbe. The American National Institute of Health Consensus Development Conference on *Helicobacter pylori* advised that antimicrobial agents should be used in addition to antisecretory drugs [45]. Fortunately, there is no discord in one sphere and that is in respect of children with *H. pylori* colonization who are asymptomatic. This group do not currently qualify for therapy. Yet, they might be infecting other family members, especially when sharing a bed.

Antibiotic monotherapy with amoxycillin or bismuth does not eradicate this infection. However, triple therapy with amoxycillin (or the acid-stable macrolide clarithromycin), bismuth subcitrate and metronidazole (or tinidazole) is one agreed option. Other workers advocate 7–10 days of a quadruple regimen, by adding the proton-pump inhibitor omeprazole, in preference to H_2-receptor antagonists. This is because there is enhancement of the antibiotic(s) activity in the presence of marked hypochlorhydria. Inevitably, triple therapy – and even more so a quadruple regimen – are associated with poor compliance.

It is usually possible to eliminate *H. pylori* after one or sometimes two treatments, because multi-drug resistance is still uncommon. In a study conducted in Dublin [46], *H. pylori* was cleared in more than 95% of children after only 1 week of treatment with the following:

- Colloidal bismuth subcitrate – 480 mg/1.73 m²/day (max. 120 mg four times day)

- Metronidazole – 20 mg/kg/day (max. 200 mg three times a day)

- Clarithromycin – 15 mg/kg/day (max. 250 mg twice a day)

If bismuth is used, the colloidal subcitrate is safer and so preferable to the subsalicylate preparation [47].

A major aspect of adequate eradication therapy in the long-term approach is the relationship between *H. pylori* and both adenocarcinoma of the stomach and mucosa-associated lymphoid tissue (MALT) gastric lymphoma [48].

DISEASE PREVENTION

A future vaccine might have a role in preventing particular disease as opposed to avoiding *H. pylori* colonization. For example, a vaccine would be appropriate in China, where gastric cancer rates are high, but not in the USA, where the incidence is low.

REFERENCES

1. Pringle MLK, Butler NR, Davie R. 11,000 seven year olds. The First Report of the National Child Development Study (1958 cohort). London: Longmans, 1966.

2. Hirsch BZ. Recurrent Abdominal Pain: Common Problems in Pediatric Gastroenterology and Nutrition. Chicago: Year Book Medical Publishers, 1989.

3. Bines JE. Chronic and recurrent abdominal pain. In: Walker-Smith JA, Hamilton JR, Walker WA, editors. Practical Pediatric Gastroenterology, 2nd ed. Ontario: BC Decker, 1996:25–6.

4. Apley J, Nalsh N. Recurrent abdominal pains. A field survey of 1000 school children. Arch Dis Child 1958;33:165–70.

5. Hotopf M, Carr S, Mayou R et al. Why do children have chronic abdominal pain, and what happens to them when they grow up? Population based cohort study. BMJ 1998;316:1196–200.

6. Akehurst R, Kaltenthaler E. Treatment of irritable bowel syndrome: a review of randomised controlled trials. Gut 2001;48:272–82.

7. Hyams JS, Treem WR, Justinich CJ et al. Characterization of symptoms in children with recurrent abdominal pain: resemblance to irritable bowel syndrome. J Pediatr Gastroenterol Nutr 1995;20:209–14.

8. Hyams JS, Burke G, Davis PM et al. Abdominal pain and irritable bowel syndrome in adolescents: a community-based study. J Pediatr 1996;129:220–6.

9. Milla PJ. Acquired motility disorders in childhood. Can J Gastroenterol 1999;13:76A–84A.

10 Smalley JR, Klish WJ, Campbell MA et al. Use of psyllium in the management of chronic nonspecific diarrhea of childhood. J Pediatr Gastroenterol Nutr 1982;1:361–3.

11. Longo WE, Vernava AM. Prokinetic agents for lower gastrointestinal motility disorders. Dis Colon Rectum 1993;36:696–708.

12. Navarro J. Abdominal pain in infants and children. In: Navarro J, Schmitz J, editors. Paediatric Gastroenterology. Oxford: Oxford University Press, 1992:436–41.

13. Brams WA. Abdominal migraine. JAMA 1922;78:26–7.

14. Albayaty M, Bentley D. Abdominal migraine in childhood. 9th Migraine Trust International Symposium, London, 1992.

15. Symon DN, Russell G. Abdominal migraine: a childhood syndrome defined. Cephalalgia 1986;6:223–8.

16. Barlow CF. Headaches and Migraine in Childhood. Oxford: Blackwell Scientific, 1984.

17. Cullen KJ, MacDonald WB. The periodic syndrome: its nature and prevalence. Med J Aust 1963;2:167–73.

18. Dignan F, Symon DN, AbuArafeh I et al. The prognosis of cyclical vomiting syndrome. Arch Dis Child 2001;84:55–7.

19. Symon DN, Russell G. The relationship between cyclic vomiting syndrome and abdominal migraine. J Pediatr Gastroenterol Nutr 1995;21:S42–3.

20. Bentley D, Kehely A, Al-Bayaty M et al. Abdominal migraine as a cause of vomiting in children: a clinician's review. J Pediatr Gastroenterol Nutr 1995;21:S49–51.

21. Fleisher DR, Matar M. The cyclic vomiting syndrome: a report of 71 cases and literature review. J Pediatr Gastroenterol Nutr 1993;17:361–9.

22. Katchburian A, Horn J, Bentley D. Abdominal migraine in childhood; food intolerance and the IgE level. Sixth International Migraine Symposium, London, 1986.

23. Michie A, Al-Bayaty M, Bentley D. Is abdominal migraine often environmentally determined? 11th Migraine Trust International Symposium, London, 1996.

24. Rings EH, Grand RJ, Buller HA. Lactose intolerance and lactase deficiency in children. Curr Opin Pediatr 1994;6:562–7.

25. Gudmand-Høyer E. The clinical significance of disaccharide maldigestion. Am J Clin Nutr 1994;59:735S–41S.

26. Johnson JD, Kretchmer N, Simoons FJ. Lactose malabsorption: its biology and history. Adv Pediatr 1974;21:197–237.

27. Walker-Smith J. Sugar malabsorption. In: Diseases of the Small Intestine in Childhood, 3rd ed. London: Butterworth, 1988:285– 314.

28. Yolken RH, Hart W, Oung I et al. Gastrointestinal dysfunction and disaccharide intolerance in children infected with human immunodeficiency virus. J Pediatr 1991;118:359–63.

29. Hyams JS, Etienne NL, Leichtner AM et al. Carbohydrate malabsorption following fruit juice ingestion in young children. Pediatrics 1988;82:64–8.

30. Warren JR, Marshall BJ. Unidentified curved bacilli on gastric epithelium in active chronic gastritis. Lancet 1983;1:1273–5.

31. Tomb JF, White O, Kerlavage AR et al. The complete genome sequence of the gastric pathogen Helicobacter pylori. Nature 1997;388:539–47.

32. Bujanover Y, Reif S, Yahav J. Helicobacter pylori and peptic disease in the pediatric patient. Pediatr Clin North Am 1996;43:213–34.

33. Blaser MJ. Helicobacter pylori and gastric diseases. BMJ 1998;316:1507–10.

34. Bourke B, Jones N, Sherman P. Helicobacter pylori infection and peptic ulcer disease in children. Pediatr Infect Dis J 1996;15:1–13.

35. Ashorn M, Mäki M, Ruuska T et al. Upper gastrointestinal endoscopy in recurrent abdominal pain of childhood. J Pediatr Gastroenterol Nutr 1993;16:273–7.

36. McCallion WA, Bailie AG, Ardill JE et al. Helicobacter pylori, hypergastrinaemia, and recurrent abdominal pain in children. J Pediatr Surg 1995;30:427–9.

37. Chong SK, Lou Q, Asnicar MA et al. Helicobacter pylori infection in recurrent abdominal pain in childhood: comparison of diagnostic tests and therapy. Pediatrics 1995;96:211–5.

38. Shepherd AJ, Williams CL, Doherty CP et al. Comparison of an enzyme immunoassay for the detection of Helicobacter pylori antigens in the faeces with the urea breath test. Arch Dis Child 2000;83:268–70.

39. Braden B, Teuber G, Dietrich CF et al. Comparison of new faecal antigen test with ^{13}C-urea breath test for detecting Helicobacter pylori infection and monitoring eradication treatment: prospective clinical evaluation. BMJ 2000;320:148.

40. Mönkemüller KE, Wilcox CM. Gastrointestinal infections in children. Curr Opin Gastroenterol 2001;17:35–9.

41. Moayyedi P, Carter AM, Catto A et al. Validation of a rapid whole blood test for diagnosing Helicobacter pylori infection. BMJ 1997;314:119.

42. Schreiber R. Disorders of the stomach. In: Walker-Smith JA, Hamilton JR, Walker WA, editors. Practical Pediatric Gastroenterology. Toronto: BC Decker, 1996:148–9.

43. Anon. Validation of a near patient test for H pylori. BMJ 1997;314.

44. Harris A, Misiewicz JJ. Treating Helicobacter pylori – the best is yet to come? Gut 1996;39:781–3.

45. NIH Consensus Conference. Helicobacter pylori in peptic ulcer disease. JAMA 1994;272:65–9.

46. Walsh D, Goggin N, Rowland M et al. One week treatment for Helicobacter pylori infection. Arch Dis Child 1997;76:352–5.

47. Sullivan PB. Helicobacter pylori in children. Current Medical Literature – Paediatrics 1994;7:63–8.

48. Marshall BJ. Helicobacter pylori: a primer for 1994. Gastroenterologist 1993;1:241–7.

chapter 10

Constipation and Encopresis

Although the term constipation suggests the infrequent passage of a stool, it is lacking a well-accepted, more comprehensive definition. Clayden describes the condition as one characterized by pain and difficulty or delay in defecation [1]. In the West, constipation is a common pediatric problem in that it affects as many as 7.5% of school children [2], although it is less evident in those beyond 12 years of age. In 55% of cases, there is a positive family history. As many as 25% of all referrals to pediatric gastroenterologists are because of constipation. Although some infants defecate only once every 4 or 5 days, 94% of preschool children pass at least one stool a day.

HISTORY AND PHYSICAL EXAMINATION

In the history taking, questions need to be focussed upon alterations in diet or fluid intake, degree of physical activity and other factors such as medication, all of which might be associated with the onset of constipation. If carers are coercive in wanting to witness early 'potty' training, this might be the explanation. One highly effective method of achieving non-verbal and negative communication with a mother is for an infant to refuse to use the 'potty'. Quite soon, stools become harder and more difficult to pass, and then cause an anal fissure with even greater pain and subsequently a genuine and somatic reason for 'hanging on'. Often, school children, for a number of reasons, are reluctant to use the school toilet. Prying eyes, teasing comments and perhaps cold and murky outside facilities might encourage the child to neglect the urge to pass a stool until his or her arrival home. Such disregard of the reflex mechanism will result in a firmer stool being formed within the colon.

During the physical examination, the clinician must carefully palpate the abdomen, searching for fecal masses or rocks, and inspect the anus for signs of abuse or anal fissures. The presence of other perianal features, such as tags, old abscesses and scars, perhaps in the scrotum, would suggest Crohn's disease. If gentle and lateral traction is applied to the anal orifice – ideally not by the examiner but by a trusted parent – then eventually, with reflex dilatation, internal tears, mucosal lesions or fissures become evident. A warm atmosphere and a good light source, but above all an unhurried examination, are essential. The clinician needs to note the size and contents of the rectal ampulla should it have been decided that this uncomfortable part of the assessment is justified. If an internal examination is too distressful, it should be promptly abandoned or carried out under sedation.

During the physical evaluation, underlying non-gastrointestinal conditions that can cause constipation must be considered by the diagnostician. Namely, one must look for features of hypothyroidism and hypercalcemia. Even celiac disease uncommonly might be accompanied by constipation. Neurological diseases that can damage the lumbosacral reflex arc, such as spina bifida and myelodysplasia, may cause sphincter dysfunction with incontinence and constipation. To exclude an underlying spinal disorder (e.g. a tethered cord) or other lesion, the skin must be inspected at the base of the spine. Clues such as an old surgical scar, lipoma, mole or tuft of hairs should be sought. More significantly, reflexes in the lower limbs must be both present and symmetric. Also, the Achilles tendons must be examined as well as gait, to ensure a primary neurological cause is not responsible for the constipation.

PATHOGENESIS AND INVESTIGATIONS

It is prudent to recall that the earlier in life the onset of the constipation, the greater the likelihood that there is a significant primary cause. In the full-term well neonate who has not passed meconium within 48 h of birth, there may be an indication to investigate. Sherry and Kramer [3] observed that 99.8% of term neonates pass a stool within 48 h of delivery and after a meconium plug has been expelled. Should the problem persist, Hirschsprung's disease and anatomic disorders need to be excluded.

Unfortunately, there is no consistent correlation between anorectal manometry findings and the symptoms of chronic childhood constipation or, indeed, encopresis [4]. Some investigators have noted a statistically significant difference in the anorectal pressure findings between those with and without constipation [1]. However, a megarectum from any cause will produce abnormal pressure results secondary to the rectal distension. Seemingly, as yet, manometry alone does not supply all the answers. Most investigators have demonstrated a decreased ability of the internal anal sphincter to relax, with rectal distension in severe constipation.

Findings that may be of consequence are those of reduced rectal sensitivity and increased rectal compliance, causing a diminution in the intensity of the urge to defecate [5].

Refractory constipation, especially in the presence of a personal or family history of atopy, might be due to milk protein [6].

MANAGEMENT

In the majority of children with constipation, given good compliance and the support of the carers as well as a pediatric dietitian, conservative measures are invariably successful.

Anal fissures, although a major deterrent to the passage of a stool, rapidly respond to topical analgesics (2% lignocaine ointment), together with a stool softener (sodium docusate or lactulose) or bulk forming agents (psyllium) such as Metamucil, Fiberall and Seraton, and a stimulant laxative such as senna. In the USA, mineral oil has traditionally been used as an emollient laxative. Unfortunately, its safety is open to debate. In our experience, nighttime administration of increasing volumes of senna is effective. At first, we prescribe only 2.5 to 5.0 ml, and subsequently increase the dose daily by aliquots of 2.5 to 5.0 ml unless spurious diarrhea intervenes, when the amount is then reduced. The symptoms are titrated against the volume of laxative, while continuing with softening agents as well as the necessary dietary guidelines.

Enemas should be avoided unless there is clinical or radiological evidence of gross fecal impaction that has failed to respond to oral sodium picosulfate (UK) or a similar agent. Their excessive use is widespread and often counterproductive. Gleghorn's group [7] successfully avoided initial enema 'cleanouts' in 98% of 45 patients. If resorted to, enemas must be isotonic. Should a Fleet enema (sodium biphosphate) be used, fluid intake must be adequate and clear written instructions issued to the carer. When manual fecal disimpaction is embarked upon, adequate sedation is obviously essential. Persistence with large volumes of senna, perhaps as much as 25 ml a time, accompanied by all the other therapeutic and dietary measures, will usually achieve the desired outcome.

Sometimes, infants and young children, especially if physically small, retain stools because they are afraid of the usual adult-type lavatory, particularly when switching from a 'potty'. They may have fears of falling into the lavatory: a special child's seat will resolve this dilemma. Another simple explanation, and one that is frequently overlooked both by parents and experts, relates to the positioning of the child when on the lavatory – because defecation depends upon an effective Valsalva maneuver to achieve rectal peristalsis, the child's feet must reach the floor. If this is the cause, a foot support will often eliminate the constipation.

The establishment of a daily regimen is, in the first instance, of considerable importance. Nevertheless, carers must not be too obsessed or curious about their child's visits to the toilet, as often it then develops into a psychologically unhealthy family theme.

An extensive study by van der Plas and colleagues [8] revealed no evidence to support the use of anal sphincter feedback training in the treatment of children with chronic constipation, and the investigators concluded that intensive conventional laxative treatment should remain the first choice in such patients.

A mixture of polyethylene glycol of high molecular weight (3,800) is now available to treat constipation in infants and children. This mixture is similar to the one used for colonic preparations prior to colonoscopy but without sodium which makes it more palatable. In the USA it is marketed under the name of Miralax.

Dietary recommendations

The intake of both fluid and fiber should be increased. Dietary fiber consists of several different components, the major distinction being the soluble forms (mostly gums and hemicellulose), found in fruits and vegetables, and the insoluble type (bran and cellulose), present chiefly in cereal foods (Fig. 10.1). The two types of fiber are treated differently in the large bowel but both have a part to play in increasing stool bulk and softness as well as stimulating colonic peristalsis.

Infants under the age of 1 year

Extra fluid can be provided in the form of unsweetened fruit juice, diluted 50:50 with water.

Over the age of 4–6 months, fiber can be introduced into the diet in the form of puréed fruit and vegetables. Later, cereal fiber such as breakfast dishes based on wholewheat (see Appendix IV.37) can be used.

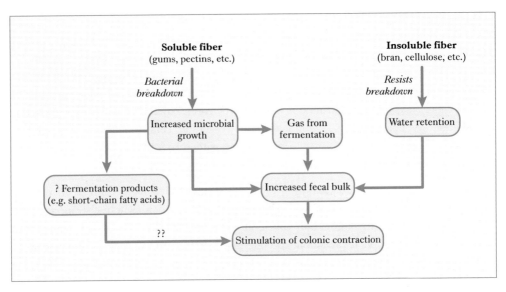

Figure 10.1 Action of dietary fiber.

Older children

Intake of high-fiber foods, particularly wholemeal breads and cereals, should be encouraged. The consumption of large quantities of confectionery and sweet foods reduces the desire to chew bulky high-fiber items. Thus, refined sugars should be avoided and instead replaced by foods such as potato-chips, savory snacks, raisins, peanuts and fruit. In the USA, recommendations have been made for fiber requirements in children and a simple formula devised to assist in meeting those requirements: age of child plus 5–10 g fiber. So, for example, a 5 year old child would require between 10 and 15 g fiber daily. It should not be necessary to add bran to the diet; indeed, there is some evidence that the mineral balance is altered when bran is given as a supplement. However, in stubborn cases, bran may be needed. Unfortunately, none of the common forms of bran – wheat, oat or soya – are particularly palatable, and, usually, children who refuse wholegrain bread and vegetables will also reject bran. It can be incorporated into home-baked cakes and cookies or mixed with gravies, savory sauces and soups. Often it is necessary to give it with a milkshake syrup or evaporated milk in order to disguise its dry texture. A coarse bran is preferable to a finely ground one because large particles are less quickly degraded within the colon and thus retain their physical properties, such as water-holding capacity, for longer.

Fluid intake is as important as dietary fiber, since the aim is to produce a soft stool with a high water content. Often, a drink of warm water or fruit juice taken immediately upon awakening will stimulate the gastrocolic reflex, providing the child has access to a toilet and sufficient time.

In some pre-school children, particularly those with a personal or family history of atopy, removal of all cow's milk proteins may resolve the constipation.

ENCOPRESIS

Originally, this term was used to describe the involuntary passage of whole bowel movements into the underwear or their deposition in an improper place [9]. However, it has since been adapted and used in a broader concept related to fecal soiling.

It is seen in 1–2% of children, and there is a three- or fourfold male dominance. The majority of encopretics do not have anal sphincter dysfunction or a neurological/ neuromuscular disease to account for this embarassing disorder. The condition usually results from constipation with 'spurious' diarrhea around the rock-like empacted stools, or from an excessive intake of laxatives. An intensive and comprehensive program, including counseling, education, initial catharsis and laxatives, can result in improvement for almost 80% of cases.

Emphatic early 'potty' training might have induced a negative response, manifested later by the deliberate withholding of feces. Upon observation, it is often evident that, paradoxically, children are straining hard, not to achieve stooling but to retain their feces. Parents frequently misinterpret the straining efforts as an endeavor to evacuate the bowel and are surprised to learn of an alternative explanation. An infant or young child with apparently little control over his or her carers may deliberately retain the stools and then soil, causing much distress. This method can be a most effective and powerful means of expressing displeasure and gaining attention. Not surprisingly, in such situations there is a greater need for a referral to a child/family psychiatrist than for the administration of laxatives. However, it must be emphasized that, before seeking a colleague's support in this scenario, it is essential to exclude an anal or underlying neuropathologic disease.

HIRSCHSPRUNG'S DISEASE

Hirschsprung's disease is characterized by an absence of ganglion cells in the bowel wall. There is always an absence of ganglion cells in the distal rectum but the aganglionosis can extend proximally for a variable distance. The rectosigmoid is involved in 70% of cases, the proximal colon in 20% and the colon with small bowel (ileum) in the remaining 10%.

Three susceptibility genes (on chromosomes 10, 13 and 20) have been identified in Hirschsprung's disease: the RET proto-oncogene, the endothelin-B receptor gene and the endothelin-3 gene. The disorder affects about one in 5000 neonates both in the USA and UK. In as many as 50% of affected infants, the diagnosis is not established in the early weeks of life. It might not be identified for years, but presents as enterocolitis that has a high mortality. A plain abdominal radiograph in the neonate may reveal a characteristic appearance of an air-distended sigmoid and colon, tapering into a smaller rectum.

A definitive diagnosis requires suction or preferably full-thickness biopsies at different levels: the standard barium enema does not exclude this disorder. Furthermore, because of the possible absence of a reflex in the neonate, rectal distension might not relax the internal sphincter and so manometry cannot be relied upon. A full-thickness biopsy enables the experienced histopathologist to search for ganglion cells in the submucosal and the intermyenteric plexuses. In Hirschsprung's disease, not only are ganglion cells absent but hypertrophied nerve trunks can be evident. In addition, immunocytochemical staining techniques for the presence of the enzyme acetylcholinesterase must be performed on fresh non-preserved biopsy specimens.

Children with the ultra-short-segment variety (seen in 9% of cases) as well as those with pseudo-Hirschprung's disease must be identified. In the latter group, anorectal manometry findings suggest Hirschsprung's but the rectal biopsy is normal.

REFERENCES

1.   Clayden GS. Is constipation in childhood a neurodevelopmental abnormality? In: Milla PJ. Disorders of Gastrointestinal Motility in Childhood. Chichester: John Wiley, 1988:111–21.

2.   Loening-Baucke V. Chronic constipation in children. Gastroenterology 1993;105:1557–64.

3.   Sherry SN, Kramer I. The time of passage of the first stool and first urine in the newborn infant. J Pediatr 1955;46:158–9.

4.   Borowitz SM, Sutphen J, Ling W et al. Lack of correlation of anorectal manometry with symptoms of chronic childhood constipation and encopresis. Dis Colon Rectum 1996;39:400–5.

5.   Loening-Baucke VA. Sensitivity of the sigmoid colon and rectum in children treated for chronic constipation. J Pediatr Gastroenterol Nutr 1984;3:454–9.

6.   Shah N, Lindley K, Milla P. Cow's milk and chronic constipation in children. N Engl J Med 1999;340:891–2.

7.   Gleghorn EE, Heyman MB, Rudolph CD. Non-enema therapy for idiopathic constipation and encopresis. Clin Pediatr 1991;30:669–72.

8.   van der Plas RN, Benninga MA, Buller HA et al. Biofeedback training in treatment of childhood constipation: a randomised controlled study. Lancet 1996;348:776–80.

9.   Weissenberg S. Über enkopresis. Z Kinderheilk 1926;40:67.

chapter 11

Inflammatory Bowel Disease

Inflammatory bowel disease (IBD) is a term used to describe a series of chronic diseases involving the bowel that are characterized by the production of inflammation and, over the course of years or decades, may be associated with extraintestinal features. The two most common disorders in this group are Crohn's disease (CD) and ulcerative colitis (UC). CD can involve any part of the gastrointestinal tract from mouth to anus, whereas UC commonly affects only the colon and rectum. However, it is likely that CD and UC are part of a single disease spectrum. Although CD differs from UC pathologically and clinically, the two diseases overlap in a number of features: both can affect the small or large bowel and be improved but not cured with medication. UC, however, can be cured with colectomy while CD cannot [1].

Both UC and CD occur more frequently in whites than blacks. Also, both diseases appear to be more common in industrialized countries such as Scandinavia, UK and North America, and less prevalent in Central and Southern Europe, Asia and Africa. Rates for the Jewish population may be slightly higher than in the non-Jewish population, but this also varies geographically. However, both diseases can affect individuals from all races.

CROHN'S DISEASE

This chronic inflammatory condition of the bowel was first described by Crohn in 1932 as a terminal ileal disorder characterized by ulcerations and scarring. In CD, the entire gastrointestinal tract, from mouth to anus, can be diseased (Table 11.1), the most common sites being the terminal ileum and proximal colon.

The overall prevalence of CD ranges from 10 to 70 cases per 100,000 population. In 25–30% of cases, there is a family history of IBD (CD and/or UC). The incidence of CD has increased in the past three decades.

ETIOLOGY

The etiology remains unclear. Viruses and bacteria have been implicated as causative agents, but, to date, no single theory can explain all cases of the disease. This disorder is more prevalent in populations living in developed countries, particularly among certain ethnic groups, with an increased incidence among family members of a proband. Such observations would seem to indicate an association between environment, genetic predisposition, autoimmunity and/or infection and/or diet.

Area affected	Percentage of patients
Ileocolitis	50–60
Small bowel only	30–35
Colitis only	10–15
Anorectal	5
Esophageal/duodenal only	<5

Table 11.1 Intestinal distribution of Crohn's disease in children based on clinical and radiologic findings.

- Abdominal pain
- Lack of weight gain or weight loss
- Diarrhea
- Blood and/or mucus in stools
- Fatigue
- Growth failure and delayed puberty
- Extraintestinal symptoms

Table 11.2 Presenting symptoms of Crohn's disease.

CLINICAL FEATURES

The most prevalent presentation is the classic triad of abdominal pain, diarrhea and weight loss. Although at the time of onset symptoms may be vague and ill defined, they can also be quite intense, to the point of mimicking acute appendicitis. In some cases, gastrointestinal symptoms may not be overt, which may delay the diagnosis by several years. Major features are listed in Table 11.2.

Up to 20% of cases presenting with abdominal pain may have an abdominal mass found by palpation, commonly in the right lower quadrant. Many of these patients will have experienced no weight gain for several months or years, or may even have suffered weight loss; consequently, impaired linear growth and delayed puberty may precede the appearance of gastrointestinal symptoms (Fig. 11.1). The reason for the weight loss is anorexia, which results from the abdominal discomfort or pain that passage of food generates as it progresses through inflamed or narrowed bowel segments. A poor caloric intake over a long term results in short stature and delayed puberty [2,3]. Sometimes, decreased caloric consumption is barely noticeable, but, as it has extended over several years, the deficit accumulates and patients just fail to meet energy needs for growth.

Inflammation produces fever and anemia consequent to a decrease of serum transferrin, although the bone marrow stores are not iron deficient. Patients may complain of tiredness much more than their peers. Hematochezia (bright-red blood per rectum) is indicative of distal colon involvement and may be associated with the presence of mucus and tenesmus

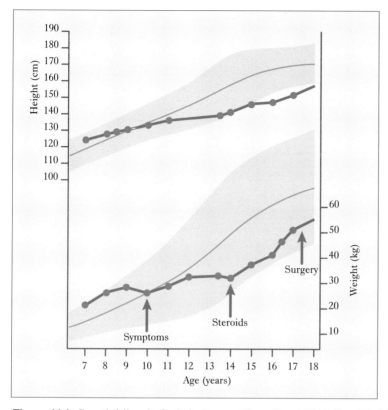

Figure 11.1 Growth failure in Crohn's disease. (From Grand RJ. Pediatr Clin North Am 1975;22:835.)

(feeling the need to defecate but not expelling any material). In some cases, diarrhea with blood, mucus and pus can be very intense.

Although perianal disease (abscess, sinus, fistula, tag, fissure) is less common in children than in adults, it is not unusual to see pediatric patients with painless symptomatology of this type. Severe, mutilating perianal CD, causing significant tissue destruction, occurs in both sexes and is extremely refractory to treatment in the majority of patients [4].

Extraintestinal manifestations of CD are listed in Table 11.3.

PATHOLOGY

Whereas UC is usually a disease of the gut mucosa, CD affects the whole thickness of the bowel wall. The distribution of this transmural disease in children (see Table 11.1) differs from that seen in adults. Duodenal and jejunal locations are less common than other sites but occur more often in children than in adults.

Features of CD include the following:

- Can involve all areas of the bowel

- Typically seen at discontinuous areas along the gut (i.e. 'skip' lesions)

- Erythema nodosum

- Pyoderma gangrenosum

- Aphthous ulcers

- Ocular disease (conjunctival ulceration, iritis, uveitis, episcleritis)

- Arthritis or arthralgia

- Ankylosing spondylitis

- Digital clubbing

- Hepatic disease (hepatitis, primary sclerosing cholangitis)

- Urinary tract disease (urolithiasis, oxaluria)

- Vascular (thromboembolic disease, seizures)

Table 11.3 Extraintestinal manifestations of Crohn's disease.

- Thickening of bowel wall (Fig. 11.2)

- Stricture formation leading to obstruction

- Microscopic fissures and ulcers pass from the mucosa into the small-bowel wall

- Granulomas (collections of transformed macrophages) are non-caseating and sarcoid-like but are not always present; there is inflammation of the submucosa (Fig. 11.3)

- Fat wrapping, thickened mesentery and enlarged regional lymph nodes

INVESTIGATIONS

If the disease is active, the erythrocyte sedimentation rate will be elevated in 50% of cases. In addition, the acute-phase proteins, particularly C-reactive protein (CRP), may be raised, as well as the platelet count. Anemia is common, which is generally a result of low serum transport proteins, as well as folic acid deficiency, rather than iron deficiency. Hypoalbuminemia can be present because of protein loss from the bowel mucosa. A number of macrcophage-derived cytokines; such as tumor necrosis factor-α, interleukin (IL)-1 and IL-6, may be elevated in active disease.

Depending on the symptom(s), endoscopic and/or radiologic examinations may be indicated. Radiologic signs of CD are listed in Table 11.4. Patients with diarrhea, tenesmus and blood and/or mucus in the stool will need a colonoscopy after parasitic and bacterial infections have been ruled out. If on colonoscopic examination the bowel appears severely ulcerated it may be preferable to abort the procedure, to avoid a risk of perforation, and instead just obtain several biopsies from the lower colon. If colonoscopy is not completed and there is evidence of obstruction of the colon, an air-contrast barium enema may be performed at a later time. To minimize the risk of bowel perforation, contrasted radiologic studies should not be performed within 48 h following large-bowel biopsies. A low-pressure barium enema may be carried out to diagnose a stricture in a patient too ill to undergo a colonoscopy but should not be undertaken in toxic patients.

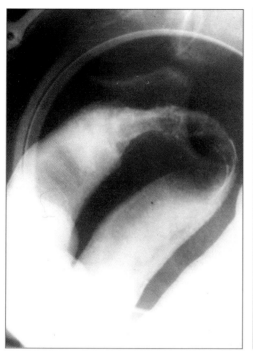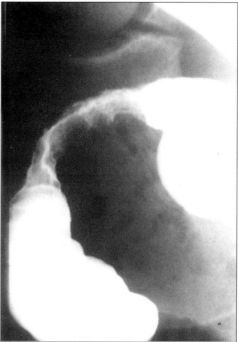

Figure 11.2 Crohn's disease — part of the colon from a 14-year-old boy who had a total colectomy. The bowel wall is greatly thickened. (Courtesy of Dr W Hyer.)

- Thickening of the mucosa (thumb printing)
- Ulceration
- Irregularities of the mucosa
- Dilatation
- Colonic pseudopolyps (cobblestone appearance)
- Narrowed segments of bowel
- Fistulous tracts
- Skip lesions in the colon
- Discrete (aphthoid) ulcers

Table 11.4 Radiologic signs of Crohn's disease.

In patients with emesis, abdominal pain, a palpable abdominal mass, poor weight gain or weight loss and/or fever, an upper endoscopy and duodenal biopsies may help to make the diagnosis. Upper gastrointestinal series with small-bowel follow-through, particularly examining the area of the terminal ileum, may show edema, spasm, narrowing, fistulas and/or mass effects caused by an abscess. Barium examination of the small and large bowel with air contrast may help determine the sites and severity of the disease. Computerized axial tomography might delineate a mass or fistulous tracts between organs.

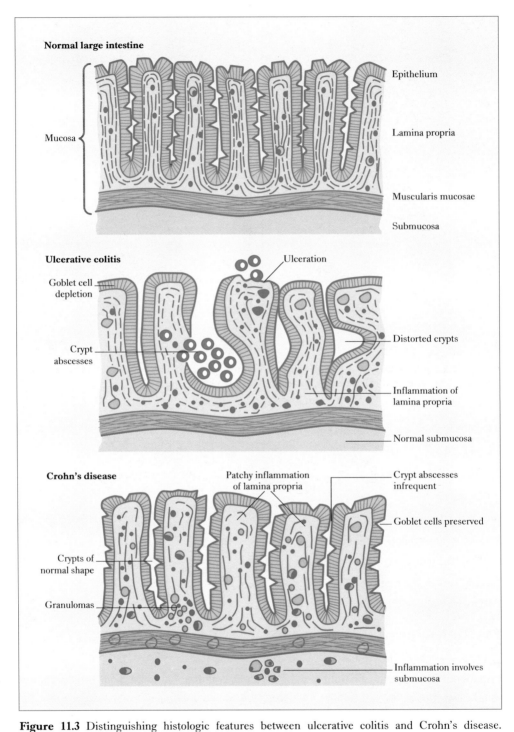

Figure 11.3 Distinguishing histologic features between ulcerative colitis and Crohn's disease. *Ulcerative colitis*: (1) goblet-cell depletion; (2) crypt abscesses; (3) ulceration; (4) inflammation of lamina propria; (5) distorted crypts; (6) normal submucosa. *Crohn's disease*: (1) goblet cells preserved; (2) crypt abscesses infrequent; (3) granulomas; (4) patchy inflammation of lamina propria; (5) crypts of normal shape; (6) inflammation involves submucosa. (By kind permission of Dr PJ Berry and Update Hospital Publications Ltd.)

In a prospective study, 357 adult patients with 606 colonoscopies, in whom the endoscopic appearances were those of IBD, were followed-up for an average period of 22 months [5]. A final, definite, endoscopy-independent diagnosis was reached by means of autopsy, surgery or histology on biopsy in 71% of patients. Accuracy of colonoscopy was 89%, with 4% errors and 7% indeterminate diagnoses. The most useful endoscopic features in this differential diagnosis were discontinuous involvement, anal lesions and cobblestoning of mucosa for CD, and erosions or microulcers and granularity for UC.

Leukocyte scanning uses autologous leukocytes labeled with ^{111}In or ^{99m}Tc-HMPAO, which are reinjected intravenously. This process may show aggregation at sites of IBD, even though CD is mediated by T cells and not neutrophils [6]. However, some authorities regard this as a poor substitute for mucosal biopsy [7].

New serologic markers of IBD include anti-*Saccharomyces cerevisiae* antibodies (ASCA) and perinuclear antineutrophil cytoplasmic antibodies (pANCA). The majority of patients with CD who have a positive ASCA result (both IgG and IgA) have small-bowel involvement and exhibit signs of obstruction and perforating/fistulizing disease. Ruemmele et al. [8] tested the diagnostic accuracy of modified assays for pANCA and ASCA in pediatric patients with either disease and in those without IBD. IgA and IgG ASCA titers were significantly greater and highly specific for CD (95% for either, 100% if both positive). pANCA was 92% specific for UC and absent in all non-IBD controls. In this and other studies [9], the majority of CD patients positive for pANCA had a UC-like presentation. Disease location, duration, activity, complications and treatment with immunosuppressive drugs did not have an impact on the ASCA or pANCA assay results. After resection, UC patients remained pANCA positive, in contrast to patients with CD, in whom ASCA titers decreased toward normal values postoperatively.

DIAGNOSIS

In some cases, diagnosis of CD can be definitive and relatively simple to make. In other instances, the diagnosis will be presumptive and more likely the result of a summation of various symptoms and findings, rather than the presence of a pathognomonic feature such as granulomas in an intestinal biopsy.

At the time of diagnosis, the patient is assigned an activity index that can be used to assess response to treatment. The Pediatric Crohn's Disease Activity Index (PCDAI) is a multi-item measure that, in contrast to the adult-derived index, includes linear growth and places less emphasis on subjectively reported symptoms and more on laboratory parameters of intestinal inflammation [10]. If the colon is the only segment affected, there may be difficulty differentiating CD from UC. Presence of microscopic inflammation in the stomach or duodenum, even without overt symptoms, veers the diagnosis toward CD. Definitive diagnosis, however, requires the presence of non-caseating granulomas in the bowel mucosa or, in cases of extraintestinal Crohn's, the skin [11]. In some cases that are typical of CD, granulomas may never be found.

The differential diagnoses of CD are listed in Table 11.5.

* Infections:
  Enteric bacterial pathogens and amebiasis
  Yersinia enterocolitica
  Clostridium difficile
  Tuberculosis

* Ulcerative colitis

* Eosinophilic colitis

* Autoimmune enteropathy

* Lymphoma

* Sarcoidosis

* Behçet's disease

* Lupus erythematosus

* Juvenile rheumatoid arthritis

* Acute appendicitis

* Gastroesophageal reflux

* Gastric/duodenal ulcer

* *Helicobacter pylori* gastritis

Table 11.5 Differential diagnosis of Crohn's disease.

COMPLICATIONS

Intestinal complications of CD include bowel obstruction, bowel perforation, fistulas and abscesses. Massive dilatation of the colon (megacolon) and rupture of the intestine are potentially life-threatening complications. Toxic megacolon is less common in CD than in UC. Fistulas may develop between any two segments of the bowel, and/or between the bowel, skin, bladder and/or vagina. Such tracts formed between the proximal and distal bowel can result in nutrient malabsorption because the absorptive area is bypassed. Perianal disease includes skin tags, anal fissures, fistulas and abscesses, which can be devastating. Markowitz et al. [12] characterized the frequency, severity and clinical course of a highly destructive form of perianal disease by reviewing a database containing records from 230 children with CD. Sixty-seven (29%) of these patients had significant perianal pathology. This included six with highly destructive disease, eight with complicated fistulas and 53 with simple perianal fistulas or abscesses. Transrectal ultrasonography is effective for the diagnosis and follow-up of patients with anorectal abscesses and fistulas.

CD of the small bowel causes an increased risk of adenocarcinoma, located most commonly in the terminal ileum and in bypassed areas of the duodenum, jejunum or ileum.

Sites of extraintestinal complications include the skin, joints, spine, eyes, liver and bile ducts (see Table 11.3). In a study by Wilschanski et al. [13], 17 of 32 children with primary sclerosing cholangitis had IBD (14 UC and 3 CD).

* Intractable bleeding

* Fixed bowel constriction

* Severe unresponsive perianal disease

* Symptomatic fistula

* Short stature with an identifiable segment of severely diseased bowel

* Intestinal perforation

* Abscess

Table 11.6 Indications for surgery in Crohn's disease.

MANAGEMENT

Management is directed to address the following:

* Reduce the inflammatory component

* Correct general and specific nutrient deficiencies

* Correct strictures, fistulas and abscesses

Medical therapy

There is no medication capable of curing the disease. Medical therapy is discussed together with that for UC on p. 193. More specific for CD, metronidazole can help patients with symptomatic perianal disease [14]. A sulfonamide combination (co-trimoxazole) and metronidazole may control bacterial overgrowth that develops proximal to areas of reduced small-bowel motility or partial bowel narrowing. Cholestyramine, an anion exchange resin that binds bile acids, may also be of help in relieving diarrhea caused by bile acid malabsorption in the presence of severe terminal ileal disease.

Surgical therapy

In CD, surgery can be performed to remove severely inflamed and/or fibrotic segments of bowel and areas of narrowing, as well as for closure of fistulous tracts. The indications for surgery in CD are listed in Table 11.6.

A child not attaining optimal growth, who is chronically ill with a diseased segment(s), might not respond to any medical or dietary treatment. The only course then is the surgical excision or bypass of the pathologic area [15]. However, about one-third of such patients will require further surgery, which increases the morbidity risks. Within 15 years of the initial operation, there will be a reoperation rate of 89%. In many cases, however, a patient may present with a partial intestinal obstruction that would appear fixed upon radiologic studies yet will respond to intravenous corticosteroids, decompression and intravenous nutrition for an extended period. Whenever a surgical resection is performed, there is usually some disease in the remaining adjacent bowel, albeit microscopic. Use of mesalamine postoperatively, even in the absence of overt disease, extends the period that a patient will remain asymptomatic after a bowel resection [16]. Repeated resections of the bowel may lead to short-bowel syndrome.

Dietary therapy

This is discussed together with that for UC on p. 193. It should be noted that several studies have demonstrated that elemental diets are capable of inducing remission in CD, although the duration of remission may be shorter than when steroids are used [17]. In some units, enteral feeding is indicated as first-line therapy in CD [18].

ULCERATIVE COLITIS

This is a serious inflammatory disorder of the large bowel, which can be accompanied by a number of non-enteric features. It was known to the ancient Greek physician Aretaeus the Cappadocian and was distinguished from epidemic dysentery by Sir Samuel Wilks in 1859.

The overall prevalence is 20–40 cases per 100,000 of the population, although it is lower in Africa and India. In Israeli Jews of European origin, HLA phenotypes AW24 and BW35 are associated with UC. The AW24 phenotype is seen more commonly in patients with early-onset and moderate-to-severe disease.

ETIOLOGY

The etiology is unknown and theories are similar to those proposed for Crohn's disease (see p. 181). Support for an autoimmune mechanism comes from the knowledge that extraintestinal signs, e.g. uveitis, arthritis and chronic active hepatitis, may accompany UC.

CLINICAL FEATURES

Most patients will experience diarrhea, with blood and/or mucus in the stools. Some may present just with cramps and intermittent blood in the feces. The most common symptoms are listed in Table 11.7. As strictures can become evident at any time during the illness, patients may present with apparent constipation.

PATHOLOGY

UC may be limited to the rectum or involve the entire length of the large bowel (pancolitis). The lamina propria is infiltrated with inflammatory cells and goblet-cell reduction is seen. Mucosal ulceration, crypt abscesses and glandular distortion are characteristic findings of this disease (Table 11.8; see also Fig. 11.3).

DIFFERENTIAL DIAGNOSIS

Typically, it is not difficult to diagnose UC, but at times the major challenge is to exclude CD, as the latter can also involve the large bowel. A number of enteric infections may present with symptoms similar to those of IBD: for example, *Campylobacter*, that has infected the colon as well as its usual site of the small bowel. In addition, the following conditions should be excluded:

- Amebiasis

- Shigellosis

- Diarrhea

- Blood and/or mucus in stools

- Abdominal pain (often left-sided)

- Weight loss

- Fever

- Tenesmus

- Fatigue

- Growth failure and delayed puberty

- Liver dysfunction (chronic active hepatitis, primary sclerosing cholangitis, pericholangitis or biliary cirrhosis)

Table 11.7 Presenting symptoms of ulcerative colitis.

Ulcerative colitis	Crohn's disease
No granulomas	Granulomas are characteristic
Crypt abscesses	Crypt abscesses are infrequent
Distorted crypts	Normal crypt shape
Inflammation of mucosa + lamina propria	Transmural inflammation
Goblet-cell depletion	Goblet-cell preservation
Mucin depletion	

Table 11.8 Histologic characteristics of ulcerative colitis and Crohn's disease.

- Salmonellosis

- Infection with *Yersinia enterocolitica*

- Tuberculosis

- Pseudomembranous colitis

- Cow or soy milk colitis (in infants)

- Behçet's disease

DIAGNOSIS

Two of the major investigations are colonoscopy with multiple mucosal biopsies and barium enema using a double-contrast technique to reveal the nature of the mucosa (Fig. 11.4). Both methods require bowel cleansing, which can be done with various commercial oral (not universally available) and rectal preparations. In milder cases, visual examination of the colon will demonstrate increased mucus and an edematous and friable mucosa with loss of the normal vascular pattern. More advanced disease will show ulcers, strictures and/or pseudopolyp formation. Colonoscopy will enable the extent of the problem to be established.

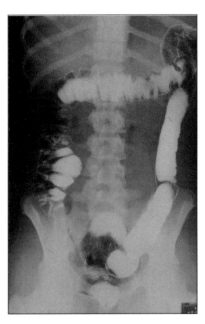

Figure 11.4 Barium enema in a 14-year-old boy with severe ulcerative colitis, showing narrowing of the colon ('lead pipe' appearance), loss of haustrations and fine spicules owing to mucosal ulceration. (Courtesy of Dr M Brueton.)

In patients with toxic megacolon or a severe pancolitis, this procedure is not without risk and should be limited to observation of the more distal segment. The introduction of air during colonoscopy could enhance bacterial translocation and a biopsy might lead to perforation. Performing a barium enema, when necessary, should be delayed until the patient is less toxic and for 48 h after a colonic biopsy, to avoid a perforation. Tests should include hemoglobin, white cell and platelet count, erythrocyte sedimentation rate, CRP (and other acute-phase proteins), interleukins (IL-1 and IL-6) and albumin. Where an infectious agent is suspected, up to seven stool specimens should be cultured for *Shigella*, *Salmonella*, *Campylobacter* and *Yersinia*. Agglutinins should also be requested for amebiasis where this is relevant or even suspected.

New serologic markers for IBD were discussed above in the section on CD. Antinuclear cytoplasmic antibody, especially perinuclear antibody (pANCA), can be found in 60–90% of adults and approximately 67% of children with UC, as opposed to 6% of patients with CD [19].

COMPLICATIONS

Problems include perforation, acute dilatation, strictures, pseudopolyps and, rarely, massive hemorrhage. One of the long-term consequences of UC is carcinoma, which is associated with the disease after 10 years of its presence and relates both to chronicity and severity. During the second decade of the disease, there is a 20% risk of cancer; by 35 years of the disease, the incidence is 43%. Colorectal carcinoma accounts for one-third of the deaths related to UC. Some advocate prophylactic colectomy after 10 years of UC. A less radical alternative is annual colonoscopy to detect dysplasia.

Extraintestinal complications include uveitis, sclerosing cholangitis and chronic active hepatitis.

TREATMENT STRATEGIES

These comprise surgery, medical therapy and dietary management. The last two are discussed together with those for CD on p. 189.

Surgical treatment

Total colectomy, removal of the rectal stump and ileostomy are curative for UC. At a later time, a rectal pull-through can be performed which re-establishes bowel continuity and so continence can be achieved. In patients with growth retardation, colectomy should be carried out before puberty or fusion of the epiphyses, to allow for catch-up growth. UC patients can undergo the construction of an ileoanal anastomosis, which will avoid the need for a colostomy. Adaptation to such is achievable, particularly in young children.

MEDICAL THERAPY FOR INFLAMMATORY BOWEL DISEASE

Sulfasalazine is recommended for colonic disease but it is not as worthwhile in CD as in UC. To induce a remission, the following should be used daily in three divided doses:

- 2 g/24 h for children under 25 kg

- 3 g/24 h for those 25–50 kg

- 4 g/24 h for those >50 kg

Sulfasalazine is not well absorbed in the small bowel. In the colon, bacteria split the bond between sulfapyridine (the carrier molecule that prevents small-bowel absorption) and 5-aminosalicylic acid (5-ASA), the active component. Many of the undesirable effects of sulfasalazine, such as headaches, itching, skin rash, diarrhea and pancytopenia, are caused by the sulfapyridine moiety. Desensitization is possible by slow, progressive increments of the dose [20]. The active component, 5-ASA, is found by itself in a series of newer compounds that, although more expensive, are associated with less intolerance: olsalazine (Dipentum) and mesalazine (Pentasa; time-released granules), Asacol (pH-released granules), mesalamine enemas and suppositories (Rowasa). Pentasa is released in the small bowel and thus is helpful in the treatment of small-intestinal disease. Balsalazide (Colazide), a prodrug, is more effective and better tolerated than mesalamine in the treatment of acute UC.

General guidelines for use of corticosteroids to initiate remission are as follows:

1. In severe cases: intravenous methylprednisolone, 1–1.5 mg/kg per day for 10 to 20 days.

2. With improvement, switch to oral prednisolone (prednisone in the USA), 1–2 mg/kg per day (maximum 60 mg/day) for 6–8 weeks.

3. Slowly wean off or switch to alternate-day maintenance steroids (7.5–15 mg/24 h).

Patients who become steroid dependent may benefit from azathioprine (AZA) or 6-mercaptopurine (6-MP), at doses of 1–2 mg/kg per day (maximum 75–100 mg/day). Some experts use a broad-spectrum antibiotic such as ciprofloxacin (Cipro) in doses of 250–500 mg every 12 h instead of, or in addition to, corticosteroids.

Budesonide, an oral corticosteroid of poor systemic absorption and thus with mainly luminal action, has been used with success both by mouth [21] and by the rectal route [22]. Disease limited to the rectum can be managed by local steroid or mesalamine enemas, but severe disease (more than six stools a day) or severe abdominal pain will justify systemic steroids.

AZA and 6-MP are used in pediatric patients with UC and CD to reduce disease activity, maintain remission, prevent relapse and lower corticosteroid dosage, but their long-term side effects remain to be studied [23,24]. Kirschner et al. [25] retrospectively reviewed the safety of AZA and 6-MP in 95 patients (mean age 14.2 years) with IBD. Overall, 54% of the patients were treated with one of these drugs without adverse reaction; 28% experienced side effects, most commonly increased aminotransferase level, that either responded to dose reduction or spontaneously resolved. Cessation of therapy was needed in 18% of patients because of recurrent fever, pancreatitis, gastrointestinal intolerance and recurrent infections. The mean prednisone dose decreased from 24.3 to 8.6 mg/day. Verhave et al. found similar positive results in a study with fewer side effects [23]. Here, 21 IBD patients (aged 3–17 years) were treated with AZA, 2 mg/kg/day, as an adjunct to their customary regimen. The median time until patients responded was less than three months for patients with UC and four months for those with CD. Reduction of corticosteroid dose was possible for all patients who responded to AZA therapy. Only minimal side effects were attributable to the drug. As leukopenia is not uncommon periodic hemograms (total and differential white cell count) are recommended. Metabolite blood levels can be monitored for active drug and potential for toxicity.

Methotrexate is another drug that can be used in patients who have chronically active CD despite steroid therapy. In a double-blind, multicenter study to determine the efficacy of this drug, 141 such patients were randomly assigned to treatment with intramuscular methotrexate (25 mg once weekly) or placebo for 16 weeks in addition to prednisone [26]. After 16 weeks, 39% of the methotrexate-treated patients were in clinical remission, as compared with 19% in the placebo group, a difference that was significant. The Crohn's Disease Activity Index after 16 weeks of treatment was significantly lower in the methotrexate group than in the placebo group.

Tumor necrosis factor (TNF) is a pivotal cytokine in intestinal inflammation. Controlled trials using a chimeric anti-TNF antibody (infliximab) have shown its efficacy in refractory CD. In a multicenter, randomized, double-blind, placebo-controlled trial including 30 patients with active CD [27], endoscopic and histologic response to infliximab was significant in most of the treated patients. This is the first therapy with demonstrable histologic improvement.

Bacteria that produce cytokines could be used to treat IBD if the results of research in mice are reproduced in humans. Belgian scientists have engineered a non-pathogenic bacterium, *Lactococcus lactis*, that produces IL-10, an anti-inflammatory cytokine that reduces inflammatory colitis. Because the genetically engineered bacterium survives stomach acid, the cytokine can be delivered direct to the target in the colon. This could reduce the dose needed and any systemic effects [28].

Codeine may relieve the severity of the diarrhea but many clinicians are reluctant to use the opiate derivatives diphenoxylate (Lomotil) and loperamide (Imodium) or even the anticholinergic preparations, particularly in acute exacerbations.

TREATMENT OF THE ACUTE PHASE

In cases of an acute presentation, particularly in UC or during a flare-up of symptoms, the main aim is to rest the bowel, avoid complications and enhance the chances of remission. A nasogastric tube for decompression may be beneficial. Total parenteral nutrition, with the withdrawal of all oral feeds, is often advocated. Intravenous methylprednisolone can be used in doses of up to 2 mg/kg per day (maximum 60 mg). Cyclosporine also plays a role in the induction of remission of fulminant colitis, but its use in chronic disease has not proven to be more advantageous than other treatments, which have fewer side effects [29]. Use of cyclosoporine is not devoid of complications: plasma drug levels need to be monitored daily, and blood pressure even more frequently. Cyclosporine has been used in combination with other drugs [30].

DIETARY MANAGEMENT OF INFLAMMATORY BOWEL DISEASE

Growth failure is a significant feature of both CD and UC, even occurring years before the onset of bowel symptoms. Consequently, children with IBD can be severely malnourished and short. This small stature is caused by anorexia, perhaps secondary endocrine abnormalities, increased caloric requirements and excessive gut loss of nutrients. Moreover, reduced somatomedin may also be a feature of malnutrition. Anorexia exists, particularly in the acute phase, resulting in an inadequate nutrient intake. A delay in height, lack of weight gain and delay in bone age and in pubertal development may be seen in 10–40% of patients. The incidence of growth failure in patients with IBD ranges between 8% and 88% for height, and between 13% and 80% for weight. Children may be below their predicted height and weight centiles for age: in order for catch-up growth to occur, the total energy intake should be appropriate for chronologic age rather than body size. Nutritional support is both corrective of the deficiencies and, for CD, could also be therapeutic [31,32].

Motil et al. [33] prospectively studied 69 children and adolescents with IBD of greater than three years duration; approximately 50% of them had CD. The prevalence of growth failure was 24%, 23% and 39% by height velocity, Z score and height-for-age criteria, respectively; deficits were equally prevalent regardless of the stage of pubertal development. Results from this study are summarized in Table 11.9. The mean caloric intake among these patients was 64 kcal/kg (269 kJ/kg) per day, which is 25% greater than the calculated requirements for normal individuals of the same chronologic age, but only 8% more than that based on height.

The importance of these deficiencies of both weight and height in children and adolescents was documented by Castile et al. [34], who observed that when these patients reach

Growth parameter	Prevalence of the anomaly			
	Crohn's disease		Ulcerative colitis	
	n	%	n	%
Waterlow				
Height for age <95%	35	23	34	56
Weight for age <90%	34	68	35	31
Weight for height <90%	34	24	35	17
Bone age >2 SD below mean	22	45	18	28
Z score from NCHS				
Height ≤1.64 SD	34	38	35	9
Weight ≤1.64 SD	34	35	35	6
Tanner I–V				
Height velocity <4 cm/year	31	32	31	16
Weight velocity <1 kg/year	31	10	31	6

SD = standard deviation; NCHS = National Center for Health Statistics.

Table 11.9 Prevalence of growth alterations in 69 children with inflammatory bowel disease. Adapted from [33] with permission.

adulthood they continue being shorter than the normal population. A daily intake of 85–95 kcal/kg (357–399 kJ/kg) is needed to correct the nutritional deficit and attain catch-up growth, which can be achieved via enteral or parenteral nutrition.

Furthermore, many studies have demonstrated that elemental diets and parenteral nutrition are capable of inducing remission of the disease, allowing in many instances reduction of the dose and duration of steroid therapy. Several studies in adults as well as in children have demonstrated that enteral nutrition is capable of causing an improvement in UC but is more effectual in CD. Modular feeding regimens tailored to the individual needs of the child should be used during acute periods (Appendix IV.14). Elemental diets have been tried with success and, providing that attention is paid to the osmolality and speed of introduction of these feeds, they can offer a very useful alternative to parenteral nutrition. In CD, their use has been reported to induce remission of symptoms and improve linear growth. However, the time until relapse seems to be shorter in patients in whom remission is induced by diet only, compared with those who receive corticosteroids.

When a patient is unable to increase his or her protein and energy intake with a regular food, the first step is to provide oral supplementation with a commercially prepared formula. If this fails, nasogastric feedings can be tried. This technique allows administration of the formula over a period of several hours, at night or even the whole day. Alternatively, peripheral or central parenteral nutrition can be used. With these methods, improved nutritional status, increased rate of growth in terms of weight and height and acceleration of puberty in patients in whom the process is delayed can be achieved.

Deficiencies of various nutrients have been reported. There is a significant protein loss from the gut, due in part to the presence of blood in the stools; consequently, a generous protein intake is required. The energy intake should be at least that which is recommended for the child's age.

In less severe cases, the use of a low-residue diet (Appendix IV.38), avoiding any foods that are noted to cause symptoms, is suggested. Children and adolescents who malabsorb lactose may experience worse symptoms than that situation causes in non-colitics.

Fat malabsorption occurs in approximately 40% of children with IBD, and the use of a low-fat regimen, perhaps with the incorporation of medium-chain triglycerides, should be considered (Appendix IV.12). Steatorrhea, as would be expected, is more common where there is disease in the upper small bowel. Reducing stool fat lowers fecal calcium losses and helps alleviate the severity of hyperoxaluria, which is associated with disease of the terminal ileum. If the child is willing to take a supplement prepared from an elemental formula, in addition to a normal diet, this may provide an optimal opportunity for absorption. However, most of these formulas are unpalatable. Nasogastric tube feeding or a gastrostomy may be a way to overcome poor oral intake.

Deficiencies of metals and vitamins (particularly the B complex and vitamin D) have been reported. A vitamin supplement should be given routinely if it is not included in the energy/protein preparation being used. Elements that are likely to be malabsorbed or lost in large quantities from the gut are calcium, magnesium and zinc. Severe magnesium depletion can occur in CD, and hypocalcemia may be caused by steatorrhea. Zinc deficiency has been reported in patients with prolonged diarrhea, which, unless supplemented, may impede catch-up growth. Consequently, it is advisable to use a mineral/trace element supplement if the child has a poor nutrient intake or is taking one that is not fortified. Suitable mineral and vitamin supplements are suggested in Appendix II.14.

There is no evidence that adhering to any particular dietary regimen (e.g. low-residue, low-fat, milk-free) offers any long-term benefit. Dietary items should only be avoided if there is clear evidence of them causing symptoms or if the patient has specific food aversions.

A balanced and nutritious diet that is adequate in calories and is unrestricted can be recommended in the absence of active disease.

REFERENCES

1. Grand RJ, Ramakrishna J, Calenda KA. Inflammatory bowel disease in the pediatric patient. Gastroenterol Clin North Am 1995;24:613–32.

2. Kanof ME, Lake AM, Bayless TM. Decreased height velocity in children and adolescents before the diagnosis of Crohn's disease. Gastroenterology 1988;95:1523–7.

3. Hildebrand H, Karlberg J, Kristiansson B. Longitudinal growth in children and adolescents with inflammatory bowel disease. J Pediatr Gastroenterol Nutr 1994;18:165–73.

4. Tolia V. Perianal Crohn's disease in children and adolescents. Am J Gastroenterol 1996;91:922–6.

5. Pera A, Bellando P, Caldera D et al. Colonoscopy in inflammatory bowel disease. Diagnostic accuracy and proposal of an endoscopic score. Gastroenterology 1987;92:181–5.

6. Shah DB, Cosgrove M, Rees JI et al. The technetium white cell scan as an initial imaging investigation for evaluating suspected childhood inflammatory bowel disease. J Pediatr Gastroenterol Nutr 1997;25:524–8.

7. Walker-Smith J, Murch S. Diseases of the Small Intestine in Childhood. Oxford: Isis Medical Media, 1999.

8. Ruemmele FM, Targan SR, Levy G et al. Diagnostic accuracy of serological assays in pediatric inflammatory bowel disease. Gastroenterology 1998;115:822–9.

9. Vasiliauskas EA, Plevy SE, Landers CJ et al. Perinuclear antineutrophil cytoplasmic antibodies in patients with Crohn's disease define a clinical subgroup. Gastroenterology 1996;110:1810–9.

10. Otley A, Loonen H, Parekh N et al. Assessing activity of pediatric Crohn's disease: Which index to use? Gastroenterology 1999;116:527–31.

11. Ploysangam T, Heubi JE, Eisen D et al. Cutaneous Crohn's disease in children. J Am Acad Dermatol 1997;36:697–704.

12. Markowitz J, Grancher K, Rosa J et al. Highly destructive perianal disease in children with Crohn's disease. J Pediatr Gastroenterol Nutr 1995;21:149–53.

13. Wilschanski M, Chait P, Wade JA et al. Primary sclerosing cholangitis in 32 children: Clinical, laboratory, and radiographic features, with survival analysis. Hepatology 1995;22:1415–22.

14. Stein BL, Gordon PH. Perianal inflammatory conditions in inflammatory bowel disease. Curr Opin Gen Surg 1993:141–6.

15. Patel HI, Leichtner AM, Colodny AH et al. Surgery for Crohn's disease in infants and children. J Pediatr Surg 1997;32:1063–7; discussion 1067–8.

16. McLeod RS, Wolff BG, Steinhart AH et al. Prophylactic mesalamine treatment decreases postoperative recurrence of Crohn's disease. Gastroenterology 1995;109:404–13.

17. O'Morain C, O'Sullivan M. Nutritional support in Crohn's disease: Current status and future directions. J Gastroenterol 1995;30(Suppl. 8):102–7.

18. Walker-Smith J. Enteral nutrition in Crohn's disease in childhood. J Pediatr Gastroenterol Nutr 2001;32:107.

19. Dubinsky MC, Ofman JJ, Urman M et al. Clinical utility of serodiagnostic testing in suspected pediatric inflammatory bowel disease. Am J Gastroenterol 2001;96:758–65.

20. Tolia V. Sulfasalazine desensitization in children and adolescents with chronic inflammatory bowel disease. Am J Gastroenterol 1992;87:1029–32.

21. Campieri M, Ferguson A, Doe W et al. Oral budesonide is as effective as oral prednisolone in active Crohn's disease. The Global Budesonide Study Group. Gut 1997;41:209–14.

22. Hanauer SB, Robinson M, Pruitt R et al. Budesonide enema for the treatment of active, distal ulcerative colitis and proctitis: A dose-ranging study. U.S. Budesonide Enema Study Group. Gastroenterology 1998;115:525–32.

23. Verhave M, Winter HS, Grand RJ. Azathioprine in the treatment of children with inflammatory bowel disease. J Pediatr 1990;117:809–14.

24. Markowitz JF. Summary of the workshop on 6 mercaptopurine/azathioprine pharmacology. Inflamm Bowel Dis 1998;4:118–20.

25. Kirschner BS. Safety of azathioprine and 6-mercaptopurine in pediatric patients with inflammatory bowel disease. Gastroenterology 1998;115:813–21.

26. Feagan BG, Rochon J, Fedorak RN et al. Methotrexate for the treatment of Crohn's disease. The North American Crohn's Study Group Investigators. N Engl J Med 1995;332:292–7.

27. D'haens G, Van Deventer S, Van Hogezand R et al. Endoscopic and histological healing with infliximab anti-tumor necrosis factor antibodies in Crohn's disease: A European multicenter trial. Gastroenterology 1999;116:1029–34.

28. Berger A. New cytokine treatment for inflammatory bowel disease. Br Med J 2000;321:530.

29. Treem WR, Cohen J, Davis PM et al. Cyclosporine for the treatment of fulminant ulcerative colitis in children. Immediate response, long-term results, and impact on surgery. Dis Colon Rectum 1995;38:474–9.

30. Ramakrishna J, Langhans N, Calenda K et al. Combined use of cyclosporine and azathioprine or 6-mercaptopurine in pediatric inflammatory bowel disease. J Pediatr Gastroenterol Nutr 1996;22:296–302.

31. Kleinman RE, Balistreri WF, Heyman MB et al. Nutritional support for pediatric patients with inflammatory bowel disease. J Pediatr Gastroenterol Nutr 1989;8:8–12.

32. Oliva MM, Lake AM. Nutritional considerations and management of the child with inflammatory bowel disease. Nutrition 1996;12:151–8.

33. Motil KJ, Grand RJ, Davis-Kraft L et al. Growth failure in children with inflammatory bowel disease: a prospective study. Gastroenterology 1993;105:681–91.

34. Castile RG, Telander RL, Cooney DR et al. Crohn's disease in children: assessment of the progression of disease, growth, and prognosis. J Pediatr Surg 1980;15:462–9.

chapter 12

Necrotizing Enterocolitis and Short-Bowel Syndrome

NECROTIZING ENTEROCOLITIS

This acute gastrointestinal disorder was first described in the German literature in 1825 [1], but is still something of an enigma. Despite years of investigation, the etiology remains unclear, and accepted prevention and treatment strategies are lacking. Necrotizing enterocolitis (NEC) predominantly affects premature infants; less commonly (10%), term neonates and, rarely, severely debilitated children. There have been instances of nursery epidemics. Some centers see this problem affecting as many as 80% of neonates born weighing less than 1.5 kg, while other units have a very low incidence of only 0.3% among their premature babies. Several countries, for example Switzerland and Scandinavia, have a very low incidence. In a study involving 52 centers in Japan [2], the incidence was only 0.3%. In the USA, the incidence is 2.4 in 1000 live births [3,4]. NEC is the most common neonatal gastrointestinal emergency in both the UK and America.

RISK FACTORS

The following factors increase susceptibility to NEC:

- Extreme prematurity [5]
- Birth weight under 2.0 kg
- Formula feeding
- Significant bacterial colonization of nursery
- History of asphyxia/respiratory distress/exchange transfusion/congenital cardiac disease

NEC is rarely seen in term babies with a weight that is appropriate for the gestational age. Many have suffered from asphyxia or the other conditions mentioned above. Some have received indomethacin for a patent ductus arteriosus (PDA).

NEC is considerably more common in formula-fed neonates than in those receiving human milk [6]. Breast milk is rich in secretory IgA, which acts on the gastrointestinal mucosa to prevent bacterial adherence and thus impedes invasion. There are many growth factors and regulatory peptides in breast milk [7], including epidermal growth factor (EGF). EGF is found in generous quantities in the milk produced by mothers of both preterm and term neonates. When breast milk is stored or frozen in a refrigerator, or heat-treated (pasteurized or boiled), many of its antibacterial properties are diminished; therefore the milk will be of less help in preventing NEC. There is some evidence that the optimal regimen is 'raw' human milk fed to a mother's own baby.

However, in a large prospective study of more than 2000 premature infants [8], the only perinatal factors associated with NEC, in contradistinction to the findings of other neonatologists, were birth weight and maternal toxemia. In addition, Rotbart et al. [9], have noted a significant correlation between NEC and birth weight.

Prenatal steroid therapy has been evaluated in a number of trials, including one large multicentered, collaborative, randomized and blinded study [10]. The latter revealed a significantly decreased incidence of NEC in infants of mothers treated with steroids, for all birth-weight and gestational groups. One possible explanation is that antenatal maternal steroid therapy, by enzyme induction, promotes intestinal maturation.

PATHOGENESIS

For details of pathogenesis, see Fig. 12.1. Experiments in animals have shown that hypoxia, particularly when combined with an artificial feed, can induce the pathologic equivalent of NEC by causing a reduction of blood flow in the mesenteric vessels. It has been postulated that the 'diving reflex' in response to hypoxia deprives the gut of its blood supply so as to protect preferentially the intracranial circulation.

PRESENTATION

The presenting symptoms commonly include the following:

- Abdominal distension
- Lethargy
- Vomiting and regurgitation
- Temperature instability
- Apnea
- Occult or gross blood in stools

Early detection is often possible by noting distension of the abdomen or a trace of blood in the stools: this may enable prompt measures to be taken to prevent a cascade of downhill events. The average mortality is approximately 30% [11], yet it can be as high as 80% [12].

DIAGNOSIS

Good observations of the symptoms and signs will enable an early diagnosis to be made. It can be confirmed by the following:

1. Radiology and imaging [13]. Radiographs of the abdomen may show pneumatosis intestinalis (intramural gas), ascites, air in the peritoneum or gas in the portal vein (Figs 12.2–12.4). Early films will show dilated loops of the bowel. Abdominal magnetic resonance imaging can assist non-invasive diagnosis of bowel necrosis.

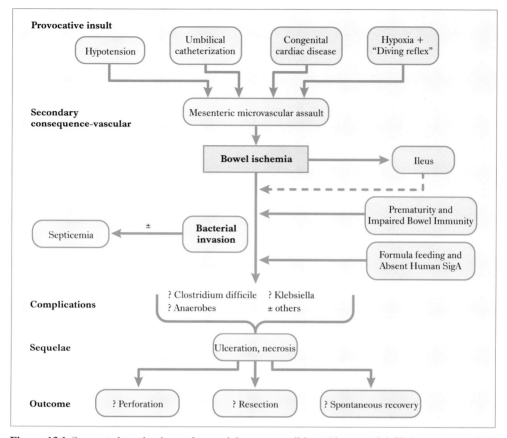

Figure 12.1 Suspected mechanisms of necrotizing enterocolitis — 'the cascade'. SIgA = secretory IgA.

2. Blood and stool culture. This may help identify aerobic or anaerobic organism(s). The platelet count and fibrinogen degradation products should be checked to exclude thrombocytopenia and disseminated intravascular coagulation (DIC).

3. Viral investigation. Serum should be examined for IgM antibodies to rotavirus. Stools can be tested for the same virus by Rotastick (Prolab Diagnostics, UK and Canada) or can be examined using electron microscopy to detect various viruses.

MANAGEMENT

1. Stop all oral feeds and start parenteral nutrition. If dehydrated, correct deficit.

2. Promptly remove umbilical catheters.

3. Decompress the gastrointestinal tract.

4. Start early antibiotics to cover both aerobic and anaerobic organisms — many advocate aminoglycosides and a penicillin, or alternatively a cephalosporin such as cefotaxime as well as metronidazole in the absence of any identified gastrointestinal pathogens sensitive to other antibiotics. Major side effects of aminoglycosides are ototoxicity and nephrotoxicity.

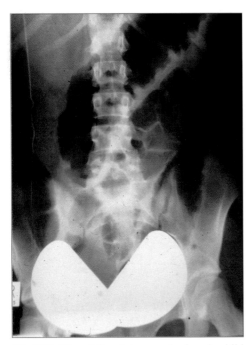 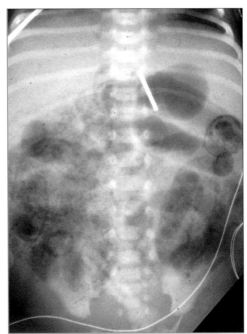

Fig 12.2 Film of the abdomen of a female child showing thickened edematous wall in distended loops of the transverse and descending colon compatible with early necrotising enterocolitis.

Figure 12.3 Film of the chest and abdomen shows massive air-distended bowel with diffuse intramural air. (Courtesy of Dr A Baker and Dr P Kane.)

If there is evidence of obstruction, suspected bowel gangrene, perforation or failure to respond to conservative measures, prompt surgery is indicated [14].

The presence of erythropoietin (Epo) in human milk and the expression of Epo receptors on intestinal villous enterocytes of neonates suggest that Epo has a role in growth and development of the gastrointestinal tract. In a retrospective cohort study of 483 very-low-birth-weight (500–1250 g) neonates, the incidence of NEC was lower in those who had received recombinant Epo [15].

COMPLICATIONS

Early complications include perforation with or without intestinal resection [16]. Late complications may involve feeding intolerance and stricture(s) leading to obstruction. Such strictures can complicate a case of NEC that has been successfully managed in the initial phase [17]. Limited ileal resection for NEC is associated with a subsequent high prevalence (24%) of cholelithiasis [18]. Due to the chronic medical and neurodevelopmental risks in some infants, long-term follow-up is often indicated [19].

SHORT-BOWEL SYNDROME [20]

Short-bowel syndrome is the malabsorptive state that results when, following surgery, there is a residual small-bowel length of <75 cm. The length of the jejunum and ileum, measured

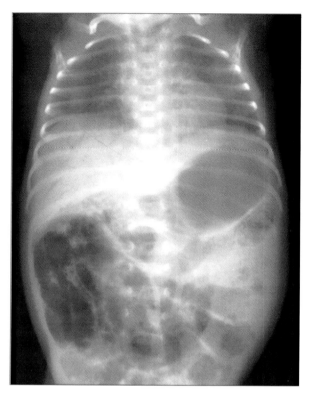

Fig 12.4 Film of the thorax and abdomen of an infant showing bowel intramural and free gas in necrotising enterocolitis. Gas is also seen in the extra- and intrahepatic portal system. (Courtesy of Dr P Kane.)

along the antimesenteric border, is approximately 250–300 cm in a term neonate, but is found to be less in a preterm baby. A short bowel can be congenital or secondary to extensive bowel resection. In neonates, the most common reasons for small-bowel resection are volvulus and NEC. In older children, it can be the result of volvulus or trauma, such as a gunshot wound or another catastrophic event impairing blood supply to the bowel. Inflammatory bowel disease is rarely a cause for a short bowel in children.

The severity of symptoms and the prevalence of short- and long-term complications relate to the site and the extent of the bowel excised, the residual surface area and gut motility. Removal of the mid small bowel gives rise to fewer problems than proximal or distal small-bowel resection. Also, the presence of the ileocecal valve is extremely important and often influences the outcome [21]. The experience of Wilmore et al. [22] suggests that, where the ileocecal valve is present, a minimal length of 15 cm of small bowel is required if the neonate is to survive; however, in the absence of this 'valve', the least length needed is 40 cm. With the use of parenteral nutrition (PN), malnutrition is not as great a problem in these children as is the liver-associated cholestasis and fibrosis (PN-induced liver disease) that frequently results from its use. Nowadays, the most common cause of death in a child with a short bowel is liver failure and not malnutrition. Intensive use of enteral feedings to provide a minimum of 20–30% of the daily caloric intake plays an important role in preventing PN-related liver disease [23,24].

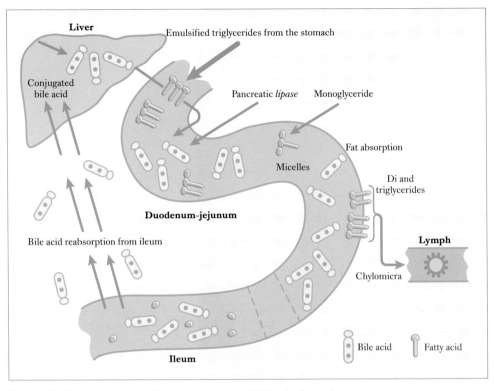

Figure 12.5 Intraluminal micelle formation, fat and bile salt absorption.

SYMPTOMS

The severity of symptoms relates directly to the length and function of the small bowel remaining after surgery. Diarrhea is the dominant feature and is caused by one or more of the following:

- Carbohydrate malabsorption
- Bile salt malabsorption
- Fat malabsorption
- Bacterial overgrowth ($>10^5$/ml)
- Intestinal inflammation
- Decreased surface area and consequent impaired salt/water transport

The transit time through the remaining bowel is usually normal or slower, but, as the bowel has been shortened, the stomach to anus or ostomy transit time is very reduced (≤ 4 h). However, in patients with a history of gastroschisis, hypoperistalsis is not an uncommon finding. With resection of short bowel segments, the malabsorption is mild, but with extensive bowel removal, bile salt depletion becomes profound and steatorrhea predominates [25]. The non-absorbed dietary fat is converted to hydroxy fatty acids by bacteria and these exacerbate the diarrhea. Hepatic synthesis of bile salts from cholesterol to replace fecal losses is controlled by a negative feedback mechanism. Bile salts facilitate the absorption of fatty acids and monoglycerides, which are derived from dietary triglycerides following lipolysis by lipase. Bile salts form aggregates called micelles (Fig. 12.5), which solubilize insoluble lipids and provide a mechanism for transport to the intestinal mucosa. If extensive resection occurs, the liver cannot compensate by synthesizing adequate amounts of bile.

Adaptation and pathophysiology

The phenomenon of compensatory enlargement of the small-gut surface area following excision surgery was first demonstrated in dogs. This is attained by mucosal villous hyperplasia and bowel dilatation. Resections of the proximal small bowel are associated with greater compensatory changes than those seen when surgery is limited to the distal small bowel. In addition, removal of the distal small gut, in contrast to the ileum, is linked to serious and chronic sequelae because of the relative failure of jejunal accommodation.

Luminal nutrients, especially fat, are essential for adaptation. The specific activity of some mucosal enzymes (Na^+/K^+ ATPase, enterokinase etc.) increases, although brush-border disaccharidases are decreased secondary to the reduced surface area.

INVESTIGATIONS

Intestinal transit time is demonstrated by noting when a colorant marker appears in stools. However, this test is of little clinical use because prokinetics (in cases of hypokinetic bowel) or drugs that slow peristalsis (e.g. loperamide) have little, if any, effect in improving nutrient and water obsorption.

Bacterial overgrowth can be suspected when baseline breath hydrogen levels are 15–20 parts per million (ppm) or greater, or increase above 20 ppm over baseline after ingestion of a dose of lactulose. Aerobic/anaerobic cultures of small-bowel contents are rarely performed in clinical practice.

Specific malabsorption studies are carried out to show impaired uptake of nutrients — e.g. carbohydrates: hydrogen breath test (see p. 166) as a test for specific substrates. Stools can be tested for pH (not reliable) and for the presence of reducing sugars with the Clinitest reaction. Vitamin B_{12} malabsorption (Schilling test, see p. 14) is common in patients who have had extensive resection of their ileum.

MANAGEMENT – MEDICAL

Specific non-nutritional problems

1. Diarrhea — cholestyramine is useful where a large bile acid loss causes watery stools; however, it impairs the absorption of several nutrients including the fat-soluble vitamins, as well as folate, iron and calcium.

2. Gastric hypersecretion — this is a common finding following resection. It does not necessarily occur in the immediate postoperative period but may take up to 1 month to develop. It responds to H_2 blockers (ranitidine, 3 mg/kg/day, administered intramuscularly or intravenously in divided doses every 6 or 8 h; famotidine,

0.5 mg/kg/day, administered intravenously as a constant infusion) and octreotide at 0.1–0.2 μg/kg/day, administered intravenously or subcutaneously, for 48 h. Oral H_2-receptor antagonists may be indicated for up to 1 year post resection.

3. Bacterial overgrowth — antibiotics against aerobic/anaerobic bacteria are required [26]. Because of the type of bacteria developed, D-lactic acid can be produced and absorbed, leading to metabolic acidosis. A routine laboratory assay determines L-lactic acid; therefore, in the presence of acidosis and a large anion gap in a patient with short bowel, plasma D-lactic acid determination should be requested.

4. Water and electrolyte imbalance following colonic resection, particularly in the immediate post-surgical period — a high fluid intake is needed, especially in hot environments. In cases of non-adapted ileostomies, sodium losses can be large. Serum sodium may be normal, but total body sodium decreased. This can be diagnosed by determining urinary sodium concentration (normally <40 mmol/l).

Parenteral nutrition

Severe malabsorption and diarrhea will necessitate parenteral feeding and this is usually the first phase of treatment. Careful monitoring is required and extra supplements of electrolytes and trace minerals are often needed to replace losses in stools. However, although poorly absorbed, it is necessary to introduce some nutrients into the bowel early on to help maintain normal mucosa (trophic effect) and gut hormones.

Oral nutrition

Although long-term parenteral nutrition may be necessary for a minority of children and can be successfully carried out at home, oral nutrition should be commenced as soon as possible. The secretion of enterogastrone requires the presence of nutrients in the gut lumen and this in turn will hasten adaptive mucosal changes. Human milk contains factors that may stimulate mucosal hyperplasia and increase the brush-border enzymes. It is important that small volumes of a hypo-osmolar feed are used. Even though adaptation to a high osmolar load does occur, episodes of abdominal distension, vomiting and diarrhea may indicate a failure to tolerate the high osmolality of the feed rather than suggest intolerance to a specific nutrient.

Controversy exists as to which formula is ideal for infants and young children with short-bowel syndrome. Breast milk is generally well tolerated and should be recommended if available. Protein hydrolysates such as Alimentum (Ross) or Pregestimil (Mead Johnson) (Appendix IV.5) are most often used with success. An amino acid based formula such as Neocate (SHS) is usually well tolerated and can be used when protein hydrolysate is not successful. Continuous nasogastric feedings are used in the early stages and lead to improved absorption. Small bolus feedings are gradually introduced. Enteral feedings need to be balanced with parenteral nutrition, and once parenteral feeding is stopped extra vitamin and mineral supplements are required. Feeds may need to be concentrated or supplemented with additional calories to provide adequate nutrition to cover for increased losses in the stools. Solids should be introduced slowly at the normal time if at all possible. Many of these children develop feeding problems.

Occasionally modular formulas may be recommended if none of the other alternatives have been successful. Appendix IV.14 discusses modular feedings [27].

The fluid requirements of infants who have undergone gut surgery may be as high as 25–50% above normal. It is difficult to achieve such an intake unless the nutrition is given by constant infusion. Bolus feeding might give rise to adverse reactions. Electrolyte losses can be high when the colon has been resected, and requirements for sodium and potassium may be increased by as much as five times the normal. The addition of sodium and potassium salts to the feed will greatly increase the osmolality. Therefore, in the immediate post-surgical period, most of the electrolyte requirement should be infused intravenously until the gut has become accustomed to the hyperosmolar feed. Calcium, magnesium, zinc and iron may need to be supplemented because long-term deficiencies of these elements have been described. Moreover, full supplements of water- and fat-soluble vitamins as well as trace elements should be given to compensate for the malabsorption. It is often necessary to place a gastrostomy button for the long-term administration of enteral feeds.

MANAGEMENT – SURGICAL

There are a number of surgical options in cases of short-bowel syndrome: stricture resection, tapering enteroplasty and bowel lengthening [28].

Intestinal transplantation [29–31]

Originally, graft rejection was common in this radical procedure, even with the use of immunosuppression. However, animal studies revealed that co-transplantation of the liver with the small intestine reduced the likelihood of rejection [32]. Later, with the introduction of the powerful immunosuppressant tacrolimus (FK506), it has been possible to carry out successful isolated intestinal transplants. Much of the American experience has been focused at the University of Pittsburg and the University of Nebraska [33].

SEQUELAE

Malnutrition during a critical period of brain growth can cause mental retardation [34] and permanent small stature. End-stage liver failure, associated with parenteral nutrition, is the principal cause of death where there has been massive small-bowel resection.

COMPLICATIONS

The major deficiencies caused by gut surgery are summarized in Figure 12.6. These can be minimized by the correct choice of feeding regimen and the addition of dietary supplements where necessary.

Renal stones may arise from the enhanced colonic absorption of oxalates after ileal resection. A high fluid intake should be maintained. In addition, the diet should contain adequate amounts of magnesium, as this is necessary to maintain the oxalate in solution. Older children should avoid foods that are high in oxalate. These comprise of rhubarb, spinach, beetroot, parsley (can be used in small amounts), cocoa, chocolate, wheatgerm, beans and nuts.

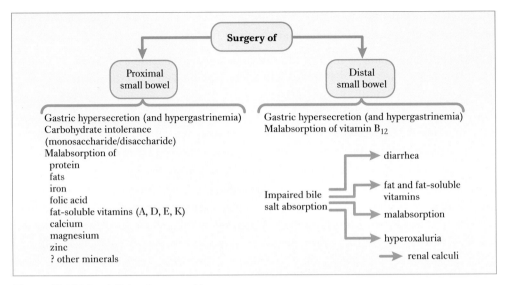

Figure 12.6 Major deficiencies caused by gut surgery.

Other sequelae include osteoporosis, and there should be a prospective awareness of rickets arising months or even years after surgery.

REFERENCES

1. Siebold JF. Gerburtshulfe, frauenziemmer und kinderkrankheiten Heft 1. Leipzig 1825;5:3.

2. Shimura K. Necrotizing enterocolitis? A Japanese survey. NICU 1990;3:5–7.

3. Kosloske AM. The epidemiology and pathogenesis of necrotizing enterocolitis. Semin Neonatol 1997;2:231–8.

4. Neu J. Necrotizing enterocolitis: The search for a unifying pathogenic theory leading to prevention. Pediatr Clin North Am 1996;43:409–32.

5. Beeby PJ, Jeffery H. Risk factors for necrotising enterocolitis: The influence of gestational age. Arch Dis Child 1992;67:432–5.

6. Lucas A, Cole TJ. Breast milk and neonatal necrotising enterocolitis. Lancet 1990;336:1519–23.

7. Zumkeller W. Relationship between insulin-like growth factor-I and -II and IGF-binding proteins in milk and the gastrointestinal tract: Growth and development of the gut. J Pediatr Gastroenterol Nutr 1992;15:357–69.

8. Kanto WP Jr, Wilson R, Breart GL et al. Perinatal events and necrotizing enterocolitis in premature infants. Am J Dis Child 1987;141:167–9.

9. Rotbart HA, Nelson WL, Glode MP et al. Neonatal rotavirus-associated necrotizing enterocolitis: Case control study and prospective surveillance during an outbreak. J Pediatr 1988;112:87–93.

10. Bauer CR, Morrison JC, Poole WK et al. A decreased incidence of necrotising enterocolitis after prenatal glucocorticoid therapy. Pediatrics 1984;73:682–8.

11. Thomas DF. Pathogenesis of neonatal necrotizing enterocolitis. J R Soc Med 1982;75:838–40.

12. Anagnostopoulos D, Valioulis J, Sfougaris D et al. Morbidity and mortality of short bowel syndrome in infancy and childhood. Eur J Pediatr Surg 1991;1:273–6.

13. Maalouf EF, Fagbemi A, Duggan PJ et al. Magnetic resonance imaging of intestinal necrosis in preterm infants. Pediatrics 2000;105:510–4.

14. Warner BW, Ziegler MM. Management of the short bowel syndrome in the pediatric population. Pediatr Clin North Am 1993;40:1335–50.

15. Ledbetter DJ, Juul SE. Erythropoietin and the incidence of necrotizing enterocolitis in infants with very low birth weight. J Pediatr Surg 2000;35:178–81.

16. Rescorla FJ. Surgical management of pediatric necrotizing enterocolitis. Curr Opin Pediatr 1995;7:335–41.

17. Tam PKH. Necrotizing enterocolitis — surgical management. Semin Neonatol 1997;2:297–305.

18. Davies BW, Abel G, Puntis JW et al. Limited ileal resection in infancy: The long-term consequences. J Pediatr Surg 1999;34:583–7.

19. Simon NP. Follow-up for infants with necrotizing enterocolitis. Clin Perinatol 1994;21:411–24.

20. Vanderhoof JA, Langnas AN. Short-bowel syndrome in children and adults. Gastroenterology 1997;113:1767–78.

21. Weber TR, Tracy T Jr, Connors RH. Short-bowel syndrome in children. Quality of life in an era of improved survival. Arch Surg 1991;126:841–6.

22. Wilmore DW, Dudrick SJ, Daly JM et al. The role of nutrition in the adaptation of the small intestine after massive resection. Surg Gynecol Obstet 1971;132:673–80.

23. Meehan JJ, Georgeson KE. Prevention of liver failure in parenteral nutrition – dependent children with short bowel syndrome. J Pediatr Surg 1997;32:473–5.

24. Simmons MG, Georgeson KE, Figueroa R et al. Liver failure in parenteral nutrition-dependent children with short bowel syndrome. Transplant Proc 1996;28:2701.

25. Goulet O. Lipid requirements in infants with digestive diseases with references to short bowel syndrome. Eur J Med Res 1997;2:79–83.

26. Vanderhoof JA, Young RJ, Murray N et al. Treatment strategies for small bowel bacterial overgrowth in short bowel syndrome. J Pediatr Gastroenterol Nutr 1998;27:155–60.

27. Samour PQ, Helm, KK, Lang CE. Handbook of Pediatric Nutrition 2nd Ed. Aspen, 2000.

28. Figueroa-Colon R, Harris PR, Birdsong E et al. Impact of intestinal lengthening on the nutritional outcome for children with short bowel syndrome. J Pediatr Surg 1996;31:912–6.

29. Thompson JS. Recent advances in the surgical treatment of the short-bowel syndrome. Surg Annu 1990;22:107–27.

30. Langnas AN, Dhawan A, Antonson DL et al. Intestinal transplantation in children. Transplant Proc 1996;28:2752.

31. Vanderhoof JA. Short bowel syndrome in children and small intestinal transplantation. Pediatr Clin North Am 1996;43:533–50.

32. Beath SV, Needham SJ, Kelly DA et al. Clinical features and prognosis of children assessed for isolated small bowel or combined small bowel and liver transplantation. J Pediatr Surg 1997;32:459–61.

33. Vanderhoof JA. Short bowel syndrome in children. Curr Opin Pediatr 1995;7:560–8.

34. Simon NP. Follow-up for infants with necrotizing enterocolitis. Clin Perinatal 1994;21:411-24.

chapter 13

Gastroesophageal Reflux

'… the infant, mewling and puking in the nurse's arms.'

William Shakespeare, *As You Like It*, Act II, Scene VII

Gastroesophageal reflux (GER) is the effortless retrograde passage of small volumes of gastric contents into the esophagus or oropharynx. GER is both a normal physiologic event that occurs in virtually everyone [1,2] and a pathophysiologic phenomenon that can result in mild to severe symptoms.

Postprandial regurgitation, a mild form of GER, is a very common pediatric problem that in most instances runs a harmless and self-limited course. Although it affects up to 50% of all babies at 2 months of age [2–4], and is still quite frequent at 3 months, it usually has resolved by 6–12 months. The incidence of regurgitation is equally distributed in boys and girls, whether breastfed or bottlefed. As the infant matures, so do the mechanisms responsible for preventing reflux, such as the subdiaphragmatic segment of the esophagus containing the distal sphincter, which elongates. The role of the physician is to determine when reassurance is the only necessary intervention, or when simple or more complex therapy is required [5]. Reflux, regurgitation and vomiting are not synonyms: reflux and regurgitation are involuntary, in contrast to rumination or vomiting, which involve an active effort.

Excessive regurgitation can result in gastroesophageal reflux disease (GERD). GERD can cause apnea, bradycardia or worsen bronchopulmonary dysplasia. This disorder is more common in low-birth-weight infants and among children with cow milk allergy, respiratory disease and some central nervous system (CNS) disorders. As a consequence of regurgitation, poor intake and even feeding refusal, GERD may result in failure to thrive.

The negative impact of regurgitation and GER should not be underestimated. Some parents may have severe difficulties in coping with such a child, even one who is growing well and is otherwise asymptomatic. In our experience, a number of infants with mild regurgitation but with other medical problems or with parental anxiety, whose reflux is not treated appropriately, may develop feeding aversion.

PHYSIOLOGY OF THE ESOPHAGUS

Although the lower esophagus functions as a sphincter, it does not have the usual configuration associated with such a structure. There is an area of increased intraluminal

Increase pressure	Decrease pressure
Gastrin	Caffeine
Cisapride	Theophylline
Metoclopramide	Alcohol
Domperidone	
Bethanechol	

Table 13.1 Effects of hormones and drugs on pressure of the lower gastroesophageal sphincter.

pressure in the distal esophagus, and, on swallowing, there is relaxation of the esophagus upon which food enters the stomach. Tone, and thus function, of the lower esophageal sphincter (LES) is influenced by hormones and drugs (Table 13.1). Several characteristics of the lower esophagus and stomach summate to create a valvular-like mechanism. Normally, the esophagus enters the stomach at an angle. Part of the LES is in the abdomen, and an increase in the intra-abdominal pressure assists in bringing the sidewalls of the esophagus into apposition, thus preventing reflux. Furthermore, the phreno-esophageal ligament helps to maintain the integrity of the LES, as does the crura of the diaphragm and other neighboring ligaments.

The term 'hiatal hernia' implies that the gastroesophageal junction is displaced into the chest, i.e. there is herniation of the stomach through a hiatus (opening) in the diaphragm (Fig. 13.1). Where there is a hiatal hernia, the negative intrathoracic pressure acting on the LES promotes reflux. Consequently, hiatal hernia is frequently associated with GER. However, the presence of an uncomplicated hiatal hernia, even with GER, is not *per se* an indication for surgical repair. The term 'partial thoracic stomach', which also results in GER, is applied to what is observed as a consequence of a hiatal hernia or a shortened esophagus (congenital or acquired). The diagnosis of these is made by contrasted radiological studies ('barium swallow') or endoscopy. A thoracic stomach can be suspected on a plain radiograph of the chest.

PATHOPHYSIOLOGY

Symptomatic GER is a common problem in infants and young children, but the mechanical events that lead to its intermittent occurrence are not well understood. Factors contributing to the high incidence of infantile regurgitation include:

- Shorter length and reduced pressure of the LES
- Transient LES relaxations (TLESRs)
- Decreased gravitational and peristaltic clearance of the refluxed material from the distal esophagus
- Slow gastric emptying

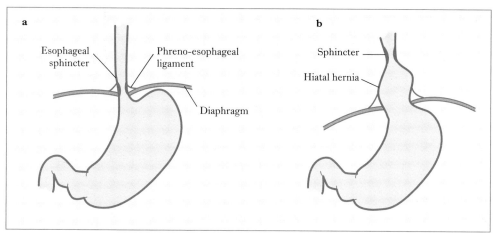

Figure 13.1 (a) The normal position of the lower esophageal sphincter — part in the abdomen, part in the thorax. **(b)** The position of the lower esophageal sphincter in hiatus hernia.

In adults with and without GERD, most reflux episodes occur during TLESRs. TLESR is different from the relaxation that is produced by swallowing, and is the normal mechanism for burping and belching [6]. Recent studies have demonstrated that TLESR is the most important cause of GER in children. Absent basal LES pressure is a relatively infrequent cause of reflux, and only in children with pathologic GER [7,8]. However, it is not the TLESR that is pathologic in GER, but the absence of the control mechanism on the phenomenon. Gradual functional maturation of the LES may explain the benign course of infantile GER [9]. GER is an important mechanism favoring additional reflux (which could lead to GERD) because of the effect of refluxate on the esophageal mucosa in exacerbating this vicious cycle.

Clinical features

The incidence of reflux is difficult to assess because the criteria to define it without relatively invasive investigations are not clear. Although about 60% of affected infants are symptom-free by 18 months, 30% have persistent troubles. The major features of uncomplicated GER are regurgitation and/or vomiting, the difference between the two being rather arbitrary: regurgitation is considered as a volume not larger than 5–10 ml. Regurgitation does not result in dehydration, failure to thrive, weight loss, feeding refusal, interruption of sleep, awaking with desperate crying spells or any other symptom. These infants have been termed 'happy spitters'.

Manifestations of GERD are failure to thrive from inappropriate energy intake (refusal due to pain from esophagitis) or lack of retention (vomiting), grimacing or posturing and the indication of the effort to swallow back regurgitated but not vomited material. Sandifer syndrome is characterized by lateral hyperextension of the neck and torsion of the head to one side in paroxysmal dystonic posturing, hematemesis from severe esophagitis, cyanosis and/or apnea and pneumonia from aspiration. GER can also be associated with acute life-threatening events (ALTEs). Esophagitis is caused by gastric acid regurgitating into an unprotected esophageal mucosa. Complications of GER are listed in Table 13.2 and symptoms of esophagitis in Table 13.3.

- Esophagitis
- Esophageal stricture
- Feeding refusal
- Failure to thrive
- Iron-deficiency anemia
- Hematemesis
- Aspiration pneumonia
- Apnea
- Dysphonia

Table 13.2 Complications of gastroesophageal reflux.

- Irritability
- Feeding refusal
- Interruption of feeding
- Awaking with intense crying
- Hematemesis
- Pounding of the chest (toddlers)
- Abdominal pain
- Chest pain (central or lateral)

Table 13.3 Symptoms of esophagitis.

Asthma can at times be caused or worsened by GER [10,11], particularly among those patients whose wheezing is worse at night. GER can be responsible for chronic hoarseness [10,12–14]. Strictures occur in 5% (Figs 13.2 and 13.3).

GER is more common in preterm infants and relatively uncommon in older children, except in association with cystic fibrosis, cerebral palsy or a debilitating illness. In infants with refusal to feed or interruption of the feed after what can be considered an insufficient volume, GER should be suspected.

INVESTIGATIONS

Simple regurgitation or even uncomplicated GER may not require any testing at all. In the young infant, vomiting can be caused by metabolic disorders or anatomic abnormalities such as pyloric stenosis or a duodenal web, and these need to be considered. The diagnosis of pyloric stenosis can be made by ultrasound, but that of a duodenal web requires a contrasted upper gastrointestinal series. Patients with Down syndrome have a higher incidence of duodenal webs than the rest of the population. Tests are needed whenever symptoms are atypical, or to obtain further information in a patient who has failed to respond to medical management. In children with a closed fontanel who develop sudden

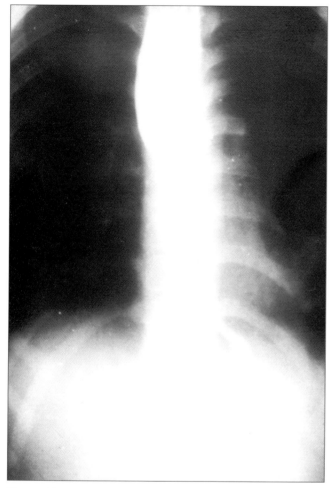

Figure 13.2 A long-segment distal esophageal stricture is present secondary to inflammatory change from gastroesophageal reflux. Note the dilated upper aspect of the esophagus with an air fluid/food level due to partial mechanical obstruction. (Courtesy of Milton Wagner, MD and Lynn Trautwein, MD.)

onset of vomiting, it is important to rule out increased intracranial pressure before an extensive work-up for GER is initiated.

There are many known tests for evaluating the presence and severity of reflux, but no single technique can consistently and infallibly detect abnormalities at the gastroesophageal junction. Children who experience an ALTE may need to have GER ruled out by means of a combination of tests such as a 24-h pH monitoring and oxymetry. Suggested tests are outlined below.

Barium swallow with fluoroscopy

The purpose of this study is more to rule out any underlying pathology – hiatal hernia, esophageal stricture (see Fig. 13.2), pyloric stenosis, duodenal or gastric web – than to demonstrate reflux. It should be noted that normal babies aged 0–12 months have been reported to experience three or four episodes of reflux during a 5-min period of intermittent fluoroscopic evaluation. In infants over the age of 12 months, this drops to less than one or

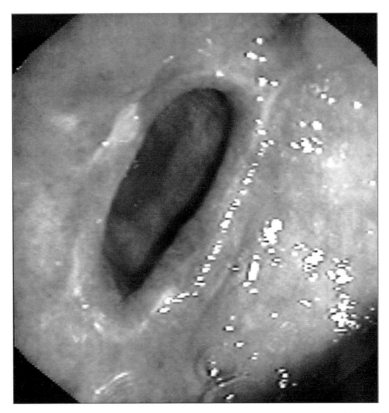

Figure 13.3 Endoscopic view of an esophageal stricture. (Courtesy of Kendall Brown, MD.)

two episodes. In a study by Balson et al. [15], there were approximately 83.3% of false positives and 46.1% of false negatives (compared to pH monitoring — see below).

Physicians may be wrongly perplexed when a child with classic postprandial regurgitation fails to show radiographic evidence of reflux.

Continuous esophageal pH monitoring

Intraesophageal pH microelectrodes have been designed with diameters less than 2 mm. Such a probe, positioned approximately 3 cm above the distal esophageal sphincter calculated by a standardized mathematical formula, is coupled with a recorder and 24 h of monitoring is carried out (Fig. 13.4) [16]. Scores have been developed that take into consideration the percentage of time in which the esophageal pH is below 4.0 in the prone and supine position and the number of reflux episodes lasting longer than 5 min, with correction for the 2-h postprandial period in which reflux is acceptable. Using the formula of Byrne and Euler, the probe data are abnormal if in 24 h the score exceeds 50, i.e. $x + 4y > 50$, where x = the number of episodes and y = the number of episodes lasting more than 5 min. A pH of less than 4.0 for more than 4% of a 24-h recording is also considered abnormal (Tables 13.4 and 13.5) [17]. Prolonged recording of intraesophageal pH can also be performed while oxygen saturation is being monitored, to detect an association between desaturation and GER.

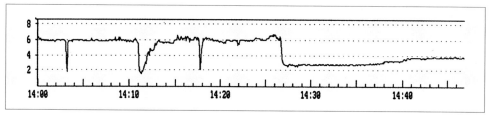

Figure 13.4 A segment of a recording of an esophageal pH monitoring: three brief episodes of reflux are followed by rapid recovery of alkaline pH. At 14:27 hours, a rapid fall in pH persists for more than 15 min.

The pH probe has indications and limitations. Not every child who regurgitates needs a pH probe. Quantification of reflux has no prognostic value and provides a limited amount of information regarding therapy. In general terms it could be said that the greatest application of the pH probe is to detect reflux whenever emesis is not present. The presence of GER detected by pH probe, however, does not necessarily mean that reflux is the cause of the symptoms in question (apnea, cyanosis, stridor, pneumonia, pain, wheezing, bradycardia and hoarseness). The relationship between abnormal pH probe results and histologic evidence of esophagitis is not always clear [18–20]. The pH probe may also be useful to document reflux in older children without prior history of regurgitation who suddenly start vomiting, in whom increased endocranial pressure has been ruled out. Positive or negative results from a pH probe in an infant with clear-cut, uncomplicated GER will add very little to the management. Simultaneous recordings, however, with a proximal and a distal pH probe may be helpful in diagnosing aspiration pneumonia caused by refluxed material from the stomach [17].

Tuttle test of acid reflux

Hydrochloric acid (0.1 N per 1.7 m²) or unsweetened apple juice (300 ml per 1.7 m²) is ingested and the esophageal pH is monitored for 30 min. A drop in pH to less than 4 on two or more occasions is considered abnormal.

Endoscopy

Modern fiberoptic equipment enables evidence of esophagitis or stricture to be observed (see Fig. 13.3). A stricture can be resolved by esophageal dilatation. Erythema of the esophageal mucosa alone is not a good indication of esophagitis, and biopsies are needed [18–20]. The presence of esophagitis in the absence of corrosive poisoning confirms significant exposure of the esophageal mucosa to acid reflux. Esophagitis is more closely related to poor esophageal clearance than to either number or duration of episodes. Although eosinophils are the characteristic cells found in peptic reflux esophagitis, neutrophils and lymphocytes can also be present (Fig. 13.5). Presence of eosinophils in the esophageal mucosa has also been linked to dietary protein hypersensitivity rather than to peptic reflux [21,22]. In addition to visualizing the lower esophagus, a biopsy and/or brushings may be taken which allows a diagnosis of monilial or herpetic disease to be made and the severity of inflammation to be determined. In Barrett's esophagus, there is metaplasia of the esophageal mucosa, with the epithelium becoming cylindric. Visualization

	Mean ± 1 SD
Episodes below pH 4	10.6 ± 8.2
Episodes >5 min	1.7 ± 2.1
Longest episode (min)	8.1 ± 7.2
Percentage time below pH 4	1.9 ± 1.6

Table 13.4 Results of continuous 24-h esophageal pH monitoring in normal infant. From Boix-Ochoa J, Lafuente JM, Gil-Vernet JM. Twenty-four hour esophageal pH monitoring in gastroesophageal reflux. J Pediatr Surg 1980;15:74–8.

Age (months)	Percentage time below pH 4
Newborn	1.16
1	1.78
2	2.53
6	3.22
8	3.85
15	2.55

Values for infants younger and older than 4 months of age are significantly different from each other (P<0.01).

Table 13.5 Results of continuous 24-h esophageal pH monitoring in 285 asymptomatic infants from 0 to 15 months of age. From [16].

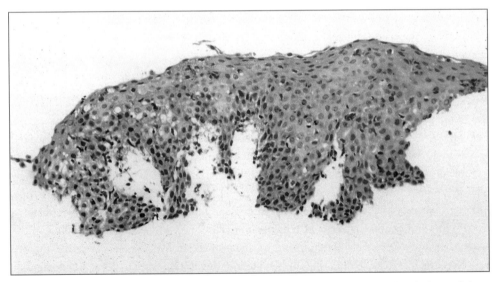

Figure 13.5 Esophageal biopsy demonstrating esophagitis. A number of eosinophils (darker stain) are seen close to the surface (top). The cells stained dark are inflammatory cells.

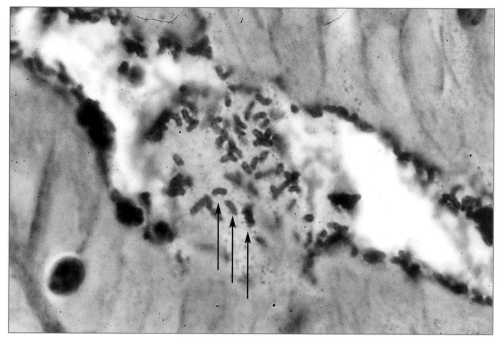

Figure 13.6 Biopsy from the antrum of the stomach, demonstrating numerous organisms identified as *Helicobacter pylori*.

and biopsies of the stomach may clinch the diagnosis of *Helicobacter pylori*, which could be the cause of epigastric pain and explain the failure of medical treatment or recurrence of symptoms (Fig. 13.6). However, in adults with duodenal ulcers, eradication of *H. pylori* has been associated with the occurrence of GER. Duodenitis (allergic or non-specific) can be the cause of delayed gastric emptying and worsening of reflux in a predisposed patient. The diagnosis is made by biopsy.

Characteristic changes in the esophageal biopsy compatible with reflux esophagitis are listed in Table 13.6.

Radioisotopic scanning ('milk scan')
A feed containing the isotope technetium-99m is ingested; then, the esophagus is scanned and the volume of refluxed fluid calculated. Aspirated technetium in the lungs might explain chronic lung disease in appropriate cases. Esophageal motility can be studied during swallowing, preferably using ^{81m}Kr or ^{99m}Tc colloid. Radiation exposure is less than with a contrasted study, but the latter will also provide information about the gross anatomy.

Manometric studies
Manometry may be useful in studying esophageal dysmotility, which can lead to GER-type symptoms in some cases [23].

- Basal cell hyperplasia
- Increased length of the papillae
- Intraepithelial eosinophils
- Lymphocytes and polymorphonuclear infiltrates

Table 13.6 Histologic characteristics of esophagitis.

MANAGEMENT

Positioning

Most infants respond to simple and conservative measures such as being held upright after feeds. Positioning, however, has become a challenging issue and much has been written about this topic. Any positioning is quite difficult to maintain, particularly in older infants, who often become slumped or change posture. Infants older than 3 months of age move too much to be kept stable. Although making parents aware of the position prevents them from moving the child unnecessarily after feedings, postprandial positioning may not be beneficial and could even be detrimental if not maintained appropriately.

For many years, specifically placing the infant in a prone position (often with the head elevated to 30°) was a cornerstone of regurgitation treatment. This was associated with less crying than when infants were placed in a seated position, although head-elevated prone was no more effective than flat prone in reducing signs of GER [24–26]. However, a case-control study conducted in the USA showed that the prone sleeping position is clearly associated with a higher incidence of sudden infant death syndrome (SIDS) [27]. In the early 1990s, parents in England, Wales, Australia and New Zealand were advised to avoid placing infants in the prone position: a significant decrease in SIDS was subsequently observed in each of these countries. Because of this relationship between prone sleeping and SIDS, postural treatment favoring the prone-flat position, despite its efficacy, is no longer recommended as first-line treatment for regurgitation [11]. The relationship between SIDS and the sleeping position of the infant is limited to the prone-flat position. To date, there is no established relationship between SIDS and the prone-elevated (30°) (anti-Trendelenburg) position.

One study demonstrated that placing the baby in a left lateral position decreased reflux [28]. This position may be an alternative to prone for the postural management of infants with regurgitation but may not be effective for all infants at risk of SIDS. Thus, placing an infant in a supine position is the current general recommendation for sleep positioning.

Feeding

Nutritional management of infants with regurgitation is the first step of treatment, but is generally recommended as an adjunct to advice on positioning.

It has been suggested that smaller-volume, more-frequent feedings that maintain adequate daily caloric intake alleviate reflux and regurgitation [29]. This recommendation is of unproven efficacy and in practice is difficult to apply. The additional burden that smaller, more-frequent feedings places on the parents may yield ineffective results and contribute to parental anxiety. Furthermore, the reduced volumes of formula may cause distress to the hungry infant who does not want to stop feeding. The feeding volume should, however, be decreased in infants who are overfed.

Thickened infant formula has been shown to relieve regurgitation and improve sleep in a significant number of bottlefed infants. Orenstein [30] found that infants fed formula thickened with dry rice cereal had both a decreased volume as well as frequency of regurgitation, compared with when the same infants were given unthickened formula. Feeding the thickened formula also resulted in decreased crying time and increased sleeping in the 90-min postprandial study period. Thickened feeds, however, can worsen cough induced by GER [31]. The two main carbohydrates used for thickening of formula are rice starch and carob bean gum. Appendices II.12 and II.13 provide details of feed thickeners and specialized formulas designed for the treatment of reflux. For breastfed infants, a gruel can be prepared by mixing expressed breast milk with infant cereal. For those on a weaning diet, it is often beneficial to increase the amount of solid food and reduce the intake of fluids. In Europe, thickened feeds are generally used early in the treatment of GER; however, this is not routine practice in the USA [31,32].

Where it is thought that regurgitation or rumination is a behavioral problem, an improvement can often be achieved if the carer stays with the child and distracts his or her attention for 20–30 min after each feed. Occasionally, the physician may need to resort to a period of 1–3 weeks of constant intragastric infusion of formula to attain an alleviation of vomiting.

Hypersensitivity to dietary protein can worsen symptoms of GER in a predisposed infant by delaying gastric emptying or possibly resulting from pain as an inflamed small bowel distends with food. In this case, or in the presence of an allergic reaction to food associated with esophagitis, the use of a hypoallergenic formula may be useful [33,34]. Allergic duodenitis can be suspected when emesis occurs several hours after a feed.

Medication

Cisapride

Cisapride, an oral prokinetic agent, facilitates acetylcholine release from myenteric nerves. Until recently, except for rare occasions, it had replaced metoclopramide in the pharmacologic management of reflux because of fewer adverse effects in the CNS [35]. However, serious cardiac arrhythmias including ventricular tachycardia, ventricular fibrillation and QT prolongation [36–40] have been reported in patients taking cisapride. In July 2000, because of major concerns about serious cardiac side effects, the drug was made available only through a limited access program in the USA, and the product licence was suspended in the UK. Nevertheless, the UK Committee on the Safety of Medicine has been asked to re-evaluate its guidelines and await findings of American trials [41].

The risk of cisapride-induced altered electric conductivity of the heart is increased in preterm infants and when high dosages are administered. In addition, pre-existing cardiac conditions (congenital or acquired) which might predispose the patient to ventricular arrhythmias, intraventricular conduction disturbances and instances of reduced hepatic function may also increase susceptibility. Recommendations have been made to perform a baseline electrocardiogram (ECG) prior to initiating cisapride and not to administer the drug to patients whose QTc interval is greater than 450 ms. Computer-assisted interpretation of the ECG should not be relied on for the determination of QTc.

The main metabolic pathway of cisapride is through cytochrome P450 CYP 3A4. The concurrent use of oral or parenteral drugs that significantly inhibit these enzymes may increase plasma levels of cisapride and cause QT prolongation, and hence is contraindicated. Major drug interactions are with the macrolide antibiotics (azithromycin, clarithromycin, and erythromycin), azole antifungals (ketoconazole, miconazole and fluconazole) and protease inhibitors (indinavir, nelfinavir and ritonavir). Many other drugs are contraindicated in those receiving cisapride. These include amiodarone, quinine, terfenadine, omeprazole, metronidazole, chlorpromazine, diltiazem, methadone and norfloxacin. In addition, grapefruit juice may increase the bioavailability of cisapride. Cisapride is also contraindicated in patients with electrolyte disorders. In children, no major side effects were identified when cisapride was used according to recommendations for patients who are not in one of the risk categories [42].

The oral dose of cisapride is 0.2 mg/kg three or four times a day (birth to 12 years) or 10 mg three times a day (12–18 years), administered 15 min before meals. It should not be administered 'around the clock' unrelated to meals, except if the infant is fed with a constant intragastric infusion.

Bethanechol

This drug is a muscarinic agonist and increases the pressure of the LES. Bethanechol is administered in a dose of 0.15 mg/kg, four times a day, 15–20 min before meals. It is not a prokinetic drug, therefore it can be used in children with diarrhea. However, it can cause agitation and may produce airway contraction.

Metoclopramide

This is a prokinetic agent with similar effects to those of cisapride but with relatively frequent adverse reactions such as extrapyramidal symptoms (torticollis-like neck rigidity and oculogyric crisis) and even tardive dyskinesia, which could be irreversible. It is a potent dopamine receptor antagonist. Metoclopramide can be given intravenously and has no side effects at the level of cardiac nerve conduction as cisapride does.

H_2 blockers and proton-pump inhibitors

These medications are important components of the treatment regimen for GER and secondary esophagitis. Improvement of esophagitis may result in a better function of the antireflux mechanisms. Ranitidine is used at a dose of 6 mg/kg/day, divided into three doses in infants under 1 year of age and into two doses in older children. The liquid form is not very palatable and some children may refuse to take it. Famotidine is prescribed at a dose of 0.5 mg/kg/day, divided into two doses, and has a better taste. Omeprazole, lanzoprazole and pantoprazole are proton-pump inhibitors, and are more potent than H_2 blockers. The dose of omeprazole is 1 mg/kg/day (max. 20 mg twice daily) [43–45].

- Failed response to adequate and prolonged medical therapy

- Esophageal stricture

- Severe esophagitis

- Recurrent aspiration pneumonia or apnea

- Barrett's esophagus

- Hiatal hernia or partial thoracic stomach

- Failure to thrive associated with GERD

Table 13.7 Potential indications for antireflux surgery.

Sucralfate

Sucralfate (Carafate) is a modified sucrose compound that is not absorbed from the gastrointestinal tract but adheres to the damaged mucosa, offering a protective coat. This medication is available in tablet form or as a suspension. In the latter preparation it is ideal for infants with esophagitis to prevent pain and distress from effort-induced GER. The dose of sucralfate is 40–80 mg/kg/24 h, given every 6 h.

Corticosteroids

These may be used in cases of allergic esophagitis and/or duodenitis [46,47].

Surgery

The surgical procedure to correct GER is a fundoplication [4]. Several techniques are available: these include the Nissen fundoplication, in which the fundus of the stomach is wrapped completely (360°) around the distal 3.5 cm of the esophagus, and the Thal partial fundoplication procedure, which is a wrap of 180°. Fundoplication can be performed as an open-surgery procedure or laparoscopically [48]. The operation creates a cinch-like action and also maintains the lower esophagus below the diaphragm, where intra-abdominal pressure assists in preventing reflux. Studies suggest that the antireflux effects of Nissen fundoplication may be based on changes of LES motor patterns that result in incomplete LES relaxation and reduction of the number of TLESRs [49]. Fundoplications are far less frequently indicated today than in former years because most cases can now be managed with appropriate medication and techniques such as nasogastric feeding. Indications for fundoplication are listed in Table 13.7. As many as 25% of patients may require reoperation after 2 years [50].

Deranged gastric motility and consequent delayed gastric emptying (DGE) are commonly implicated in the pathophysiology of GERD [51]. DGE is common in neurologically impaired children with GER and may affect the outcome of fundoplication. Amelioration of DGE by pyroplasty improves the outcome of fundoplication in such cases [52]. Either procedure, but more commonly pyroplasty, may be associated with dumping syndrome (rapid gastric emptying) [53]. This can be improved by the addition of pectin to the formula.

Besides the potential complications resulting from any type of major bowel surgery, fundoplication can lead to retching. This problem, which can last several months, is annoying to the parents and very difficult to manage. It is particularly common in children with neurodevelopmental delays. Gas bloat syndrome is the consequence of a tight fundoplication and prevents burping. This problem is more common among children with severe CNS damage because frequently they are mouth-breathers and air-swallowers.

Patients with poor oral intake will benefit from a feeding gastrostomy placed at the time of the fundoplication. Whether patients who do not have overt emesis but have evidence of regurgitation and need a gastrostomy also require a fundoplication, particularly if they are developmentally impaired, is a controversial issue [54]. It has been postulated that placement of a percutaneous gastrostomy can create or worsen GER, particularly in children with neurological disorders [55,56]. Non-nutritive oral stimulation or partial oral feeds need to be continued after placement of a gastrostomy, to avoid atrophy of the suck reflex and oral aversion.

REFERENCES

1. Orenstein SR. Controversies in pediatric gastroesophageal reflux. J Pediatr Gastroenterol Nutr 1992;14:338–48.

2. Vandenplas Y. Gastroesophageal reflux in children. Scand J Gastroenterol 1995;213:31–8.

3. Milla PJ. Reflux vomiting. Arch Dis Child 1990;65:996–9.

4. Fonkalsrud EW, Ament ME. Gastroesophageal reflux in childhood. Curr Probl Surg 1996;33:1–70.

5. Orenstein S. What are the boundaries between physiologic and pathologic reflux in relation to age in infancy? In: Giuli R, Tytgat G, DeMeester T et al. editors. The Esophageal Mucosa: 300 Questions...300 Answers. Amsterdam: Elsevier Science, 1994:741–5.

6. Mittal RK, Holloway RH, Penagini R et al. Transient lower esophageal relaxation. Gastroenterology 1995;109:601–10.

7. Cucchiara S, Staiano A, DiLorenzo C et al. Pathophysiology of gastroesophageal reflux and distal esophageal motility in children with gastroesophageal reflux disease. J Pediatr Gastroenteral Nutr 1988;7:830–6.

8. Kawahara H, Dent J, Davidson G. Mechanisms responsible for gastroesophageal reflux in children. Gastroenterology 1997;113:399–408.

9. Boix-Ochoa J, Canals J. Maturation of the lower esophagus. J Pediatr Surg 1976;11:749–56.

10. Bauman NM, Sandler AD, Smith RJ. Respiratory manifestations of gastroesophageal reflux disease in pediatric patients. Ann Otol Rhinol Laryngol 1996;105:23–32.

11. Vandenplas Y, Belli DC, Dupont C et al. The relation between gastro-oesophageal reflux, sleeping-position and sudden infant death and its impact on positional therapy. Eur J Pediatr 1997;156:104–6.

12. Putnam PE, Orenstein SR. Hoarseness in a child with gastroesophageal reflux. Acta Paediatr 1992;81:635–6.

13. Meer S, Groothuis JR, Harbeck R et al. The potential role of gastroesophageal reflux in the pathogenesis of food-induced wheezing. Pediatr Allergy Immunol 1996;7:167–70.

14. Yellon RF. The spectrum of reflux-associated otolaryngologic problems in infants and children. Am J Med 1997;103:125S–129S.

15. Balson BM, Kravitz EK, McGeady SJ. Diagnosis and treatment of gastroesophageal reflux in children and adolescents with severe asthma. Ann Allergy Asthma Immunol 1998;81:159–64.

16. Vandenplas Y, Sacre-Smits L. Continuous 24-hour esophageal pH monitoring in 285 asymptomatic infants 0-15 months old. J Pediatr Gastroenterol Nutr 1987;6:220–4.

17. Cucchiara S, Salvia G, Rea B et al. Simultaneous prolonged recordings of proximal and distal intraesophageal pH in children with gastroesophageal reflux disease and respiratory symptoms. Am J Gastroenterol 1995;90:1791–6.

18. Black DD, Haggitt RC, Orenstein SR, Whitington PF. Esophagitis in infants: morphometric histologic diagnosis and correlation with measures of gastroesophageal reflux. Gastroenterology 1990;98:1408–14.

19. Cucchiara S, D'Armiento F, Alfieri E et al. Intraepithelial cells with irregular nuclear contours as a marker of esophagitis in children with gastroesophageal reflux disease. Dig Dis Sci 1995;40:2305–11.

20. Vandenplas Y. Reflux esophagitis: Biopsy or not? J Pediatr Gastroenterol Nutr 1996;22:326–7.

21. Kelly KJ, Lazenby AJ, Rowe PC et al. Eosinophilic esophagitis attributed to gastroesophageal reflux: Improvement with an amino acid-based formula. Gastroenterology 1995;109:1503–12.

22. Khoshoo V, Zembo M, King A et al. Incidence of gastroesophageal reflux with whey- and casein-based formulas in infants and in children with severe neurological impairment. J Pediatr Gastroenterol Nutr 1996;22:48–55.

23. Cucchiara S, Campanozzi A, Greco L et al. Predictive value of esophageal manometry and gastroesophageal pH monitoring for responsiveness of reflux disease to medical therapy in children. Am J Gastroenterol 1996;91:680–5.

24. Orenstein SR, Whitington PF, Orenstein DM. The infant seat as treatment for gastroesophageal reflux. N Engl J Med 1983;309:760–3.

25. Orenstein SR. Prone positioning in infant gastroesophageal reflux: is elevation of the head worth the trouble? J Pediatr 1990;117:184–7.

26. Orenstein SR. Effects on behavior state of prone versus seated positioning for infants with gastroesophageal reflux. Pediatrics 1990;85:765–7.

27. Ponsonby AL, Dwyer T, Gibbons LE et al. Factors potentiating the risk of sudden infant death syndrome associated with the prone position. N Engl J Med 1993;329:377–82

28. Tobin JM, McCloud P, Cameron DJ. Posture and gastro-oesophageal reflux: A case for left lateral positioning. Arch Dis Child 1997;76:254–8.

29. Vandenplas Y, Belli D, Benhamou P et al. A critical appraisal of current management practices for infant regurgitation — recommendations of a working party. Eur J Pediatr 1997;156:343–57.

30. Orenstein SR, Magill HL, Brooks P. Thickening of infant feedings for therapy of gastroesophageal reflux. J Pediatr 1987;110:181–6.

31. Samour PQ, Lang CE, Helm KK. Handbook of Pediatric Nutrition. 2nd ed. Gaithersburg, MD: Aspen, 1999.

32. Groh-Wargo S, Thompson M, Cox JH, editors. Nutritional care for high-risk newborns. 3rd rev. ed. Chicago: Precept Press, 2000.

33. Hill DJ, Heine RG, Cameron DJ et al. Role of food protein intolerance in infants with persistent distress attributed to reflux esophagitis. J Pediatr 2000;136:641–7.

34. Orenstein SR, Shalaby TM, Putnam PE. Thickened feedings as a cause of increased coughing when used as therapy for gastroesophageal reflux in infants. J Pediatr 1992;121:913–5.

35. Vandenplas Y, Deneyer M et al. Gastroesophageal reflux incidence and respiratory dysfunction during sleep in infants: Treatment with cisapride. J Pediatr Gastroenterol Nutr 1989;8:31–6.

36. Lewin MB, Bryant RM, Fenrich AL et al. Cisapride-induced long QT interval. J Pediatr 1996;128:279–81.

37. Scott RB, Ferreira C, Smith L et al. Cisapride in pediatric gastroesophageal reflux. J Pediatr Gastroenterol Nutr 1997;25:499–506.

38. Vandenplas Y, Belli DC, Benatar A et al. The role of cisapride in the treatment of pediatric gastroesophageal reflux. The European Society of Paediatric Gastroenterology, Hepatology and Nutrition. J Pediatr Gastroenterol Nutr 1999;28:518–28.

39. Levine A, Fogelman R, Sirota L et al. QT interval in children and infants receiving cisapride. Pediatrics 1998;101:E9.

40. Semama DS, Bernardini S, Lous S et al. Effects of cisapride on QTc interval in term neonates. Arch Dis Child Fetal Neonatal Ed 2001;84:F44–6.

41. Markiewicz M, Vandenplas Y. Should cisapride have been 'blacklisted'? Arch Dis Child Fetal Neonatal Ed 2000;82:F3–4.

42. Shulman RJ, Boyle JT, Colletti RB et al. The use of cisapride in children. The North American Society for Pediatric Gastroenterology and Nutrition. J Pediatr Gastroenterol Nutr 1999;28:529–33.

43. Cucchiara S, Minella R, Campanozzi A et al. Effects of omeprazole on mechanisms of gastroesophageal reflux in childhood. Dig Dis Sci 1997;42:293–9.

44. De Giacomo C, Bawa P, Franceschi M et al. Omeprazole for severe reflux esophagitis in children. J Pediatr Gastroenterol Nutr 1997;24:528–32.

45. Israel DM, Hassall E. Omeprazole and other proton pump inhibitors: Pharmacology, efficacy, and safety, with special reference to use in children. J Pediatr Gastroenterol Nutr 1998;27:568–79.

46. Liacouras CA, Wenner WJ, Brown K et al. Primary eosinophilic esophagitis in children: successful treatment with oral corticosteroids. J Pediatr Gastroenterol Nutr 1998;26:380–5.

47. Walsh SV, Antonioli DA, Goldman H et al. Allergic esophagitis in children: A clinicopathological entity. Am J Surg Pathol 1999;23:390–6.

48. Meehan JJ, Georgeson KE. The learning curve associated with laparoscopic antireflux surgery in infants and children. J Pediatr Surg 1997;32:426–9.

49. Kawahara H, Imura K, Yoneda A et al. Mechanisms underlying the antireflux effect of Nissen fundoplication in children. J Pediatr Surg 1998;33:1618–22.

50. Dalla Vecchia LK, Engum SA, Scherer 3rd LR et al. Reoperation after Nissen fundoplication in children with gastroesophageal reflux: Experience with 130 patients. Ann Surg 1997;226:315–21.

51. Cucchiara S, Riezzo G, Campanozzi A et al. Gastric electrical dysrhythmias and delayed gastric emptying in gastroesophageal reflux disease. Am J Gastroenterol 1997;92:1103–8.

52 Alexander F, Wyllie R, Jirousek K et al. Delayed gastric emptying affects outcome of Nissen fundoplication in neurologically impaired children. Surgery 1997;122:690–7.

53. Samuk I, Afriat R, Horne T et al. Dumping syndrome following Nissen fundoplication, diagnosis, and treatment. J Pediatr Gastroenterol Nutr 1996;23:235–40.

54. Sullivan PB. Gastrostomy feeding in the disabled child: When is an antireflux procedure required? Arch Dis Child 1999;81:463–4.

55. Launay V, Gottrand F, Turck D et al. Percutaneous endoscopic gastrostomy in children: Influence on gastroesophageal reflux. Pediatrics 1996;97:726–8.

56. Short TP, Patel NR, Thomas E. Prevalence of gastroesophageal reflux in patients who develop pneumonia following percutaneous endoscopic gastrostomy: A 24-hour pH monitoring study. Dysphagia 1996;11:87–9.

14

Hepatobiliary Disease

Hepatobiliary disease is characterized by the presence of one or more of the following:

- Jaundice
- Acholia
- Choluria
- Fatigue
- Itching
- Hepato(spleno)megaly
- Hematemesis

The features presented above and their sequence vary amongst different diseases and individuals. The first step in the investigation of jaundice is to determine whether the bilirubin is in the conjugated or unconjugated form (Table. 14.1). Unconjugated hyperbilirubinemia – except for that seen in the neonatal period in Crigler–Najjar syndrome types I and II – is not the result of liver disease, and hence is not reviewed in this chapter. The causes of direct hyperbilirubinemia are listed in Table 14.2.

HEPATITIS

Hepatitis [1] can be caused by several factors, for example:

- Viruses – hepatitis A, B, C, D, E and G (Table 14.3)
- Toxic agents – alcohol, drugs or other chemicals
- Autoimmune disorders

Usually, acute hepatitis resolves and the liver architecture reverts to a normal pattern. However, sometimes it leads to fulminating hepatitis, which is life threatening and, without a liver transplant, has a mortality rate as high as 80%. Hepatitis is characterized by jaundice, pale stools, dark bile-containing urine and often an enlarged liver. More commonly, infections are subclinical and anicteric. Infections that may be accompanied by jaundice are listed in Table 14.4. *Listeria* species, *Toxoplasma* species and syphilis are important to diagnose as they can be treated.

Aspartate aminotransferase	Albumin	Urine succinylacetone
Alanine aminotransferase	Glucose	Serum aminoacids
Alkaline phosphatase	Prothrombin time	Serum α1-antitrypsin
γ-glutamyl transpeptidase	Partial thromboplastin time	Ceruloplasmin
Cholesterol	TORCH titers, hepatitis screen	Abdominal ultrasound
Triglycerides		Radionuclide scan
T4, TSH	Urine organic acids	Percutaneous (or open) liver biopsy
	Urine reducing sugars	

Table 14.1 Work-up of neonatal jaundice with predominantly direct hyperbilirubinemia.

Infectious	*Metabolic*
Hepatitis A, B, C, D, E, G	Galactosemia
Herpes, cytomegalovirus, *Toxoplasma gondii*, Epstein–Barr virus, rubella	Tyrosinemia
	Toxic
Neonatal hepatitis (infectious?)	Acetaminophen
Syphilis	Hydrocarbons
Affected bile flow	*Others*
Extrahepatic biliary atresia	α₁-antitrypsin deficiency
Paucity of intrahepatic bile ducts	Wilson's disease
Choledochal cyst	Peroxisomal disorders (Zellweger's syndrome)
Familial intrahepatic cholestasis	Disorders of bile acid metabolism
Cystic fibrosis	Hypothyroidism
Intrahepatic or extrahepatic mass (tumor, cysts)	
Congenital hepatic fibrosis	

Table 14.2 Causes of direct hyperbilirubinemia.

HEPATITIS A

Hepatitis A is caused by an RNA agent that is a member of the picornavirus family. It is transmitted by person-to-person contact, generally via fecal/oral contamination and, less often, as is common with hepatitis B, through blood or blood products. Immunoglobulin given before exposure or during the incubation period of hepatitis A (15–50 days) is protective against clinical illness. Water-borne, milk-borne and food-borne (especially raw shellfish) epidemics have been reported. Better sanitation with safe drinking-water supplies and improved socioeconomic conditions will result in a decreased exposure to hepatitis A. An attack of hepatitis A produces permanent immunity. However, in older children, hepatitis A (or hepatitis non-A–G) is the commonest cause of fulminant hepatitis, with an incidence ranging from 1.5% to 31%. Children with hepatitis A remain contagious until 1 week after the onset of illness or jaundice and therefore should be excluded from daycare settings during that period. Indications for hospital admission of patients with hepatitis A include vomiting leading to dehydration and prolonged clotting studies.

Virus type	A Picorna (RNA)	B Hepadna (DNA)	C Flavi (RNA)	D Delta (RNA)	E Calci (RNA)
Mean incubation period (days)	30	80	50	?	40
Transmission mode:					
Orofecal	+ve	?	-ve	-ve	+ve
Blood	rare	+ve	+ve	+ve	-ve
Chronic infection	-ve	+ve	+ve	+ve	-ve

Table 14.3 Types of human hepatitis virus.

TORCH*	Causative organism
T	*Toxoplasma gondii*
O	Hepatitis A, B, C, D, E and G Coxsackie B virus Varicella virus Zoster virus *Treponema pallidum* *Listeria* species
R	Rubella virus
C	Cytomegalovirus
H	Herpes simplex

*In the 'TORCH' syndrome, the 'O' stands for other diseases.

Table 14.4 Infectious causes of hepatitis syndrome in infancy.

Different vaccines are approved for use in children. In the US, these comprise Havrix (SmithKline Beecham) and Vaqta (Merck & Co.). Depending on the vaccine used, two or three intramuscular doses are required. In some countries, a combined A and B vaccine is now available, e.g. Twinrix (SmithKline Beecham Biologicals), for those 1–15 years of age.

HEPATITIS B

The hepatitis B virus (HBV), a DNA virus, is a major cause of acute and chronic hepatitis, cirrhosis and primary hepatocellular carcinoma (HCC). Hepatitis B infection may produce no clinical symptoms or appear as rapid, fulminant liver disease. HBV can be transmitted through blood and its products, contaminated needles or sexual intercourse. The combined use of hepatitis B vaccine and immunoglobulin will result in greater than 90% protection in children born to mothers of high infectivity (i.e. 'e' antigen positive, hepatitis B surface antigen [HBsAg] carriers – Table 14.5). In some communities, the risk of a neonate becoming a carrier is as high as 80–90%, and an infant may remain infected indefinitely, with only about 1–2% reverting to HBsAg negativity.

Hepatitis B antigen/antibody status	Significance
Surface antigen (HBsAg)	Carrier has acute infection
Antibody to surface antigen (anti-HBs)	Previous HBV infection; or immunity post vaccination
'e' antigen (HBeAg)	Carrier at high risk of transmitting HBsAg
Antibody to 'e' antigen (anti-HBe)	HBsAg carrier at low risk of transmitting infection
Antibody to core antigen (anti-HBc)	Previous HBV infection (not due to immunization)
IgM antibody to core antigen (IgM anti-HBc)	Current or recent HBV infection

Table 14.5 Hepatitis testing and interpretation.

The incidence of HBV infection is increasing globally and there is a significant prevalence within institutions for handicapped children, especially those with Down's syndrome. A major obstacle to immunization is the high cost of the vaccine for a course of three injections and the availability as well as the expense of hepatitis B immune globulin. However, now there is an opportunity to significantly reduce the likelihood of vertical transmission of hepatitis B by using an immunization regimen (Table 14.6).

HCC has a male predominance and is closely related to HBV infection. Following an immunization program in Taiwan, the boy–girl incidence ratio dropped from 4.5 in 1981–1984 (before the program was introduced) to 1.9 in 1990–1996 (6–12 years post program). The incidence of HCC in boys born after 1984 was significantly reduced in comparison with those born before 1978 [2].

Treatment

Available therapy is interferon-α (IFN-α); however, more than 50% of children with chronic HBV infection do not respond to this treatment and are prone to progressive liver disease [3]. It would seem that IFN-α treatment accelerates seroconversion but does not change the proportion of responders [4]. In a study performed in children, a second cycle of IFN-α during the 3 years following the first treatment in non-responders with chronic hepatitis B did not increase HBeAg/anti-HBe seroconversion compared with the spontaneous rate of patients without retreatment [5]. IFN-α retreatment with a higher dose may be an alternative modality for therapy of children with chronic hepatitis B infections who have failed to respond to previous IFN-α, especially in those with favorable predictive factors, i.e. low baseline titers of HBV DNA and elevated transaminase values (>100 IU/l) [6].

An additional therapeutic possibility is the nucleoside analog lamivudine, which is a potent inhibitor of hepatitis B viral DNA replication.

DELTA HEPATITIS

This form of hepatitis, first identified in 1977, cannot occur by itself but as a superinfection in HbsAg carriers.

Initial	1 month	6 months
0.5 ml*	0.5 ml	0.5 ml
(10 μg)	(10 μg)	(10 μg)
(at birth + immunoglobulin**)		

*That marketed by SmithKline Beecham (UK and USA) is a 0.5 ml dose containing 10 μg of vaccine, that by Aventis Pasteur (UK) is a 0.5 ml dose containing 5 μg of vaccine, and that by Merck Sharp & Dohme (UK) is a 0.5 ml dose containing 10 μg of vaccine.
**Administer the vaccine and immunoglobulin at different sites.
Specific dosage details of the immunoglobulin are available in the UK from the Public Health Laboratory Service and in the US from the American Academy of Pediatrics Red Book.

Table 14.6 Hepatitis B vaccine immunization regimen in infants born to HBsAg positive mothers.

The hepatitis delta virus is an incomplete RNA-containing virus with a worldwide distribution. Maternal-to-infant transmission is uncommon. In both North America and Northern Europe the pattern of infection is non-endemic.

HEPATITIS C

This form of hepatitis – caused by an RNA virus – accounts for 20% of all cases of acute hepatitis. Up to 0.7% (400,000 individuals) of the adult population of the UK are infected with hepatitis C virus (HCV) [7]. HCV is responsible for 80–90% of the previously called 'non-A, non-B' (or 'NANB') cases of hepatitis. HCV can be transmitted by blood transfusion, contaminated needles (drug use or accidental injury) or by sexual contact. In the USA, acute infection is more common among Hispanics but the chronic disease is more prevalent among African-Americans. The average risk of exposure to HCV after an accidental needle stick is 3.5%, but the hazard after transfusion has been reduced with screening to 1 in 100,000 units transfused. There is an average transmission rate from an infected mother to her infant of 6%. Breastfeeding has not been reported as being associated with transmission of HCV.

Progression of HCV infection is variable and may occur over 20 or 30 years in 85% of patients. Furthemore, hepatitis C is the leading reason for liver transplantation among adults in the USA. A UK study in men and boys with HCV infection secondary to blood product contamination has shown a risk of death from both liver disease and hepatic cancer [8].

So far, there is no effective vaccine to prevent HCV infection. Following initial exposure, HCV RNA can be detected in blood within 3 weeks. Despite remaining anicteric and asymptomatic, in an average of 50 days, patients experience some hepatocyte damage, as indicated by an elevation of ALT. Fewer than 35% develop a febrile-like syndrome and become jaundiced. Fulminant liver disease caused by acute hepatitis C is rare.

Treatment

IFN-α induces sustained remission of chronic hepatitis C in approximately 25% of patients. In patients who are non-responders to the first course of therapy, retreatment with IFN-α is of limited efficacy. A logistic regression in a study performed in adults identified five independent factors significantly associated with response to IFN-α:

- Genotype 2 or 3

- Viral load <2 million copies/ml

- Age ≤40 years

- Minimal fibrosis stage

- Female sex [9,10]

Ribavirin has also been used to treat chronic hepatitis C, but it induces only a transient response. However, a combination of IFN-α2b plus ribavirin for 24 or 48 weeks has been shown to be more effective than 48 weeks of IFN-α2b monotherapy and has an acceptable safety profile [10]. Long-acting pegylated interferons have better responses than standard preparations. Attaching polyethylene glycol (pegylation), a large inert molecule, reduces clearance thereby prolonging the half life of the drug [11,12].

HEPATITIS G

The hepatitis G virus (HGV) – also currently known as GB virus C (GBV-C) – an RNA agent, is transmitted mainly through the parenteral route. Approximately 2% of pregnant women are HGV antibody positive. There is a higher mother-to-infant transmission (30–50%) of this virus than HCV. A neonatal source can cause a persistent infection.

Children undergoing open-heart surgery are at greater risk of acquiring HGV infection than adults. However, over a 5-year follow-up period, no child developed clinical hepatitis from HGV [13].

AUTOIMMUNE HEPATITIS

This disorder predominantly affects young females, and, in the majority of them, there is the presence of the HLA antigen B8 DR3. Characteristically, a preadolescent or adolescent female may present with fatigue, anorexia, weight loss and/or jaundice. Patients may have evidence of a low-grade hemolytic anemia, and elevated serum titers of anti-smooth-muscle, antimitochondrial and/or anti-liver and kidney microsomal antibodies. A biopsy (Fig. 14.1) is necessary to better characterize the disease and should be performed prior to initiation of treatment. Liver biopsy shows necrosis, blurring of the limiting plate (which separates the portal tract from the hepatic parenchyma) and 'bridging' between portal tracts and the hepatic veins and lobules. The necrosis bridges adjacent portal areas and the central vein or portal areas of neighboring lobules. Similar changes can be produced by Wilson's disease, α_1-antitrypsin deficiency and hepatotoxic drugs.

The cause of this chronic hepatitis is unknown, but the markedly elevated IgG levels and the presence of autoantibodies as well as reduced complement would suggest an impaired immunoregulatory mechanism. Early diagnosis is important because of the need to introduce prompt immunosuppressive treatment. The main therapeutic agents are prednisone and/or azathioprine. A combined drug regimen might give the best results. Once clinical and biochemical remission has been achieved, an alternate-day steroid program will avoid some of the complications of long-term usage.

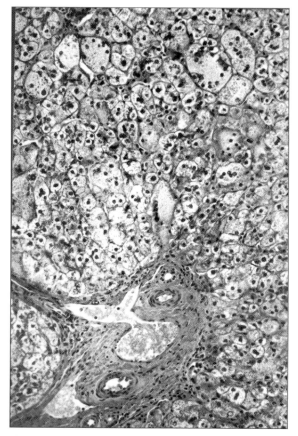

Figure 14.1 Chronic active hepatitis – needle biopsy of liver. Note portal inflammatory infiltrate, with mild fibrosis, eroded margins of hepatocyte lobules and preserved architecture. Hematoxylin & eosin, ×150. (Courtesy of Dr P Lewis.)

NEONATAL HEPATITIS

This term includes different types of liver disease. The most common etiologies are intrauterine infections and inherited metabolic diseases. Often no particular cause can be determined, but the most frequently identifiable are listed below:

Cytomegalovirus (CMV) infection: Infants are small for gestational age, with hepatosplenomegaly, and may have microcephaly, chorioretinitis and/or thrombocytopenia. Diagnosis is based on IgM antibodies and virus culture. The liver disease is frequently self-limited, but the neurosensory sequelae can be devastating. Treatment with ganciclovir is rarely necessary.

Rubella: This can present with neonatal hepatitis, cataracts, congenital heart disease and sensorineural deafness. It has almost disappeared since immunization became available.

Toxoplasmosis: This rare disease can present with neonatal jaundice, failure to thrive, hepatosplenomegaly and central nervous system involvement (chorioretinitis, microcephaly and intracranial calcifications). Treatment is with spiramycin.

Herpes simplex: This comprises a multi-system disorder with encephalitis and acute liver failure in the neonate. Early antiviral treatment with acyclovir may be successful.

Congenital syphilis: This is now rare in the USA and western Europe, but not in parts of eastern Europe, and appears to be re-emerging in Russia. It may cause a multi-system disease with hepatitis, intrauterine growth retardation, anemia, thrombocytopenia, nephrotic syndrome, skin rash and generalized lymphadenopathy.

Most infants with neonatal hepatitis present displaying one or more of the following features:

- Small for gestational age
- Hepatosplenomegaly
- Neurological manifestations
- Pigmented stools and choluria
- Dysmorphic features (Alagille's syndrome or Zellweger's syndrome – see p. 238)
- Conjugated bilirubin >100 μmol/l (>6 mg/dl)
- Alkaline phosphatase 600–800 IU/l
- Aspartate aminotransferase (AST) and ALT 200–300 IU/l

Diagnosis

The major differential diagnosis is with extrahepatic biliary atresia. If a radionuclide scan demonstrates excretion into the intestine, this probably rules out extrahepatic biliary atresia; otherwise, a liver biopsy is necessary. The nuclear imaging scan can produce both false-positive and false-negative results. The false-positive rate is due to the fact that many patients without biliary atresia will not excrete because of significant liver parenchymal disease. However, the magnitude of error depends on how the test is interpreted. If visualization of the biliary tract and gallbladder is required, the false-positive rate will be exceedingly high. Histology of neonatal hepatitis is non-specific and demonstrates giant multinucleated cells, in general without fibrosis, and extramedullary hematopoiesis, with or without cholestasis.

INFANTILE OBSTRUCTIVE CHOLANGIOPATHY

This can be caused by:

- Biliary atresia
- Choledochal cyst
- Intrahepatic cholestasis

Extrahepatic biliary atresia accounts for at least 50% of all cases of prolonged obstructive jaundice in the neonate [14]. Also, absence or hypoplasia of the intrahepatic bile ducts is responsible for persistent obstructive jaundice in almost 10% of such affected neonates.

It has been suggested that biliary atresia and neonatal hepatitis are different stages of one disease process and that they be grouped under a single heading; however, the exact cause

GGT	AP <300 IU/l	AP >600 IU/l
<300 IU/l	No obstructive process; probable neonatal hepatitis	Probable PFIC or inborn error of metabolism
>600 IU/l		Probable obstruction; about 90% predictive for biliary atresia but also seen in α_1-antitrypsin deficiency
>1500 IU/l	Unusual finding; possible diagnoses include Alagille's syndrome, neonatal sclerosing cholangitis and granulomatous hepatitis.	
Mid-level GGT elevations of 300–600 IU/l are all too common and do not help in the diagnosis		
AP = alkaline phosphatase; GGT = γ-glutamyl transferase; PFIC = progressive familial intrahepatic cholestasis		

Table 14.7 Possible interpretation of laboratory values in infantile cholestatic disease. Adapted from Allen K, Whitington PF. Evaluation of liver function. In: Polin R, Fox W, editors. Fetal and Neonatal Physiology. Philadelphia: WB Saunders, 1997.

is not known. A variety of pathogenic mechanisms for the development of biliary atresia have been postulated. An infectious cause, such as a virus, would seem most plausible in many cases [15]. The fact that biliary atresia is rarely encountered in premature infants would support an agent acting late in gestation. Genetic mechanisms likely play important roles, even regarding susceptibility to other specific causes, but no gene whose altered function would result in obstruction or atresia of the biliary tree has been identified. Biliary atresia, when untreated, is fatal within 2 years, with a median survival of 8 months.

It is important to distinguish biliary atresia from neonatal hepatitis because early intervention (with a Kasai portoenterostomy) may make a difference in the prognosis of the former. It is imperative that expert surgery is offered no later than 8 weeks of age. The incidence of biliary atresia is 1 in 12,000–14,000. There is no single non-invasive test that will definitively distinguish biliary atresia from hepatitis (intrahepatic cholestasis). The following diagnostic tests are recommended:

1. Gamma-glutamyl transpeptidase. This is usually more markedly elevated in extrahepatic biliary atresia (Table 14.7).

2. Biliary scintigraphy with a radioactive marker such as PIPIDA or DISIDA. ^{99m}Tc-diisopropyliminodiacetic acid given intravenously after oral phenobarbital (5 mg/kg/day for 3 days) will determine whether there is excretion into the duodenum. The marker behaves as a bile acid: it is taken up by the liver and excreted in the biliary tract. In cases of severe cholestasis or very impaired conjugation by the liver, the marker will not concentrate sufficiently in the biliary tree and thus, even if permeable, the test will give a false-positive result (for biliary atresia).

3. Ultrasound to exclude a choledochal cyst.

Diagnosis requires whenever possible a percutaneous, or otherwise surgical, liver biopsy. Liver biopsy will show proliferating duct formation and bile plugs in cases of extrahepatic biliary atresia. In neonatal cholestasis, multinucleated giant cells and inflammation are the typical findings.

PROGNOSIS IN EXTRAHEPATIC BILIARY ATRESIA

Of those children operated upon successfully, i.e. in whom bile flow can be established, 30–40% will remain jaundice-free until adulthood [16]. In one-third of the cases, illness will be palliated, and these patients have extended survival, delaying liver transplantation to later childhood (2 to 15 years). The remaining 30–40% will not benefit from the Kasai operation and will die of liver failure in infancy unless they undergo a transplant. The annual need of liver transplantation for biliary atresia is one case per million people in countries where liver transplant is performed routinely. This indication represents 35–67% of the reported series of pediatric liver transplantation and between 5% and 10% of the indications for liver transplantation, all ages included. Using newer transplant techniques, the 5-year survival rate for children who receive transplants with a primary diagnosis of biliary atresia is 82% [17]. This yields an overall survival rate of 86% in this entire study population.

INTRAHEPATIC CHOLESTASIS

Benign recurrent intrahepatic cholestasis (BRIC)

BRIC is a form of cholestasis, of obscure etiology, characterized by recurrent episodes of jaundice and itching associated with a morphological picture of pure intrahepatic cholestasis. No effective treatment has yet been found among the many that have been proposed for this invariably benign condition.

Alagille syndrome

This is a dominantly inherited disorder of variable expressivity, characterized by liver disease in combination with heart, skeletal, ocular, facial, renal and pancreatic abnormalities. The prevalence is 1:100,000. The Alagille syndrome gene has been identified as Jagged1 (*JAG1*), mapped to chromosome 20, band p12 [18]. Siblings and parents of probands are often found to have mild expression of the presumptive disease gene, with abnormalities of only one or two systems.

Emerick et al. [19] studied 92 patients with Alagille syndrome to determine the frequency of clinical manifestations and to correlate findings with outcome. Liver biopsy specimens showed paucity of the interlobular ducts in 85% of patients and cholestasis was seen in 96%. Cholestasis was present in 96%, cardiac murmur in 97%, butterfly vertebrae in 51%, posterior embryotoxon in 78%, characteristic facies in 96%, renal disease in 40% and intracranial bleeding or stroke occurred in 14%. The presence of intracardiac congenital heart disease was the only clinical feature statistically associated with increased mortality and characteristic facial appearance.

Treatment consists of ursodeoxycholic acid (UDCA), given orally at a level of 20–30 mg/kg/day [20]. Response is variable. Pruritus may diminish or even disappear. Biliary diversion has not been very helpful in patients with Alagille syndrome. In one series, liver transplantation for hepatic decompensation was necessary in 21% (19/92) of patients [19]. Another study indicated that the most common factors contributing to the decision for transplantation were bone fractures, pruritus and severe xanthoma [21].

The 20-year predicted life expectancy is 75% for all patients, 80% for those not requiring liver transplantation and 60% for those who are transplanted.

Progressive familial intrahepatic cholestasis (PFIC)

PFIC is a useful term for a syndrome that consists of inheritable (possibly by an autosomal recessive mechanism) chronic progressive hepatocellular cholestasis. The characteristics are cholestasis and persistently low γ-glutamyl transpeptidase. The first reports of such involved the Byler kindred and the condition became known as Byler's disease (ByD). ByD is a disorder in which cholestasis of onset in infancy leads to hepatic fibrosis and death [22]. Children who have a clinically similar disorder, but are not members of the Amish community in which ByD was described, are said to have Byler syndrome (ByS). Controversy exists as to whether ByD and ByS (subtypes of PFIC) represent one clinicopathologic entity.

Recent molecular and genetic studies have identified genes responsible for three types of PFIC and have shown that the latter are related to mutations in hepatocellular transport system genes involved in bile formation. These findings now provide the basis for the investigation of children with PFIC and should allow prenatal diagnosis in the future. The gene for ByD has been mapped to a region of the 18q21–q22 chromosome. PFIC caused by a lesion in this region, including ByD, can be designated PFIC-1. This chromosomal region also harbors the locus for BRIC, a related phenotype. Linkage analysis in six consanguineous PFIC pedigrees from the Middle East has previously excluded linkage to chromosome 18q21–q22, indicating the existence of locus heterogeneity within the PFIC phenotype [23]. By use of homozygosity mapping and a genome scan in these pedigrees, a locus designated 'PFIC2' has been mapped to chromosome 2q24.

In a review of 84 liver biopsy specimens from 28 patients with PFIC [24], hepatocanalicular cholestasis and disruption of the liver cell plate arrangement were early, uniform findings. Giant cell transformation was found in 56% of initial biopsies. Duct loss was a prominent finding; 70% of patients had ductal paucity and many had abnormal bile duct epithelium, suggesting degeneration. Fibrosis was seen in the samples from 16 patients, including bridging fibrosis in specimens obtained from six patients during the first 2 years of life.

INHERITED AND METABOLIC HEPATOCELLULAR DISORDERS

ALPHA₁-ANTITRYPSIN DEFICIENCY

Alpha₁-antitrypsin (AAT), a glycoprotein synthesized in the liver, inhibits several proteolytic enzymes that can destroy certain tissues (Fig. 14.2). Its specificity is directed against elastase. AAT deficiency accounts for a significant number of infants with obstructive jaundice in the newborn period and is the commonest cause of chronic liver disease in childhood. Cirrhosis and carcinoma of the liver affect at least 25% of AAT-deficient adults over the age of 50 years. Its prevalence is comparable to that of cystic fibrosis (1:2000 to 1:7000).

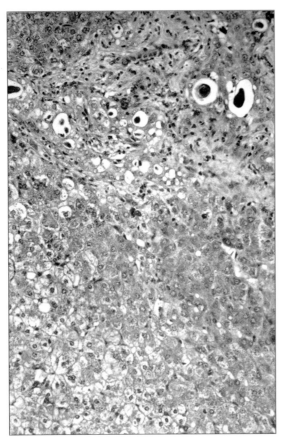

Figure 14.2 Alpha$_1$-antitrypsin deficiency: percutaneous liver biopsy from an infant 4 months of age who had been jaundiced from the third week of life (Pi phenotype PiZZ). Occupying part of the lower figure is a broad band of relatively acellular fibrous tissue which contains prominent bile ducts. No distinct portal tracts or hepatic veins are seen. The hepatocytes, in double cell plates which are normal in this age group, are deranged and cholestatic. The picture is compatible with cirrhosis. The infant died of liver failure at 9 months of age. With liver transplantation, the infant might have survived. Hematoxylin & eosin. (By permission of the late Alex Mowat, London.)

AAT is a major α_1-globulin that has been studied by various electrophoretic techniques. It migrates before albumin in acid starch gel electrophoresis, forming eight distinct bands. These bands have different speeds of migration depending on the protease inhibitor (Pi) system. The pattern seen in 95% of the normal population is that of an intermediate speed. Abnormal systems can move faster or slower. The phenotype nomenclature uses letters relating to the velocity of migration, e.g. PiMM for a homozygous normal, M being a letter from the center of the alphabet. F is used for fast-moving zones, and S and Z for slow-moving zones. Thus, we have patterns of abnormal AAT such as PiFF, PiSS and PiZZ, or any heterozygous combinations of these with the normal or with each other, e.g. PiSZ. The disease occurs as a result of inheritance of two protease inhibitor deficiency alleles from the *AAT* gene locus on chromosomal segment 14q32.1. The most common deficiency allele is PiZ and a large majority of individuals with severe AAT deficiency are Pi type ZZ. Yet, in a big Swedish screening survey (n = 200,000), it was found that only 47% of infants with the PiZ (or Pi nul) expression had abnormal liver function [25]. Hence, deficiency of AAT may lead to transient liver injury and, rarely, cirrhosis. A subsequent 8-year follow-up showed that the prognosis for PiZ infants with neonatal liver disease is more optimistic than was previously thought [26,27].

Prenatal diagnosis has been achieved by analysis of material obtained at amniocentesis or chorionic villus biopsy. Recombinant DNA technology has enabled the development of synthetic probes specific to the M and Z alleles. Liver disease in PiZZ children shows a strongly positive intrafamilial correlation; consequently, if one sibling is severely affected, the risk to a subsequent one is such that prenatal testing is justifiable.

Management depends on the degree of compromise. When cirrhosis develops, fluid and sodium restriction may become necessary. Ultimately, patients with cirrhosis will require a liver transplant.

WILSON'S DISEASE (HEPATOLENTICULAR DEGENERATION)

This rare inborn error of copper metabolism, inherited as an autosomal recessive trait, results in a potentially fatal liver and nervous system disorder. The carrier frequency is 1:200–1:500, with a disease prevalence of 1:66,000–1:100,000. It is seen mainly in whites. Although a very uncommon illness, pediatricians need to be aware of it because a delay in treatment is associated with the development of cirrhosis and irreversible neurological involvement. The Wilson's disease gene is localized on chromosome 13 and codes for a copper-transporting P-type ATPase, ATP7B [28]. About one hundred mutations occurring throughout the whole gene have been documented so far [29]. Molecular genetic testing is now the standard for investigating asymptomatic siblings.

Dietary copper is essential for a variety of enzymes such as cytochrome oxidase and dismutase as well as ceruloplasmin (the major binding protein of copper); however, if this metal accumulates excessively in the cells, it inhibits ATPase and may be deposited in many organs, especially the liver, brain, kidneys and eyes. The deposits of copper cause tissue damage, necrosis and scarring, which results in decreased functioning of the organs affected. Liver failure and damage to the central nervous system are the predominant, and most dangerous, effects of the disorder. Copper is deposited in the caudate–lenticular nuclei and in the cornea, forming Kayser–Fleischer rings, which are greenish brown in color [30]. There are also renotubular defects. The pathophysiology is that copper enters the cell but is unable to exit.

Symptoms

The onset of symptoms is rare under 6 years of age, but can present as early as 2 years. Some patients may have a transient cholestasis in the newborn period, which then will clear and reoccur at an older age. Modes of presentation are variable and include acute hepatitis, chronic liver disease, cirrhosis, hepatic failure, hemolytic anemia, neurological impairment [31], and psychiatric and behavioral abnormalities [32]. A fulminating form can appear as ascites and advance to hepatic coma. Central nervous system features can include clumsiness, poor handwriting, tremor, slurring of speech and athetosis. Any child presenting with a deteriorating scholastic performance at school must be considered as a possible case of Wilson's disease. Some children find their way to the psychiatrist because the organic diagnosis has eluded the clinician.

Diagnosis

This is based on the following [33]:

- Abnormal liver function tests

- Ophthalmoscopic examination by slit lamp to show Kayser–Fleischer rings within the limbus of both eyes (not always present)

- Urinary copper excretion following chelation challenge (1 g of penicillamine) – collect urine in copper-free containers; controls excrete less than 30–50 μg of copper per 24 h; values above 50 μg per 24 h are considered abnormal and frequently reach 1000 μg (12.5 μmol) per day in Wilson's disease

- Serum ceruloplasmin – this is usually low in Wilson's disease (<20 mg/dl; 1.25 μmol/l) but can be normal (25 mg/dl)

- Serum copper – this can be low in Wilson's disease (<20 μg/dl), but, as normal (60–160 μg/dl) or high values are also observed, it is of limited use in establishing the diagnosis

- Liver biopsy – histopathology will show cirrhosis, and the copper content exceeds 250 μg per gram dry weight; if there has been no chronic cholestasis, a hepatic copper concentration greater than 400 μg/g is diagnostic

Treatment

Drinking water should be analyzed because of copper pipes. If the copper content is greater than 0.1 mg/l, distilled or bottled water should be used. Alternatively, potassium sulfide, 30–40 mg three times a day, will bind intestinal copper.

Chelation therapy is very effective and must be continued indefinitely. D-Penicillamine, 10 mg/kg/day increased after 2 weeks to 20 mg/kg/day in divided doses before meals, will cause copper and zinc to be excreted in the urine. Patients intolerant of penicillamine can be chelated with triethylene tetramine hydrochloride, 25 mg/kg/day in three divided doses. Another option is zinc sulfate, which is seemingly non-toxic. Penicillamine can cause leukopenia, immune complex nephritis, nephrotic syndrome, a lupus-like syndrome and hemolytic anemia. Pyridoxine (5–10 mg/day) should be given to prevent vitamin B$_6$ deficiency. Supplemental iron is indicated because chelation is non-selective and will remove iron as well as copper, zinc and other metals.

Dietary management

The dietary copper should be restricted to the safe and adequate quantity recommended by the National Academy of Sciences (Appendix II.14). This ranges from 0.5–1.0 mg for infants to 1.0–3.0 mg daily for older children. In practice, this means that, during chelation therapy, the patient can have a fairly normal diet although avoiding foods with a particularly high

Wheatbran	Dried fruits	Malted-milk-type beverages
Wholemeal bread	Olives	Egg yolk
Wholegrain cereals	Nuts	Shellfish
Peas	Cocoa	Game meats (e.g. pheasant, hare, venison)
Beans	Chocolate	Meat and meat extracts
Lentils	Liquorice	Stock cubes
Mushrooms	Fruit gums and pastilles	Sauces and ketchup

Note: Block salt, iodized and sea salt may contain copper; table salt should be used instead.
Water from copper pipes (or other sources likely to be contaminated) containing more than 0.1 mg/l should be avoided, and distilled or mineral water used.

Table 14.8 Foods with a high copper content.

copper content. Examples of such foods are given in Table 14.8. The copper content of milks and formulas is given in Table 14.9. It should be noted that infant formulas, particularly those formulated for premature infants, have a high copper content and hence may need to be avoided in neonates who are suspected of having the disease.

Prevention
Siblings of patients should be investigated.

Prognosis
If untreated, all patients will eventually die unless given a liver transplant.

DEFECTS OF TYROSINE METABOLISM
Tyrosine in plasma is derived from the amino acid phenylalanine and dietary proteins (Fig. 14.4). Disorders of tyrosine metabolism may arise from inherited enzyme deficiencies or as the result of liver damage. Secondary disturbances of tyrosine metabolism can be associated with untreated galactosemia or fructosemia.

Neonatal tyrosinemia
Neonatal tyrosinemia is a disorder due to reduced hepatic p-hydroxyphenylpyruvate oxidase activity and is seen in preterm infants. A high protein intake (>5 g/kg/day) represents too large a tyrosine load. This phenomenon is usually transient and will respond to a lower protein regimen (2–2.6 g/kg/day) or to ascorbic acid (50–100 mg/day), the cofactor of p-hydroxyphenylpyruvate oxidase. Although the outlook is very good, impaired mental development has been described.

Hereditary tyrosinemia
Hereditary tyrosinemia (a better term than 'tyrosinosis') may present in an acute or chronic manner. In the acute type, which is seen in the first year of life, there is often hepatomegaly, anorexia, vomiting and diarrhea. Later, jaundice may develop and progressive liver failure occur. Hepatomas may arise in those who do not die from liver failure. The chronic type is seen later in infancy or childhood with cirrhosis and renal tubular lesions causing

Milk	Copper content (mg Cu per 100 ml milk)
Human breast milk (mature)	0.04
Cow milk	0.02
Infant formula (whey-based)	0.05
Premature formula	0.07

Table 14.9 Copper content of milk and formulas.

hypophosphatemic rickets. Plasma concentrations of tyrosine and phenylalanine are elevated, with or without increased levels of methionine. Excessive amounts of tyrosine metabolites (mainly *p*-hydroxyphenyl-lactic acid and succinyl acetone) will be found in the urine. Renal tubular damage causes generalized aminoaciduria, glycosuria, proteinuria and phosphaturia. Hypoglycemia is common.

The site of the enzyme block is not completely understood. The accumulating metabolites imply two distinct enzyme deficiencies. It is thought that the fulminating neonatal presentation may occur with a relatively larger deficit of the distal enzyme (from tyrosine), fumarylacetoacetase, while the chronic disorder may be accompanied by a greater deficiency of *p*-hydroxyphenylpyruvate oxidase (much closer to tyrosine), which limits the amount of substrate reaching the second block (fumarylacetoacetase). The diagnosis can be established by assaying one of the compounds that has accumulated because of the metabolic block (e.g. succinyl acetone). Prenatal diagnosis is now possible by determination of fumarylacetoacetase in cultured amniotic fluid cells.

The introduction of the pharmacologic agent NTBC holds the hope of significantly alleviating some of the burdens of this disease [34]. Other potential modalities include self-induced correction of the genetic defect [35].

REYE'S SYNDROME

Reye's syndrome refers to an acute non-infectious encephalopathy and hepatomegaly. Pathologically, there is fatty infiltration of the liver. Small lipid droplets are seen through the lobule and there are significant ultrastructural changes within the mitochondria. However, inflammation is minimal and there is no cholestasis. When first described, Reye's syndrome was associated with a high mortality rate (>50%); consequently, there is now heightened professional and parental awareness of this disease. Early diagnosis is associated with a better prognosis. The age range is 3 months to 16 years and invariably there has been an antecedent or accompanying illness such as a mild respiratory infection (influenza-like) or chickenpox. Any child with severe vomiting, drowsiness and an enlarged liver must be regarded as a possible case.

The most important development in the understanding of Reye's syndrome is the observation of a dose–response relation between the risk of Reye's syndrome and the amount

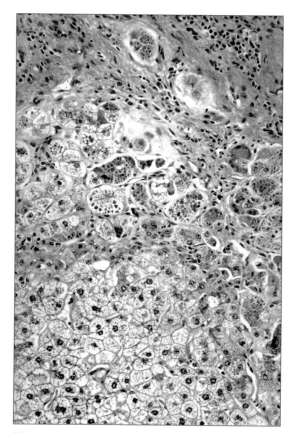

Figure 14.3 Alpha$_1$-antitrypsin deficiency. Features of a mild inflammatory infiltrate are present with expansion of the portal area with fibrosis. Globules of the anomalous alpha$_1$-antitrypsin are seen deposited prominently in peri-portal hepatocytes.

of aspirin ingested during the antecedent illness. Additional evidence for this association is provided by the marked decline in the use of aspirin among children in the USA, which has been accompanied by a dramatic fall in the incidence of Reye's syndrome there. In contrast to experience in the USA, Reye's syndrome affecting primarily children aged 5–15 years has been relatively rare in the UK and Australia, where acetaminophen rather than aspirin is the primary analgesic/antipyretic used. With the declining use of aspirin in the USA, the incidence of Reye's syndrome among children aged 5–15 years for 1982 was only 0.33 cases per 100,000 population; in 1988, only 20 cases were reported. During 1991–1994, there were an estimated 284 hospitalizations, giving an annual incidence of 0.2–1.1 cases per million population aged less than 18 years in the USA [36].

PATHOLOGY AND PATHOPHYSIOLOGY

Liver biopsy will show diffuse, severe, microvesicular fatty infiltration. Necrosis and inflammation are absent or minimally present; however, electron microscopy reveals expansion of the mitochondrial matrix, loss of matrix density and dense bodies and irregularities of the limiting membrane.

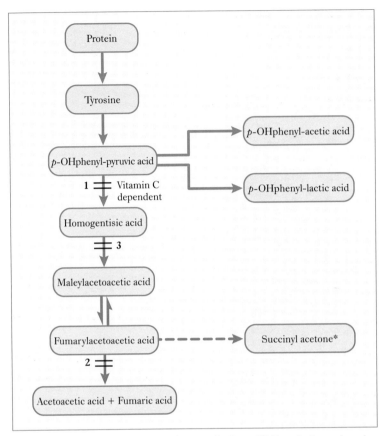

Figure 14.4 Inborn errors of tyrosine metabolism. (1) Para-hydroxyphenylpyruvate oxidase deficiency in transient neonatal tyrosinemia. Overcome in premature infants with vitamin C and a reduction in protein intake. (2) Fumarylacetoacetase deficiency present in hereditary tyrosinemia together with block (1). The accumulating metabolites are marked *. (3) The block in alkaptonuria – the first inborn error to be studied and described by Garrod in 1909.

SYMPTOMS

Typically, the disease presents acutely in a previously well child who is recovering from an upper respiratory tract infection or varicella. Vomiting is the dominant feature. Usually, the child is anicteric but there is hepatomegaly. Tachypnea or apnea may occur. Hyperventilation of central origin can result in respiratory alkalosis. Neurological sequelae range from lethargy to coma; seizures may develop, particularly in young children.

Clinical staging of hepatic encephalopathy is as follows:

- Grade 1 – lethargic
- Grade 2 – agitated
- Grade 3 – decorticate
- Grade 4 – decerebrate
- Grade 5 – flaccid

DIAGNOSIS AND LABORATORY FINDINGS

In addition to the findings of an encephalopathy and enlarged liver, the following are strongly indicative of the diagnosis:

- Sterile cerebrospinal fluid (<10 white cells/ml)

- Elevated serum hepatocellular enzymes (AST, ALT)

- Blood ammonia over 1.5 times normal (well above 100 μg/dl)

- Prolonged prothrombin time (greater than two standard deviations from the mean)

- Hypoglycemia is a common but not constant finding and the serum bilirubin is usually less than 68 μmol/l (4.0 mg/dl)

If the diagnosis is in question, a liver biopsy will confirm the syndrome (see above).

TREATMENT AND PROGNOSIS

Cases of Reye's syndrome must be managed in highly specialized, preferably pediatric, units. Supportive measures include correction of hypoglycemia and of the hyperammonemia. Monitoring intracranial pressure with a bolt helps prevent irreversible brain damage. Of survivors, 34–61% have a permanent neuropsychiatric disorder. If a recurrence arises, it is important to exclude ornithine transcarbamylase and carbamyl phosphate deficiency because these biochemical disorders have caused Reye-like syndromes. Outcome is related to the depth of coma as well as blood ammonia levels. Few who reach stage IV coma (i.e. deep coma unresponsive to painful stimuli) will survive.

DIETARY MANAGEMENT OF HEPATITIS AND ACUTE LIVER DISEASE

In the absence of hyperammonemia or ascites, the aim of dietary treatment is to maintain the nutritional status.

The provision of an adequate energy intake is of prime importance, with carbohydrate providing at least 60% of the energy. In the presence of severe cholestasis, there may be steatorrhea and diarrhea and a low-fat diet will be beneficial. Jaundice in itself does not mean that a low-fat diet is needed. Fat intake should only be reduced if feeding gives rise to abdominal pain or if steatorrhea is so severe that the patient is unable to gain weight. If a low-fat diet is prescribed, the energy deficit should be compensated for by an increased use of glucose polymers or by the introduction of medium-chain triglycerides (MCTs). Some infant formulas, such as Portagen or Pregestimil (Appendix IV.7), include MCTs. The protein intake in uncomplicated hepatitis should be moderate for the size of the child based on the UK/USA recommendations for weight. Hypoalbuminemia is not an indication for a high-protein diet because of the risks of hyperammonemia and hyperaminoacidemia. A moderate protein intake with a high energy content should result in the correction of low albumin levels. Whenever possible, infants should continue to be given breast milk, in addition to an MCT formula, because of the immunological benefits.

In severe cases, because of anorexia or feeding intolerance, infants may require enteral nutrition delivered via a nasogastric tube as a bolus or constant infusion, and older children dietary supplements in the form of drinks, or nasogastric supplements. Examples of drinks for older children are given in Appendix IV.13 and those providing an energy supplement in the form of glucose are listed in Appendix IV.19. A formula containing a protein hydrolysate (Appendix IV.5) may be beneficial.

Whenever a patient with acute liver disease is too sick (emesis, fullness, discomfort, unconsciousness) to receive nutrition through the enteral route, intravenous nutrition should be implemented.

LIVER DISEASE DUE TO PARENTERAL NUTRITION

Hepatic dysfunction is a common metabolic complication of parenteral nutrition in infants and this is caused by intrahepatic cholestasis [37]. Although the underlying mechanism of this is not completely known, it probably involves a number of factors, including imbalances of administered nutrients, and seems to be related to infection. Hepatic dysfunction is nearly always self-limited and resolves following cessation of parenteral nutrition. However, in some cases it progresses to cirrhosis and, if the patient does not receive a transplant, can prove fatal.

CIRRHOSIS

Cirrhosis describes a histopathologic change and is the end-stage of chronic hepatic disease in which there is widespread irreversible liver damage, fibrosis and the presence of regenerating nodules to replace normally arranged hepatocytes. It may be of unknown cause or secondary to extrahepatic biliary atresia, hepatitis, cystic fibrosis, Wilson's disease, galactosemia, α_1-antitrypsin deficiency, hemochromatosis or congenital (hepatic fibrosis). Cirrhosis can be a consequence of prolonged intravenous nutrition or drugs such as methotrexate, used for treatment of leukemia or juvenile rheumatoid arthritis [38].

Clinical features

Signs of chronic liver failure and portal hypertension are the chief characteristics. Hematemesis from bleeding esophageal varices could be the presenting symptom. Physical signs will depend upon the underlying cause, e.g. Kayser–Fleischer rings in Wilson's disease; pulmonary disease in cystic fibrosis; acne and striae in chronic active hepatitis. Hepatic coma (portal systemic encephalopathy) can be precipitated by:

- Gastrointestinal bleeding
- Renal failure
- Excessive dietary protein
- Infection
- Constipation
- Diuretics
- Sedation

Diagnosis

Imaging (ultrasound, computerized tomography or magnetic resonance imaging) can provide some indication of an altered hepatic density or even fibrosis. Biopsy is the principal means of diagnosis. Although liver function tests may be normal, elevation of the transaminases and γ-globulin with hypoalbuminemia are commonly seen in cirrhosis. Several non-invasive tests have been developed to assess the functional aspects of the hepatocytes, but none has proved to be practical, inexpensive and reliable.

MEDICAL AND SURGICAL MANAGEMENT OF CHRONIC LIVER DISEASE

Prevention of bleeding from esophageal varices requires neutralization of gastric pH in patients with gastroesophageal reflux and avoidance of medications such as acetylsalicylic acid. Propranolol has been shown to be effective in the avoidance of the first bleeding episode but less effective in preventing rebleeding. Endoscopic banding and sclerosis of esophageal varices are the methods of choice to treat bleeding sites and to prevent rebleeding [39]. In the presence of hypersplenism, thrombocytopenia may arise. Because of this and impaired coagulation resulting from reduced activity of vitamin K-dependent factors, therapy with vitamin K (5–10 mg) should be considered in patients with cholestasis. If ascites is present, an aldosterone antagonist such as spironolactone (3 mg/kg/day) will mobilize the ascitic fluid. In the presence of tense ascites, paracentesis will reduce both the respiratory and abdominal distress. If large volumes of ascitic fluid are removed, infusion of albumin is recommended to avoid rapid re-accumulation and pre-renal kidney failure. Such fluid frequently becomes infected and the patients present with atypical symptoms of peritonitis (abdominal discomfort, fever, worsening of the cholestasis or clotting abnormalities). Whenever portal hypertension becomes unmanageable, there are several procedures available: portocaval shunt, mesocaval shunt or a transjugular intrahepatic portosystemic shunt (TIPS).

Hepatocyte transplantation

Hepatocyte transplantation has been attempted in patients with end-stage liver disease and certain liver-based metabolic disorders [40] such as Crigler–Najjar syndrome type I [41], urea cycle defects and familial hypercholesterolemia. The rationale behind the technique is that donated hepatocytes will support the failing liver, thus bridging patients to whole organ transplantation or, in some cases, avoiding transplantation while the native liver regenerates. The transplanted cells produce the missing enzyme in patients with inborn errors of metabolism, correcting the underlying defect. The advantages of hepatocyte transplantation over the conventional method are:

- Non-surgical procedure
- Better utilization of donor organs, as cells from one donor could be used for more than a single patient
- Native liver is still present as a safety net
- Future option of gene therapy, as the native liver cells will be available for genetic manipulation
- Much cheaper procedure

The hepatocytes are isolated from donor livers not used for transplantation. The donated cells are transplanted as a suspension into the portal vein via a transhepatic approach and integrate into the recipient liver cell plates. Liver cells have to be blood-group matched and there is also a need for lifelong immunosuppression as in conventional liver transplantation.

NUTRITIONAL MANAGEMENT OF CHRONIC LIVER DISEASE

Energy

The energy intake in all forms of liver disease needs to be generous in order to protect the damaged organ from the effects of tissue catabolism. The UK or USA energy recommendations for age should be used, even if the child is small for chronological age. Carbohydrate is generally well tolerated and should be used as the major energy source; generous carbohydrate will alleviate hypoglycemia. Glucose polymers can be incorporated into drinks and food or given *per se* as a drink (Appendix IV.19).

Lipids may be malabsorbed: MCTs, whose absorption is independent of bile salts, can be used to replace up to 75% of ordinary dietary fat. The introduction of MCT as a milk formula for infants is described in Appendix IV.17. For older children, a water-miscible MCT emulsion can be used in drinks or MCT oil in cooking, though care must still be taken to introduce these products slowly in order to avoid gastrointestinal symptoms. A recipe for a suitable high-energy drink incorporating MCTs is given in Appendix IV.9. If there is portal hypertension and shunting of the products of digestion into the systemic circulation, MCTs should be used with caution as they might induce ketosis.

Protein

Protein intake should depend upon the clinical findings. Where there is a low serum albumin, a moderately high protein intake may be indicated using UK/USA recommendations for age. A higher protein load should be used with caution and reduced if the blood ammonia rises or hepatic coma develops. When tissue catabolism is increased, a low-protein diet may be necessary and intakes similar to the WHO recommendations for weight (Appendix I) can be followed. As a last resort, a minimum protein diet as described in Appendix V.11 can be used for short periods.

For adults with hepatic failure, supplementation of low-protein diets with branched-chain amino acids has achieved some success. Some of the symptoms of encephalopathy are thought to be due to the passage of aromatic amino acids across the blood–brain barrier; branched-chain amino acids inhibit the transport of aromatic amino acids. While few improvements in psychometric parameters have been described, it has been suggested that nutritional status is profited by this type of supplementation, due to the increase in the total nitrogen intake. As most children with long-standing liver disease are malnourished, they may benefit from the use of such supplements, but this is as yet unproven.

Sodium

If ascites is present, reduction of the dietary sodium intake to 10–20 mmol a day may be indicated. Details of the sodium content of foods are given in Appendix V.4. However, with advanced liver disease, patients are usually anorexic and there may be difficulty in persuading the child to consume any food if salt restriction is severe. Children with ascites require frequent small feeds or meals throughout much of the day and night where practical, due to the discomfort caused by gastric distension.

Vitamins and minerals

The problems of children requiring a modified diet for hepatic disease are very similar to those with chronic renal failure.

Supplementation with fat-soluble vitamins is very important and includes: vitamin A (5000–15,000 IU/day), vitamin E (100–500 mg/day), vitamin D (Alfacalcidol in the UK, Calcitriol in the USA; 50 ng/kg daily) and vitamin K (1–10 mg/day). Iron or blood is indicated if hypochromic anemia is present secondary to blood loss.

Fat-soluble vitamins are poorly absorbed if there is lipid malabsorption, and double the normal supplement of vitamins A and D may be needed. The requirement for vitamin D is increased not only as a consequence of impaired absorption but also because much of the vitamin is converted into the inactive hydroxylated cholecalciferol. In addition, if barbiturates are used, requirements for vitamin D are further elevated because of the enzyme induction property of such medications. Large doses of vitamin D (e.g. 1.25–5 mg/day) may be needed to correct osteomalacia (rickets).

Malabsorption and deficiency of vitamin E causing neurological degeneration are common consequences of chronic cholestatic liver disease in childhood and constitute a major problem. Data suggest that low intraluminal bile acid concentrations are the cause. The frequency of biochemical vitamin E deficiency and of the clinical signs of the associated neurological syndrome were studied in children with chronic forms of intrahepatic neonatal cholestasis and with extrahepatic biliary atresia [42]. Based on serum vitamin E concentrations and the ratios of serum vitamin E to total serum lipid concentration, 64% of the intrahepatic and 77% of the extrahepatic cholestasis groups were classified as vitamin E deficient. Prior to age 1 year, neurological function was normal in all children. Between ages 1 and 3 years, neurological abnormalities were present in approximately 50% of the vitamin E-deficient children; after age 3 years, neurological abnormalities were present in all vitamin E-deficient children. Areflexia was the first abnormality to develop between the ages of 1 and 4 years; truncal and limb ataxia, peripheral neuropathy and ophthalmoplegia developed in those aged from 3 to 6 years. Neurological dysfunction progressed to a disabling combination of findings by the age of 8–10 years in the majority of vitamin E-deficient children.

The long-term efficacy and safety of d-α-tocopheryl polyethylene glycol 1000 succinate (TPGS) in correcting vitamin E deficiency has been investigated in 60 children with chronic cholestasis who were unresponsive to oral vitamin E (70–212 IU/kg/day) [43]. All children responded to TPGS with normalization of vitamin E status. Neurological function, which had deteriorated before entry in the trial, improved in 25 patients, stabilized in 27, and worsened in only two, after a mean of 2.5 years of therapy. Thus, TPGS (20–25 IU/kg/day) appears to be a safe and effective form of vitamin E for reversing or preventing vitamin E deficiency during chronic childhood cholestasis.

REFERENCES

1. Ryder SD, Beckingham IJ. ABC of diseases of liver, pancreas, and biliary system: acute hepatitis. BMJ 2001;322:151–3.

2. Chang MH, Shau WY, Chen CJ et al. Hepatitis B vaccination and hepatocellular carcinoma rates in boys and girls. JAMA 2000;284:3040–2.

3. Narkewicz MR, Smith D, Silverman A et al. Clearance of chronic hepatitis B virus infection in young children after alpha interferon treatment. J Pediatr 1995;127:815–8.

4. Bortolotti F, Jara P, Barbera C et al. Long term effect of alpha interferon in children with chronic hepatitis B. Gut 2000;46:715–8.

5. Ballauff A, Schneider T, Gerner P et al. Safety and efficacy of interferon retreatment in children with chronic hepatitis B. Eur J Pediatr 1998;157:382–5.

6. Ozen H, Kocak N, Yuce A et al. Retreatment with higher dose interferon alpha in children with chronic hepatitis B infection. Pediatr Infect Dis J 1999;18:694–7.

7. Foster GR, Chapman R. Combination treatment for hepatitis C is not being given. BMJ 2000;321:899

8. Darby SC, Ewart DW, Giangrande PL et al. Mortality from liver cancer and liver disease in haemophilic men and boys in UK given blood products contaminated with hepatitis C. Lancet 1997;350:1425–31.

9. Nowicki MJ, Balistreri WF. The hepatitis C virus: identification, epidemiology, and clinical controversies. J Pediatr Gastroenterol Nutr 1995;20:248–74.

10. Poynard T, Marcellin P, Lee SS et al. Randomised trial of interferon alpha2b plus ribavirin for 48 weeks or for 24 weeks versus interferon alpha2b plus placebo for 48 weeks for treatment of chronic infection with hepatitis C virus. International Hepatitis Interventional Therapy Group. Lancet 1998;352:1426–32.

11. Davis GL. Treatment of chronic hepatitis C. BMJ, 2001;323:1141-2.

12. Fried MW, Shiffman ML, Reddy RK et al. Pegylated (40 kDa) (PEGASYS) interferon alfa-2a in combination with ribavirin: efficacy and safety results from a phase III, randomized, actively-controlled, multicenter study (abstract). Gastroenterology 2001;120:A55.

13. Chen HL, Chang MH, Ni YH et al. Hepatitis G virus infection in normal and prospectively followed posttransfusion children. Pediatr Res 1997;42:784–7.

14. Balistreri WF, Grand R, Hoofnagle JH et al. Biliary atresia: current concepts and research directions. Summary of a symposium. Hepatology 1996;23:1682–92.

15. Bates MD, Bucuvalas JC, Alonso MH et al. Biliary atresia: pathogenesis and treatment. Semin Liver Dis 1998;18:281–93.

16. Otte JB, de Ville de Goyet J, Reding R et al. Sequential treatment of biliary atresia with Kasai portoenterostomy and liver transplantation: a review. Hepatology 1994;20:41S–48S.

17. Ryckman FC, Alonso MH, Bucuvalas JC et al. Biliary atresia – surgical management and treatment options as they relate to outcome. Liver Transpl Surg 1998;4:S24–33.

18. Oda T, Elkahloun AG, Pike BL et al. Mutations in the human Jagged1 gene are responsible for Alagille syndrome. Nat Genet 1997;16:235–42.

19. Emerick KM, Rand EB, Goldmuntz E et al. Features of Alagille syndrome in 92 patients: frequency and relation to prognosis. Hepatology 1999;29:822–9.

20. Balistreri WF. Bile acid therapy in pediatric hepatobiliary disease: the role of ursodeoxycholic acid. J Pediatr Gastroenterol Nutr 1997;24:573–89.

21. Hoffenberg EJ, Narkewicz MR, Sondheimer JM et al. Outcome of syndromic paucity of interlobular bile ducts (Alagille syndrome) with onset of cholestasis in infancy. J Pediatr 1995;127:220–4.

22. Bull LN, Carlton VE, Stricker NL et al. Genetic and morphological findings in progressive familial intrahepatic cholestasis (Byler disease [PFIC-1] and Byler syndrome): evidence for heterogeneity. Hepatology 1997;26:155–64.

23. Strautnieks SS, Kagalwalla AF, Tanner MS et al. Identification of a locus for progressive familial intrahepatic cholestasis PFIC2 on chromosome 2q24. Am J Hum Genet 1997;61:630–3.

24. Alonso EM, Snover DC, Montag A et al. Histologic pathology of the liver in progressive familial intrahepatic cholestasis. J Pediatr Gastroenterol Nutr 1994;18:128–33.

25. Sveger T. Liver disease in alpha-1-antitrypsin deficiency detected by screening of 200 000 infants. N Engl J Med 1976;294:1316–21.

26. Sveger T. Prospective study of children with α-1-antitrypsin deficiency: eight-year-old follow-up. J Pediatr 1984;104:91–4.

27. Sveger T. The natural history of liver disease in alpha-1-antitrypsin deficient children. Acta Paediatr Scand 1988;77:847–51.

28. Cox DW. Review: molecular approaches to inherited liver disease. Focus on Wilson disease. J Gastroenterol Hepatol 1997;12:S251–5.

29. Riordan SM, Williams R. The Wilson's disease gene and phenotypic diversity. J Hepatol 2001;34:165–71.

30. Rodman R, Burnstine M, Esmaeli B et al. Wilson's disease: presymptomatic patients and Kayser-Fleischer rings. Ophthalmic Genet 1997;18:79–85.

31. Schlaug G, Hefter H, Engelbrecht V et al. Neurological impairment and recovery in Wilson's disease: evidence from PET and MRI. J Neurol Sci 1996;136:129–39.

32. Akil M, Brewer GJ. Psychiatric and behavioral abnormalities in Wilson's disease. Adv Neurol 1995;65:171–8.

33. Brewer GJ. Recognition, diagnosis, and management of Wilson's disease. Proc Soc Exp Biol Med 2000;223:39–46.

34. Russo PA, Mitchell GA, Tanguay RM. Tyrosinemia: a review. Pediatr Dev Pathol 2001;4:212–21.

35. Holme E, Lindstedt S. Diagnosis and management of tyrosinemia type I. Curr Opin Pediatr 1995;7:726–32.

36. Sullivan KM, Belay AD, Durbin RE et al. Epidemiology of Reye's syndrome, United States, 1991–1994: comparison of CDC surveillance and hospital admission data. Neuroepidemiology 2000;19:338–44.

37. Balistreri WF, Bove KE. Hepatobiliary consequences of parenteral alimentation. Prog Liver Dis 1990;9:567–601.

38. Hashkes PJ, Balistreri WF, Bove KE et al. The long-term effect of methotrexate therapy on the liver in patients with juvenile rheumatoid arthritis. Arthritis Rheum 1997;40:2226–34.

39. Price MR, Sartorelli KH, Karrer FM et al. Management of esophageal varices in children by endoscopic variceal ligation. J Pediatr Surg 1996;31:1056–9.

40. Strom SC, Chowdhury JR, Fox IJ. Hepatocyte transplantation for the treatment of human disease. Semin Liver Dis 1999;19:39–48.

41. Fox IJ, Chowdhury JR, Kaufman SS et al. Treatment of the Crigler–Najjar syndrome type I with hepatocyte transplantation. N Engl J Med 1998;338:1422–6.

42. Sokol RJ, Guggenheim MA, Heubi JE et al. Frequency and clinical progression of the vitamin E deficiency neurologic disorder in children with prolonged neonatal cholestasis. Am J Dis Child 1985;139:1211–5.

43. Sokol RJ, Butler-Simon N, Conner C et al. Multicenter trial of d-alpha-tocopheryl polyethylene glycol 1000 succinate for treatment of vitamin E deficiency in children with chronic cholestasis. Gastroenterology 1993;104:1727–35.

chapter 15

Pancreatic Exocrine Insufficiency

CYSTIC FIBROSIS

Cystic fibrosis (CF) is a multi-organ disease that is characterized by the triad of malabsorption, failure to thrive and chronic sinopulmonary infections. The many potential features of CF include pancreatic insufficiency (approximately 85%), liver dysfunction (15–30%) and raised concentrations of sodium and chloride in the sweat (Table 15.1), as well as obstructive azoospermia in postpubertal males. In the past decade, a cascade of long-awaited developments in molecular research has resulted in the identification of the so-called CF gene. Cloning of this gene has fostered the recognition of a broader disease spectrum [19].

LIFE EXPECTANCY

CF is the most common chronic hereditary disease in whites that is potentially lethal. Fifty years ago, only one baby in five with this condition survived the first years of life. Earlier diagnosis and better management, however, have extended survival considerably in the USA, Canada, Australia and the UK (Fig. 15.1a). For affected children born in 1990 in the UK, the median life expectancy was estimated at 40 years, double that of those born in the 1970s (Fig. 15.1b) [20]. Surveys have shown that longevity is associated with attendance at specialized centers, leading to the WHO and the International Cystic Fibrosis Association endorsing such establishments.

EPIDEMIOLOGY

This life-limiting recessively inherited disorder is seen in about 1:2000 live births in most Western European countries and in 1:3200 neonates in the United States. In UK whites, one in 20 carries the CF gene; therefore, theoretically, in one in 400 couples both of the partners will be carriers. In African-Americans, one survey demonstrated that the prevalence of CF was only 1:17,000 [21]; another, using the CF Foundation National Registry, found it to be 1:15,000 [22]. The figure ranges from 1:377 in Brittany [23], through 1:620 in south-west Africa [24] and 1:640 in the American Amish, to 1:90,000 in Hawaii [25].

PATHOGENESIS

The disease is caused by a mutation of the cystic fibrosis transmembrane conductance regulator (CFTR) gene, which is present on the long arm of chromosome 7. This CF gene

Feature	Comments
Failure to thrive	Malabsorption occurs in approximately 85% of patients and is due to defective production of pancreatic amylase, trypsin, chymotrypsin, lipase (and co-lipase) and bicarbonate; those with sufficient pancreatic enzymes may eventually become insufficient; there is a close correlation between ΔF508 and pancreatic insufficiency
Salty sweat	This observation has, in rare instances, resulted in a carer suspecting the diagnosis
Bulky, very malodorous stools	The classic stools are seen in older infants and children, while in younger patients the feces are watery and foul-smelling; this feature is also seen in celiac disease, Shwachman–Diamond syndrome, lipase deficiency, enterokinase deficiency, etc.
Heat stroke	Suggestive of CF although less so in hot climates
Raised intracranial pressure and night blindness	Due to vitamin A deficiency
Hemolytic anemia	Due to vitamin E deficiency; characteristically occurs in newly diagnosed cases
Bruising and bleeding	Due to vitamin K deficiency
Edema	Results from hypoproteinemia; seen in 5–15% of infants (especially in newly diagnosed cases)
Ear, nose and throat	Purulent sinusitis, mild conductive hearing loss (27%); nasal polyps (histologically different from non-CF polyps) seen in 18% of patients aged >6 months
Skin reactions and atopy	Many CF patients have a history of adverse reactions to various allergens, including house dust, June grass (US) and ragweed, with both positive skin testing and a raised IgE; >50% have a positive reaction to *Aspergillus fumigatus*
Delayed puberty and retarded growth	Delayed puberty is seen in males and females – linked with both poor nutrition and the impaired respiratory reserve; menarche begins 1–2 years later than in non-CF subjects; amenorrhea is associated with advanced pulmonary disease and malnutrition
	Growth failure, though not inevitable, is associated with difficulty in achieving adequate nutritional requirements because of suboptimal intake, malabsorption and poor nutrient utilization
Chronic pain	In the last 6 months of life there is a high incidence of headaches (55%), chest pain (65%), back pain (19%), abdominal pain (19%) and limb pain (16%) [1]; pain is due to hypercarbia, hypoxia, migraine, sinusitis, pleurisy and musculoskeletal joint sources [2,3]
Psychosexual problems/quality-of-life issues	Consequences of a chronic, disabling and demanding disease with a high risk and trauma/stress of organ transplantation
Gastrointestinal tract/biliary tree and hepatic aspects of CF	
Meconium peritonitis	If the bowel of the fetus is perforated from meconium, then ileus and peritonitis develop; the peritoneal cavity may calcify and be evident radiologically
Meconium plug syndrome	Seen in 10–20% of CF cases
Meconium ileus	This is the earliest (non-*in-utero*) gastrointestinal manifestation of CF; one in five cases present with this feature; meconium has a high albumin content and reduced water concentration; atresia and volvulus may be associated with meconium obstruction

Distal intestinal obstruction syndrome (DIOS) – formerly known as a 'meconium ileus equivalent'	Occurs in 10–40% of patients; seen in adolescents and adults when viscous stools form in the ileum, cecum and proximal colon to obstruct the bowel; may be difficult to distinguish from other conditions such as fibrosing colonopathy
Celiac disease	Increased incidence in CF – prevalence of 1:75 in some white communities
Lactose intolerance	The disaccharidase value in CF reflects the normal ethnic and age-related distribution
Giardiasis	Increased incidence (28%) in CF
Gastroesophageal reflux	Significantly more common in CF, including the newly diagnosed [4]; seen in >25% and often associated with esophagitis; symptoms are non-specific and the patient may present with deteriorating lung disease
Crohn's disease	Prevalence of 1:404 cases (=11 times greater than in non-CF subjects) [5]
Intussusception	Occurs in 1%; regarded as a complication of DIOS
Vitamin B_{12} malabsorption	Very rare in CF
Cancer of the gastrointestinal tract	With increasing survival, there is now evidence of a rise in digestive tract cancers [6]
Rectal prolapse	Seen in 18.5%; precedes the diagnosis of CF in 43% of cases
Fibrosing colonopathy [7]	There is an apparent dose-related association between high-content pancreatic lipase microspheres and this recently described serious colonic condition [8–10]; lipase must be between 500 and 2500 units/kg per meal [11] – for infants, 2000–4000 lipase units per 120 ml of formula or breast milk; a toxic effect from Eudragit L30D-55 enteric-coated pancreatin (a methacrylic acid and ethyl acrylate copolymer) might be the causative agent [12,13]; thickness of the CF colon, as determined by ultrasound, is age related [14]; bowel wall thickening is said to predict colonopathy
Pancreatic exocrine insufficiency	Steatorrhea, failure to thrive
Pancreatic endocrine insufficiency	30% have glucose intolerance but diabetes mellitus is seen in 13% of those aged >25 years – at this stage there is fatty degeneration of islets of Langerhans; there is also insufficient secretion of a stimulator of insulin production – a gastric inhibitory peptide; glycosylated hemoglobin A1c is elevated before the development of diabetes mellitus
Recurrent pancreatitis	Eventually, pancreatic insufficiency may develop; in adults (American whites) there is a strong association between mutations in the *CFTR* gene and idiopathic pancreatitis [15]
Biliary and liver disease	
Liver diseases	Focal biliary cirrhosis (40%); portal hypertension (5%); esophageal varices
	Multilobular biliary cirrhosis (<10%); CF patients with pancreatic insufficiency and mutations associated with a severe or a variable genotype (G85E and/or 5T allele) are at an increased risk of liver disease [16]
	Prolonged jaundice in neonates (inspissated plugs) – infantile cholestasis associated with meconium ileus [17]
Biliary tree	Non-functioning small gallbladder in 30–50%; bile acid malabsorption because of reduced bile pool; cholelithiasis in <10% – risk increases with age (seen in 24% of CF adults at postmortem); distended gallbladder (20%)
Renal tract	Increased urinary excretion of oxalate and glycolate – both products of vitamin C metabolism [18]

Table 15.1 Features of cystic fibrosis.

product, comprising 1480 amino acids, functions as a cyclic adenosine monophosphate (cAMP)-regulated chloride channel at the apical surface of epithelial cells (Fig. 15.2). It is therefore involved in the secondary process of sodium and water reabsorption mechanisms. The commonest mutation of CFTR – occurring in 70% of cases [26] – is known as ΔF508; however, in all there are more than 500 recognized mutations of this gene. In some cases of CF, CFTR is absent; in others, it fails to reach the cell membranes or is dysfunctional even when located to its correct site at the opening to a cell channel.

INVESTIGATIONS

To address the question "What is a diagnosis of CF?" the American Cystic Fibrosis Foundation convened a conference of experts in 1998 to formulate a consensus statement [19]. The panel of experts proposed the diagnosis should be expanded to include identification of *CFTR* mutations and abnormal bioelectrical properties of nasal epithelium, in addition to the sweat test, a family history of CF or a positive result on neonatal screening [27].

Sweat test

Despite the discovery of the *CFTR* gene, the initial diagnosis is still dependent upon an adequate sweat test. It is mandatory that the physician requesting such a test is well acquainted with details of methodology as well as reference laboratory values. Providing that the uncommon causes for a positive result are excluded (Table 15.2) and the test is skillfully performed by well-trained and experienced staff using a standardized and audited technique, the sweat test remains the diagnostic gold standard.

Sweat mass and electrolyte content

Pilocarpine iontophoresis-stimulated sweat collection continues to be the prime method used to establish the diagnosis [28–30]. The mass of sweat must be at least 100 mg and the test should always be performed at two different sites on the limbs and then repeated. It must not be carried out until after the third day of life because of elevated electrolyte values before then. Normally, in well children, the mean sweat sodium and chloride levels are about 30 mmol/1; in contrast, in CF, the concentrations exceed 60 mmol/1 (>70 mmol/1 in adolescents and adults), with a mean value of 100 mmol/1. The relationship between sweat sodium and chloride is very close, with a gap usually within 5 mmol/1 – a wider discrepancy suggests a technical error and invalid result.

About 10% of normal adolescents have a raised sweat sodium exceeding 60 mmol/1 – in such circumstances, the fludrocortisone suppression test will clarify the diagnosis. In the normal sweat duct, sweat electrolytes are reduced following the administration of oral 9-α-fludrocortisone (3 mg/m^2/day) for 2 days, but this is not so in CF.

To avoid a false-positive or a false-negative result, it is essential that the label of CF is never made unless it is confirmed on at least two occasions within an expert and appropriate tertiary referral or accredited CF care center. In the United States, there is an established external quality assessment (EQA) program which is administered by the College of Pathologists. However, as yet there is no such comparable system with national standards in the UK [31]. Technical errors and poor expertise are not uncommon failings.

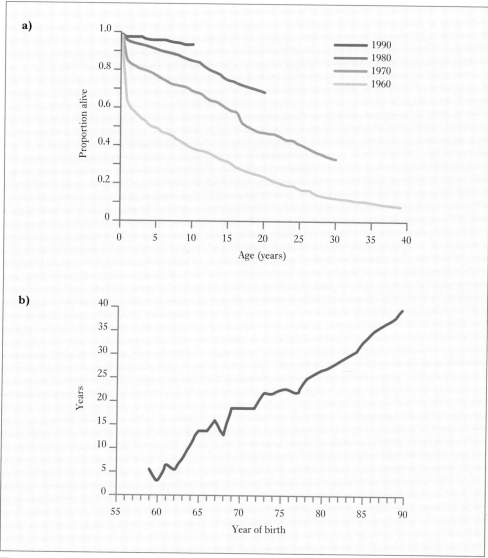

Figure 15.1 (a) Survival curves for cohorts born at the beginning of each decade, extrapolated to the year 2000. (b) Median survival by year of birth from 1959 to 1990. (Reproduced with permission from [20].)

An alternative to the traditional pilocarpine method is that of measuring sweat osmolality (or conductivity) using a Macroduct coil collection system. In CF, values are 220–416 mmol/kg. This option is not as time consuming nor as susceptible to operator error as the traditional technique. Although the Macroduct method is more costly in capital outlay, it is rapid.

Serum immunoreactive trypsin (IRT)

Diagnosis in neonates is based on IRT and gene analysis. IRT is 10 times higher in the serum of the neonate with CF. This is a very sensitive test, but the cut-off level of 60 μg/1 (99th percentile of normal) is critical. The specificity of the IRT test has been improved by a

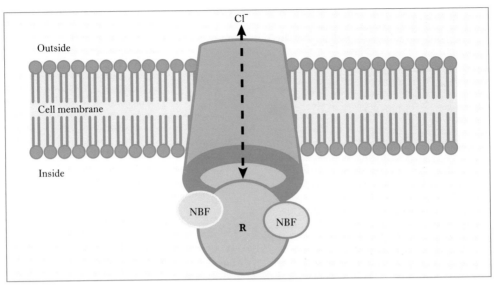

Figure 15.2 Schematic representation of the different function domains of the CFTR protein and the proposed structure of CFTR in the cell. NBF = nucleotide-binding fold; R = regulatory domain; Cl⁻ = chloride.

human trypsinogen monoclonal antibody assay. However, not all infants with CF have an elevated IRT. In addition, beyond 1–2 months of age, the test is unreliable and so cannot then be used. In New South Wales, Australia, IRT was assayed in more than one million neonates during a 13-year period [32]. Initially, only the dried blood spots from the neonates were used. In those with a positive result, direct gene analysis, solely for the common mutation ΔF508, was carried out on the original specimen. An early diagnosis was achieved in 92% of the cases. The false-positive rate was 0.7% with IRT alone, but only 0.05% when IRT was combined with DNA testing. Despite the shortcomings of early screening for IRT followed by gene analysis, this approach has been described as 'reasonably sensitive and highly specific' for neonates [33].

Studies have estimated the cost per affected birth avoided by antenatal screening to be between US$450,000 and US$860,000. This staggering figure is derived from the cost of an educational component, DNA testing, genetic counseling and the screening program. Setting aside the ethical and social aspects of antenatal population programs, it is evidently less costly to screen than to treat over a lifetime.

Nasal transepithelial potential difference

This test is based on the recognition that CF respiratory epithelia conduct sodium and chloride ions abnormally, causing hyperpolarization of the membrane. Reduced chloride secretion through the cAMP-regulated chloride channel (CFTR) and increased sodium resorption via the epithelial sodium channel are manifested by a potential difference. Therefore, when collecting supportive data for a diagnosis, measuring the transepithelial voltage in the nasal mucosa of the turbinates can provide corroborative evidence in that it provides a good index of tissue integrity. This technique is usually confined to CF centers.

- Anorexia nervosa
- Adrenal insufficiency (untreated)
- Atopic dermatitis
- Celiac disease
- Cystic fibrosis
- Ectodermal dysplasia
- Fucosidosis
- Glycogen storage disease (type 1)
- Hypoparathyroidism
- Hypothyroidism
- Hypogammaglobulinemia
- Malnutrition
- Mucopolysaccharidosis
- Nephrogenic diabetes insipidus

Table 15.2 Causes of elevated sweat electrolytes in childhood.

Ancillary investigations

Fecal enzymes – stool trypsin or chymotrypsin test

This can be carried out on fresh stools or by sending a dried fecal smear to a central laboratory. The chymotrypsin 'tubeless' test has been described as both simple and reliable.

Stool porcine enzyme or chymotrypsin is a means of confirming the patient has been complying with treatment (P Durie, personal communication, 1997) and taking an undetermined quantity of pancreatic enzymes. Other stool markers of CF include fecal pancreatic elastase-1 and the steatocrit test.

Three-day fat collection

It is necessary to ensure an adequate fat intake during the study (>35% of dietary energy). Markers (e.g. carmine) should be used at the beginning and end of collection to qualify that it is over a period of 72 h. However, not all investigators adopt this practise. If the stool fat is greater than 10%, it is considered excessive. The findings should be expressed as a coefficient of absorption (CA).

$$CA = \frac{\text{dietary fat} - \text{fecal fat}}{\text{dietary fat}}$$

The CA relates to age as follows:

- Term infant: 80–85%
- 10 months to 3 years: 85–90%
- Above 3 years: 95%

Stool smear

A quick but crude screen for the detection of steatorrhea is to measure the number of fat globules present in a stool smear that has been stained. A count greater than 100 per high-power field is abnormal, but diet and transit time will influence the findings.

Steatocrit

This method is the counterpart to the creamatocrit, which can be used to quantify fat present in a capillary sample of breast milk.

Method

1. Take 0.5 g of fresh stool and homogenize with 2.5 ml of water and 0.6 g of fine sand.

2. Draw the suspension into a capillary tube.

3. Seal the tube with wax and centrifuge at 1300 revolutions per minute to separate the fatty (F) and solid (S) segments.

4. Steatocrit $= \dfrac{\text{length of F}}{\text{length of F} + \text{length of S}}$

$$\text{Steatocrit (\%)} = \dfrac{F \times 100}{(F + S)}$$

A steatocrit result greater than 2% is abnormal.

Inevitably, clinicians are no more enthusiastic about inspecting stools for steatorrhea than are laboratory technicians faced with the daunting task of quantifying the total fat contained in a 3-day collection of homogenized feces. Therefore, non-invasive and alternative pancreatic function tests have been sought, both to aid the diagnosis of CF and to evaluate the efficacy of treatment. However, it is still occasionally necessary to perform duodenal intubation to examine the proximal small-bowel aspirate.

Secretin–pancreozymin test

Ideally, this sophisticated test of stimulation should be performed using a triple-lumen tube to prevent contamination of pancreatic juices with gastric acid. Alternatively, but less satisfactorily, a single intraduodenal tube can be used. Secretin is responsible for bicarbonate secretion; pancreozymin (cholecystokinin) stimulates the release of trypsin (initially as trypsinogen – Fig. 15.3), chymotrypsinogen, carboxypeptidase and pancreatic amylase and lipase.

Method

Give intravenous pancreozymin (1.5 IU/kg) slowly, followed by intravenous secretin (1.5 IU/kg), again slowly. It is important that the patient is tested for adverse reactions to both these hormone preparations before the investigation is undertaken. The duodenal aspirate must be collected in ice-cooled flasks and analyzed promptly for volume and for content of bicarbonate, trypsin, chymotrypsin, lipase and amylase (Table 15.3). The addition of glycerol and storage at −20°C will delay degradation of lipase and trypsin [34].

	Birth	One month	Normal	Cystic fibrosis	Pancreatic insufficiency
Volume (ml/kg per 50 min)					
Premature	4.4 (4–15)	8.96 (3.4–18.7)	3.9 (1.8–81)	0.3–2.7	1.8–3.9
Term	5.39 (1.6–9.7)				
Bicarbonate (mequiv/1 per 50 min)			0.19 (0.08–0.37)	0.001–0.04	0.008–0.19
Trypsin (μg/kg per 50 min)					
Premature	60 (0–482)	196.1 (0.9–660)	765 (215–2100)	0–450	0.9–320
Term	66.1 (1.2–350)				
Lipase (IU/kg per 50 min)					
Premature	77.4 (3–343)	283.6 (11–730)	1464 (350–5000)	0–270	0–68
Term	143.9 (2.2–785)				
Chymotrypsin (mg/kg per 50 min)			860 (252–1900)	0–126	0–105
Amylase (IU/kg per 50 min)					
Premature	0.88 (0–3.6)	1.67 (0–4.6)	665 (160–2150)	0–117	0–31
Term	3.20 (0.1–9.8)				

Table 15.3 Pancreatic function after the secretin–pancreozymin test. From Gryboski J, Walker WA. Gastrointestinal Problems in the Infant. London: WB Saunders, 1983.

Non-invasive tests

Fecal pancreatic elastase 1 (E1) is a reliable test of exocrine pancreatic function. Nissler [35] measured E1 concentration of 148 healthy infants under 12 months of age and observed that 96.8% had E1 concentrations greater than an adult lower limit after two weeks of life, independent of gestational age. The adult reference value for pancreatic E1 of greater than 200 mg/g feces can be applied to infants older than two weeks, independent of gestational age, birth weight and the type of nutrition. Furthermore, Luth et al [36] demonstrated that fecal elastase 1 is highly sensitive in the diagnosis of severe and moderate exocrine pancreatic insufficiency and has a significantly higher sensitivity than fecal chymotrypsin estimation, but neither test is suitable for screening. Perhaps E1 is destined to become the 'gold standard' of indirect pancreatic function tests?

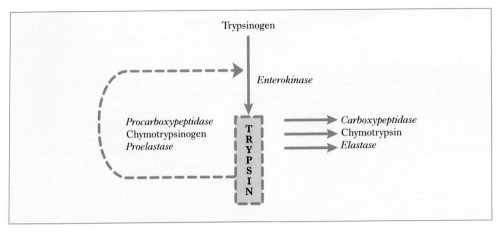

Figure 15.3 The activation of pancreatic zymogens.

Enzymatic cleavage of a compound and urine recovery
This test of pancreatic function involves the ingestion of a non-absorbable compound that is broken down by a specific enzyme. The absorbed residue is then identified in the urine.

Chymotrypsin substrate test (Bz-Tyr-PABA test; bentiromide test)
N-benzoyl-L-tyrosyl-p-aminobenzoic acid (Bz-Tyr-PABA) is cleaved by the proteolytic enzyme chymotrypsin to benzoyl-tyrosyl, releasing p-aminobenzoic acid (PABA). As the latter is absorbed and then excreted in the urine, its presence reflects the activity of chymotrypsin. The 6-h urinary recovery is usually between 60% and 90% in the presence of normal renal function.

Carbon-13 (^{13}C) mixed triglyceride (MTG) breath test
This is a non-invasive, breath-test method of measuring intraluminal lipolysis both before commencing treatment with pancreatic enzymes and after, to evaluate the effectiveness of such therapy. Labeled carbon dioxide present in the expired breath is measured [37]. Expiratory breath sampling is not readily accomplished in infants or young children, however, as a satisfactory technique necessitates patient cooperation. A $^{13}CO_2$ facility is not confined to a pediatric gastroenterology department, as samples can be directed to a laboratory with access to mass spectrometry.

DIAGNOSIS

A positive family history of CF is found only in a minority of cases. Furthermore, as respiratory symptoms may be minimally evident, and the pancreas and growth initially normal, there needs to be a low threshold on the part of clinicians to request a sweat test. Conversely, even in those with steatorrhea and respiratory problems, there may be a delay of almost 2 years before the diagnosis is made. The average age for diagnosis is highly variable between different countries and their regions. American data have demonstrated, not surprisingly, that patients in metropolitan and urban areas are diagnosed at an earlier age than are those from rural and farming communities. Moreover, in the clinic population, 15%

of the patients have growth percentiles for height and weight exceeding the 75th percentile. Therefore, good stature does not exclude the diagnosis.

The expression of the gene is very variable, with hundreds of mutations: some patients are seriously handicapped physically, whereas others, who are experiencing minimal symptoms, are not identified until later in adulthood. Moreover, there are patients in whom a single clinical feature (e.g. electrolyte abnormalities, pancreatitis, liver disease, sinusitis or obstructive azoospermia and infertility) is the dominant finding. As long ago as 1975, the late Harry Shwachman reported 70 patients from his Boston clinic who were not diagnosed until over the age of 25 years.

Bowling and colleagues in Brisbane, Australia, have shown in a matched study of 28 patients and a cohort of 23 that early diagnosis reduces the morbidity in the first 2 years of life [38].

NUTRITIONAL ASSESSMENT AND MANAGEMENT [39]

Improvement in the nutritional state of those with CF is likely to correct the depressed immune system and increase both respiratory muscle strength and exercise tolerance. In addition, healthier nutrition will enhance growth, appearance and morale. Therefore, an aggressive approach to this aspect of management, using a diet high in both energy and fat, is fully justified and is associated with enhanced survival. The 85% of CF children who have impaired pancreatic function show a picture similar to that of protein–energy malnutrition (PEM); that is, they have a decreased body fat content and muscle mass, as well as a raised rate of muscle catabolism. Furthermore, in addition to pancreatic insufficiency, there are abnormalities of bile salt metabolism. Nutritional problems in CF are multifactorial, including increases in intestinal losses and high caloric requirements. There are a number of reasons for the elevated energy expenditure, such as lung infections, inflammation and the increased work of breathing. If diabetes is either unrecognized or inadequately controlled, there will be further energy depletion secondary to the glycosuria.

Dietary assessment

The pediatric CF dietician needs to carry out at least an annual assessment of the nutritional intake over 3 consecutive days using a diary [40].

Anthropometry

In adherence with the American Cystic Fibrosis Foundation guidelines, children should be seen routinely every 3–4 months and infants weekly or even bi-weekly until normal weight gain is established. At each visit, anthropometric measurements should be plotted, including weight and height for age, head circumference (in the first 2 years of life) and triceps skinfold thickness and mid-arm circumference to assess body fat and lean body mass. Energy balance is calculated by determining the energy intake and expenditure, then the coefficient of fat absorption.

Biochemical indices

The following biochemical indices should be used to assess the nutritional state of the patient:

* Plasma vitamin A
* Plasma vitamin E

- Plasma zinc

- Serum electrolytes

- Serum iron

- Albumin

- Prothrombin time

- Essential fatty acids

Weakness and muscle fatigue may be due in part to hypomagnesemia secondary to fat malabsorption or the consequence of aminoglycosides causing renal tubular loss of magnesium. If this is suspected, magnesium must be quantified.

Pancreatic enzyme replacement

Steatorrhea is not totally remedied by pancreatic enzyme enteric-coated microspheres (ECMP), but 90% fat absorption can be achieved. A range of products with varying amounts of pancreatic enzymes are available:

- Creon (Solvay; UK/USA)

- Nutrizym (Merck; UK)

- Pancrease (Janssen-Cilag; UK, OrthoMcNeil; USA)

- Ultrase (Scandipharm; USA)

In most preparations, the enzymes are derived from the porcine pancreas. pH-sensitive enteric-coated microspheres minimize oral ulceration in that they are not released in the mouth. These enteric-coated preparations are more effective than conventional pancreatic powder and enteric-coated capsules.

In some patients, H_2-receptor antagonists have a role in that they reduce postprandial jejunal 'hyperacidity' and thus inhibit acid–peptic inactivation of the supplemented enzymes. These agents improve lipid solubilization and achieve a better pH environment in the proximal small intestine. Ranitidine or cimetidine can be offered 30 min before each meal if ECMP alone does not adequately correct the fat loss. However, the long-acting H_2-receptor antagonist famotidine has the advantage of needing only once-daily administration and has been successfully used in adults with active duodenal disease. Unfortunately, side effects have been reported and the question has been raised as to whether there are too many H_2-receptor antagonists.

An alternative would be to decrease gastric acid secretion by inhibiting the proton pump H^+/K^+ ATPase. This can be achieved using omeprazole, a substituted benzimidazole. However, should this approach be adopted, it would be prudent to limit it to a short time only, because achlorhydria will predispose a vulnerable patient to an enteric infection such as salmonellosis.

Sodium bicarbonate (15 g/m^2/day) given with pancreatic enzymes may improve their efficacy. Some pancreatic enzyme preparations incorporate a bicarbonate buffer.

For maximum efficiency, pancreatic preparations should be taken with all meals as well as snacks. Many children from an early age swallow the tablets either immediately before or during the meal. For infants and children who cannot swallow tablets, the contents of the capsules should be mixed with soft acidic food such as apple sauce and taken immediately prior to the meal or snack. The enzymes should never be mixed with food on the plate as this makes the meal unappetizing and so will diminish the appetite. The quantity of the preparation given will depend upon the child's size, diet and extent of pancreatic function.

Protein

Fecal losses of nitrogen are as high as 30% in untreated CF patients and the correct use of a pancreatic enzyme supplement does not result in normal absorption. The greater the amount of fat in the stools, the higher the nitrogen loss. Total serum protein levels are generally slightly elevated owing to a raised globulin level, while albumin levels are low. Body protein stores are decreased, with a low muscle mass and increased muscle catabolism. The requirements for protein are thus greater than normal. Children should receive an intake of 120–150% of the recommended daily allowance (RDA) on a per kilogram body weight basis. The use of high-protein, high-calorie snacks or drinks as a supplement to the diet can improve the nutrient intake.

Fat

Fat malabsorption is the most striking of the gastrointestinal symptoms (Fig. 15.4). In former years, a low-fat diet was recommended for CF; however, fat is a major high-density source of calories and is now used generously. Serum levels of some essential fatty acids, such as arachidonic and linoleic acid, as well as phospholipid and cholesterol levels are low in CF. The daily administration of essential fatty acids in the form of 1 ml/kg of corn or safflower oil has been advocated. This must be taken with pancreatic enzyme cover. A significant positive correlation has been found between linoleic acid levels and height in some patients, and supplements of linoleic acid monoglycerides have been used.

Carbohydrate

In CF, carbohydrate is the most important source of digestible energy in the diet. In older children, starch can give rise to abdominal pain and distension because of bacterial fermentation with gas production in the large bowel. It is important that pancreatic enzyme supplements are administered with all starchy snacks.

A glucose polymer preparation can be used in place of sucrose to improve energy intake. The advantages are that there is less risk of dental caries and the polymer does not have such a sweet taste.

Energy

Children with CF clearly have an energy requirement that is greater than normal. An intake of at least 100% RDA for chronological age or 130–150% RDA for height-age is needed. When indicated, energy intake can be increased by 20–30% of the total caloric need by increasing the quantities of fat and sugar consumed.

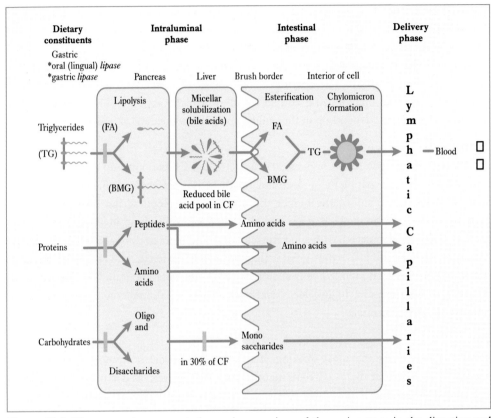

Figure 15.4 Diagrammatic representation and comparison of the major steps in the digestion and absorption of dietary fat, protein and carbohydrate. These include: the lipolysis of dietary triglycerides (TG) by pancreatic enzymes; micellar solubilization of the resulting long-chain fatty acids (FA) and β-monoglycerides (BMG) by bile acids; absorption of the fatty acids and β-monoglycerides into the mucosal cells with subsequent re-esterification and formation of chylomicrons; and movement of the chylomicrons from the mucosal cells into the intestinal lymphatic system. ▌ = block in cystic fibrosis. (Modified and reproduced with permission from Roy CC, Silverman A, Cozzetto FJ. Pediatric Clinical Gastroenterology, 2nd ed. St Louis: CV Mosby, 1975.)

Fiber

The production of soft, bulky stools, flatus and reduced bile salt reabsorption are features both of CF and of a high-fiber diet. Currently recommended CF diets have a poor content of fiber. It has been suggested that this low-residue diet might be responsible for some gastrointestinal symptoms in CF [41], which are often – and perhaps falsely – attributed to pancreatic enzyme insufficiency.

Minerals

Sodium

There is no evidence that, in temperate climates, children with CF have an increased requirement for salt. However, in older children, because of the high content of sodium in their sweat, any situation that increases sweating, such as fever, physical exercise or a high environmental temperature, may necessitate the addition of salt tablets supplying an extra

2–3 mmol/kg daily. If an infant is on a normal low-electrolyte formula, anorexia and poor growth may result from chronic salt depletion.

Calcium

Children with CF rarely have rickets, although suboptimal serum concentrations of vitamin D metabolites have been reported.

Iron

Some studies report diminished iron absorption in CF with pancreatic enzyme therapy, but others do not endorse this observation. Anemia is a rare finding in CF even though low plasma iron levels are seen.

Trace metals

Impairment of zinc absorption and retention has been shown and low levels of zinc noted in plasma. The normalizing of body zinc levels by the addition of an oral supplement is recommended. However, zinc absorption is improved by exocrine pancreatic enzyme replacement [42]. High levels of copper in the fingernails and plasma have been described, with plasma copper levels rising as the disease progresses.

Fat-soluble vitamins

Vitamin A

Decreased levels of vitamin A have been reported in 40% and low carotene levels in 90% of CF patients. Symptoms of vitamin A deficiency are seen in patients with untreated CF.

The recommended intake for vitamin A ranges from 1500 μg to 3000 μg (4000–8000 IU) daily; the high dose may not be necessary if zinc is administered. However, CF patients who are supplemented with vitamin A have almost a 3.5-fold liver reserve compared with controls. Despite low serum vitamin A concentrations, it has been suggested that the accumulation of this vitamin might cause hepatic toxicity [40].

Vitamin D

Malabsorption of oral vitamin D and reduced bile salt reabsorption results in diminished body stores and low plasma levels of 25-hydroxyvitamin D_3. Osteomalacia and demineralization of bone have been demonstrated in CF adolescents, and a reduced cortical thickness shown in younger children. A daily dose of 10–20 μg (400–800 IU) is recommended.

Vitamin E

Vitamin E is an antioxidant that may have a role in the protection of lung tissue against oxidative damage. Tissue vitamin E levels are low in patients with CF who do not receive supplements, but can be normalized in most children by taking daily supplements of vitamin E as listed below [43].

0–12 months of age	25–50 IU
1–4 years of age	100 IU
4–10 years of age	100–200 IU
>10 years of age	200–400 IU

Vitamin K

Hypoprothrombinemia responsive to vitamin K therapy has been described. The vitamin supplement should provide at least the RDA. Those with liver disease are at greater risk of experiencing vitamin K deficiency.

Water-soluble vitamins

These are more readily absorbed than the fat-soluble variety. Provided that an adequate diet containing the RDA is available, supplementation is not indicated.

Nutritional options

Several regimens have been tried in order to improve the nutritional status of older children, and these may have a role in the treatment of CF at particular times. An 'artificial' or elemental diet consisting entirely of amino acids, peptides, MCTs, glucose polymers, vitamins and minerals has been used at many centers to replace normal foods.

Various modes of administration have been used: the oral route, via a nasogastric tube, parenteral nutrition and short-term peripheral hyperalimentation. More recently, percutaneous gastrostomy feeding has been advocated [44].

When a child has persistently failed to gain weight, enteral feeding may become an increasingly attractive option, but it is not without risk of complications. For example, a nasogastric, nasojejunal or gastrostromy tube might exacerbate gastroesophageal reflux, which is common in CF. The choice of enterostomy tube and the technique for placement should be based upon local factors and the particular expertise at a given CF center. Advantages and disadvantages are associated with the siting of a nasogastric versus a jejunal/duodenal tube. If the patient's weight is less than 85% of that expected for height or has been static for 3 months [45], enteral feeding is a valid alternative. Enteral feeding can be administered continuously during the night, with a gap of 1–2 h before the morning session of physical therapy.

An energy-dense polymeric feed providing more than 1.5 kcal/ml (6.3 kJ/ml) is well tolerated in those heavier than 20 kg – others prefer an elemental chemically defined formula. A number of investigators have demonstrated the continuing benefits of long-term enteral feeding [46]. Feeds suitable for such administration are described in Appendix III.

NON-NUTRITIONAL ASPECTS OF MANAGEMENT

Nearly all the mortality and much of the morbidity in CF are the result of chronic lung disease. Reversible airway obstruction is common and bronchopulmonary aspergillosis is a potential complication. Fifty percent of patients with an FEV_1 of less than 30% will die within 2 years [47]. Physical therapy is a major component of the treatment regimen. A therapeutic team ideally should include a nurse specialist [48], a dietician/nutritionist, CF counselors, a physical therapist and a clinical psychologist. All have key roles to play.

Developments in correcting ion transport and in organ transplantation

Different agents aimed at correcting the impaired ion transport are being evaluated. Examples include 'ion channel drugs' to switch on non-functioning CFTR, and 'synthetic chaperones' to transport CFTR to the cell when there is an error in its carriage mechanism.

Drugs have been developed to stimulate fluid secretion via a calcium-dependent channel, but this activity is inhibited by the naturally occurring enzyme inositol 3,4,5,6-tetrakisphosphate. However, okadaic acid, an analog of a shellfish toxin, can prevent the inhibition of these chloride channels [49] and may have a place in CF therapy.

Heart–lung transplantation for CF was first successfully carried out in the early 1980s. Pulmonary infection is the commonest cause of postoperative morbidity. One group in France has demonstrated an actuarial survival of 64.2% at 5 years [50]. The declining survival after the first year following surgery is partly the result of obliterative bronchiolitis.

SHWACHMAN–DIAMOND SYNDROME

(pancreatic exocrine insufficiency, bone marrow dysfunction, and metaphyseal chondrodysplasia)

This rare, multi-organ, autosomal recessive syndrome, of unknown pathogenesis, constitutes the next most common cause of pancreatic exocrine insufficiency (PEI) after CF. It was first described by Shwachman et al. in 1964 [51]: PEI was reported in children with neutropenia or pancytopenia but in whom sweat electrolytes and lungs were both normal.

FEATURES
Manifestations include:

- Short stature (growth hormone deficiency) [52] – most are on the 3rd centile
- Metaphyseal chondrodysplasia (femur, tibia and knees), evident radiologically
- 'Cup'-shaped deformities of the ribs
- Hypoplasia of the iliac bones
- Susceptibility to infection and orthopedic complications with sepsis
- Neutropenia with impaired chemotaxis (intermittent in two-thirds but constant in one-third)
- Pancreatic exocrine insufficiency (but, with advancing age, 50% become sufficient)
- Anemia in 66% (and HbF present in 80%)
- Thrombocytopenia in 24%
- Myelodysplastic syndrome (MDS) in 33% (24% of MDS cases transform to acute myeloid leukemia [53]; previously it was suspected that only 5–10% underwent this change)
- Skin disorders (eczema or ichthyosis in 50–65%)
- Hepatic dysfunction (not commonly seen)
- Cardiac failure with myocardial fibrosis has been reported in a few patients
- Hirschsprung's disease, diabetes mellitus and hepatosplenomegaly may be present

In-depth immunological studies have revealed humoral defects, with absent serum thymulin. IgA and IgM deficiency have been noted in some patients.

Fat loss in stools decreases with age because of an increase in lipase secretion. The gastrointestinal symptoms may appear by 3 months of age; however, not infrequently, they are noted in the early weeks after birth.

Mental retardation was reported in 18 (85%) of 21 patients reviewed by Aggett et al. [54]. Furthermore, children with this syndrome may have particular psychological characteristics [55]. Glycosuria and galactosuria may become evident secondary to renal tubular defects. Hip dysostosis can cause coxa vara with an abnormal gait. The syndrome can prove fatal in as many as 25%, the main cause being infection with overwhelming sepsis. Fortunately, with advancing age, this risk declines.

INVESTIGATIONS
These include the following:

- Sweat test (to exclude CF)
- Fecal fat studies
- Pancreatic stimulation tests to assay trypsin, amylase and lipase
- Bone survey to identify skeletal anomalies
- Hemoglobin electrophoresis
- Immunoglobulin concentrations
- White cell function tests
- Bone marrow aspiration

DIAGNOSIS
The Shwachman–Diamond syndrome should be considered if there is a combination of failure to thrive and radiologic evidence of metaphyseal dysostosis, or if there is thrombocytopenia or an elevated fetal hemoglobin level. Ultrasonography revealing a uniformly hyperechogenic pancreas combined with a negative sweat test and a low IRT are diagnostic of this condition. Bone marrow examination is necessary to exclude MDS and leukemia. Pancreatic stimulation tests, which not all experts agree are necessary, will demonstrate very low enzyme secretions (<2% of normal values), but a normal level of bicarbonate, in the duodenal fluid.

TREATMENT
This is symptomatic. Enzyme replacement is necessary for those with pancreatic insufficiency.

ISOLATED ENZYME DEFICIENCIES

TRYPSINOGEN DEFICIENCY
The presence of trypsinogen in the pancreas is essential for normal proteolytic activity. Inactive trypsinogen is converted to the active form (trypsin) by the intestinal enzyme

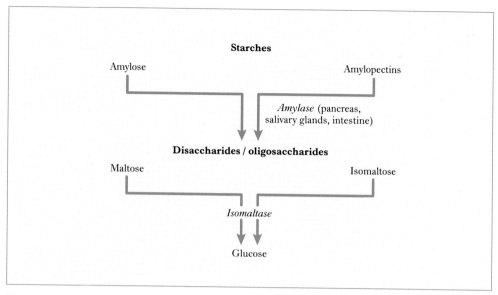

Figure 15.5 The metabolism of starches.

enterokinase (see Fig. 15.3). Activated trypsin is then able to catalyze other proenzymes – procarboxypeptidase (to carboxypeptidase) and chymotrypsinogen (to chymotrypsin) – and, furthermore, convert more trypsinogen to trypsin.

Isolated trypsinogen deficiency is a very rare inborn error of metabolism associated with hypoproteinemia, edema, failure to thrive and/or anemia. For diagnosis, a secretin–pancreozymin test should be performed, then repeated after adding exogenous enterokinase. In the presence of isolated trypsinogen deficiency, there is no trypsin activity following stimulation.

Treatment
Therapy involves an elemental diet containing a protein hydrolysate. Older children tolerate a fairly normal diet, but growth is improved if a supplement of an elemental or predigested drink is given.

CONGENITAL ENTEROKINASE DEFICIENCY
Enterokinase is a duodenal mucosal enzyme that activates the zymogen proenzyme trypsinogen [56]. The clinical features of enterokinase deficiency are similar to those of CF: loose, frequent stools from birth and failure to thrive. To establish the diagnosis, duodenal trypsin and chymotrypsin are assayed before and after the addition of exogenous enterokinase. Small-bowel biopsy reveals normal mucosal histology but the enzyme enterokinase is absent from the homogenate.

Treatment
Replacement therapy is not yet used, but an adequate response is seen with pancreatic preparations. Alternatively, the disorder can be managed by using protein hydrolysate.

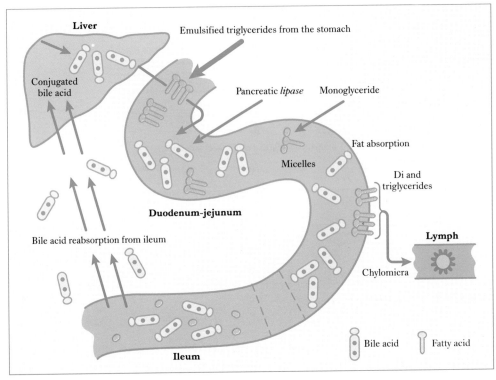

Figure 15.6 Intraluminal micelle formation, fat and bile salt absorption.

PRIMARY INTESTINAL ENTEROPEPTIDASE DEFICIENCY

A rare case has been described [57]. Proteolytic activity is very low in the duodenal juice, but normal levels are induced *in vitro* with porcine enteropeptidase.

PANCREATIC AMYLASE DEFICIENCY

This very rare enzyme deficit disorder is a physiologic phenomenon seen in immature neonates and is a potential problem in infants given a disproportionately large intake of starch for their amylase capacity (Fig. 15.5). It is questionable as to whether a true permanent amylase deficiency does exist.

COMBINED LIPASE–CO-LIPASE DEFICIENCY [58]

The role of co-lipase is to facilitate the attachment of lipase to its substrate. To date, this deficiency has been reported in only three patients, who presented with steatorrhea. Management is with pancreatic enzymes.

CONGENITAL LIPASE DEFICIENCY

In this condition, steatorrhea is present from birth and a characteristic feature is the passage of fat from the bowel. Although pancreatic lipase – but not co-lipase – is deficient, a functioning gastric source of this lipolytic enzyme is present (Fig. 15.6). There is also

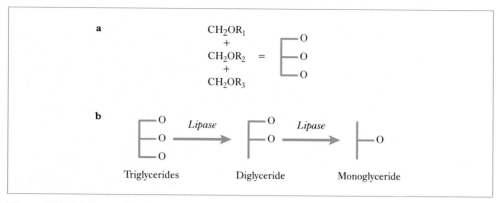

Figure 15.7 (a) Fatty acids; (b) the action of lipase.

evidence of lingual/pharyngeal lipase activity. The differential diagnosis includes CF and the Shwachman–Diamond syndrome.

Neutral fats (triglycerides) are composed of the carbohydrate glycerol and three fatty acids ($R_1R_2R_3$) (Fig. 15.7a). Lipase releases fatty acids from glycerol by hydrolysis (Fig. 15.7b).

The diagnosis is confirmed by the secretin–pancreozymin test, which demonstrates normal proteolytic and amylolitic enzymes.

Treatment
Large amounts of pancreatic extracts should be used for this lipase deficit.

REFERENCES

1. Ravilly S, Robinson W, Suresh S et al. Chronic pain in cystic fibrosis. Pediatrics 1996;98:741–7.

2. Turner MA, Baildam E, Patel L et al. Joint disorders in cystic fibrosis. J R Soc Med 1997;S31:13–20.

3. Wulffraat NM, de Graeff–Meeder ER, Rijkers GT et al. Prevalence of circulating immune complexes in patients with cystic fibrosis and arthritis. J Pediatr 1994;125:374–8.

4. Heine RG, Button BM, Olinsky A et al. Gastro-oesophageal reflux in infants under 6 months with cystic fibrosis. Arch Dis Child 1998;78:44–8.

5. Lloyd–Still JD. Crohn's accounts for increased prevalence of inflammatory bowel disease (IBD) in cystic fibrosis. Pediatr Pulmonol 1992;S8:307–8.

6. Neglia JP, Fitzsimmons SC, Maisonneuve P et al. The risk of cancer among patients with cystic fibrosis. Cystic Fibrosis and Cancer Study Group. N Engl J Med 1995;332:494–9.

7. Cohn JA. Epidemiological studies of fibrosing colonopathy in cystic fibrosis. In: Rudmann MA, editor. Pancreatic Enzymes in Cystic Fibrosis. A Risk–Benefit Analysis. Hannover: Solvay Pharma Deutschland, 1995:11–17. (Series in Gastroenterology, No. 4).

8. Smyth RL, Ashby D. Epidemiological studies of fibrosing colonopathy in cystic fibrosis. In: Rudmann MA, editor. Pancreatic Enzymes in Cystic Fibrosis. A Risk–Benefit Analysis. Hannover: Solvay Pharma Deutschland, 1995:19–22. (Series in Gastroenterology, No. 4).

9. Fitzsimmons SC, Burkhart GA, Borowitz D et al. High-dose pancreatic-enzyme supplements and fibrosing colonopathy in children with cystic fibrosis. N Engl J Med 1997;336:1283–9.

10. Stevens JC, Maguiness KM, Hollingsworth J et al. Pancreatic enzyme supplementation in cystic fibrosis patients before and after fibrosing colonopathy. J Pediatr Gastroenterol Nutr 1998;26:80–4.

11. Borowitz DS, Grand RJ, Durie PR. Use of pancreatic enzyme supplements for patients with cystic fibrosis in the context of fibrosing colonopathy. Consensus Committee. J Pediatr 1995;127:681–4.

12. Powell CJ. Colonic toxicity from pancreatins: a contemporary safety issue. Lancet 1999;353:911–5.

13. Connett GJ, Rolles CJ. Pancreatic enzymes and fibrosing colonopathy. Lancet 1999;354:249–50.

14. Connett GJ, Lucas JS, Atchley JT et al. Colonic wall thickening is related to age and not dose of high strength pancreatin microspheres in children with cystic fibrosis. Eur J Gastroenterol Hepatol 1999;11:181–3.

15. Cohn JA, Friedman KJ, Noone PG et al. Relation between mutations of the cystic fibrosis gene and idiopathic pancreatitis. N Engl J Med 1998;339:653–8.

16. Wilschanski M, Rivlin J, Cohen S et al. Clinical and genetic risk factors for cystic fibrosis-related liver disease. Pediatrics 1999;103:52–7.

17. Lykavieris P, Bernard O, Hadchouel M. Neonatal cholestasis as the presenting feature in cystic fibrosis. Arch Dis Child 1996;75:67–70.

18. Turner MA, Goldwater D, David TJ. Oxalate and calcium excretion in cystic fibrosis. Arch Dis Child 2000;83:244–7.

19. Wilmott RW. Making the diagnosis of cystic fibrosis. J Pediatr 1998;132:563–5.

20. Elborn JS, Shale DJ, Britton JR. Cystic fibrosis: current survival and population estimates to the year 2000. Thorax 1991;46:881–5.

21. Kulczycki LL, Schauf V. Incidence of cystic fibrosis in black children – revisited. J Pediatr 1978;92:855.

22. Hamosh A, Fitz-Simmons SC, Macek M Jr et al. Comparison of the clinical manifestations of cystic fibrosis in black and white patients. J Pediatr 1998;132:255–9.

23. Welsh MJ, Tsui L-C, Boat TF et al. Cystic fibrosis. In: Scriver CR, Beaudet AL, Sly WS, Valle D (eds). The Metabolic and Molecular Basis of Inherited Disease, 7th edn. New York: McGraw-Hill, 1995:3799–876.

24. Super M. Cystic fibrosis in the South-West African Afrikaner. An example of population drift, possibly with heterozygote advantage. S Afr Med J 1975;49:818–20.

25. Wright SW, Morton NE. Genetic studies on cystic fibrosis in Hawaii. Am J Hum Genet 1968;20:157–69.

26. Wallis C. Diagnosing cystic fibrosis: blood, sweat and tears. Arch Dis Child 1997;76:85–8.

27. Rosenstein BJ, Cutting GR. The diagnosis of cystic fibrosis: a consensus statement. J Pediatr 1998;132:589–95.

28. Andersen DH. Cystic fibrosis of the pancreas and its relation to celiac disease. A clinical and pathological study. Am J Dis Child 1938;56:344–99.

29. Di Sant'Agnese PA, Darling RC, Perera GA et al. Abnormal electrolyte composition of sweat in cystic fibrosis of the pancreas: significance and relationship to disease. Pediatrics 1953;12:549–63.

30. Gibson LE, Cooke RE. A test for concentration of electrolytes in sweat in cystic fibrosis of the pancreas utilizing pilocarpine by iontophoresis. Pediatrics 1959;23:545–9.

31. Kirk JM. Inconsistencies in sweat testing in UK laboratories. Arch Dis Child 2000;82:425–7.

32. Wilcken B, Wiley V, Sherry G et al. Neonatal screening for cystic fibrosis: a comparison of two strategies for case detection in 1.2 million babies. J Pediatr 1995;127:965–70.

33. Stockman JA III . Year Book of Pediatrics 1997. St Louis: Mosby, 1997.

34. Puntis JW. Assessment of pancreatic exocrine function. Arch Dis Child 1993;69:99–101.

35. Nissler K, Von Katte I, Huebner A et al. Pancreatic elastase 1 in feces of preterm and term infants. J Pediatr Gastroenterol Nutr 2001;33:28–31.

36. Luth S, Teyssen S, Forssmann K et al. Fecal elastase-1 determination: 'gold standard' of indirect pancreatic function tests? Scand J Gastroenterol 2001;36:1092–9.

37. Amarri S, Harding M, Coward WA et al. 13Carbon mixed triglyceride breath test and pancreatic enzyme supplementation in cystic fibrosis. Arch Dis Child 1997;76:349–51.

38. Bowling F, Cleghorn G, Chester A et al. Neonatal screening for cystic fibrosis. Arch Dis Child 1988;63:196–8.

39. Ramsey BW, Farrell PM, Pencharz P. Nutritional assessment and management in cystic fibrosis: a consensus report. Consensus Committee. Am J Clin Nutr 1992;55:108–16.

40. MacDonald A. Nutritional management of cystic fibrosis. Arch Dis Child 1996;74:81–7.

41. Gavin J, Ellis J, Dewar AL et al. Dietary fibre and the occurrence of gut symptoms in cystic fibrosis. Arch Dis Child 1997;76:35–7.

42. Easley D, Krebs N, Jefferson M et al. Effect of pancreatic enzymes on zinc absorption in cystic fibrosis. J Pediatr Gastroenterol Nutr 1998;26:136–9.

43. Ramsey BW, Farrell PM, Pencharz P. Nutritional assessment and management in cystic fibrosis: a consensus report. The Consensus Committee. Am J Clin Nutr 1992;55:108–116.

44. Rosenfeld M, Casey S, Pepe M et al. Nutritional effects of long-term gastrostomy feedings in children with cystic fibrosis. J Am Diet Assoc 1999;99:191–4.

45. Jackson A. Clinical guidelines for cystic fibrosis care. J R Coll Physicians London 1996;30:305–8.

46. Steinkamp G, von der Hardt H. Improvement of nutritional status and lung function after long-term nocturnal gastrostomy feedings in cystic fibrosis. J Pediatr 1994;124:244–9.

47. Kerem E, Reisman J, Corey M et al. Prediction of mortality in patients with cystic fibrosis. N Engl J Med 1992;326:1187–91.

48. Dyer J. Cystic fibrosis nurse specialist: a key role. J R Soc Med 1997;31:21–5.

49. Xie W, Solomons KR, Freeman S et al. Regulation of Ca^{2+}-dependent Cl conductance in a human colonic epithelial cell line (T84): cross-talk between Ins (3,4,5,6) P4 and protein phosphatases. J Physiol 1998;510:661–73.

50. Couetil JP, Soubrane O, Houssin DP et al. Combined heart–lung–liver, double lung–liver and isolated liver transplantation for cystic fibrosis in children. Transp Int 1997;10:33–9.

51. Shwachman H, Diamond LK, Oski FA et al. The syndrome of pancreatic insufficiency and bone marrow dysfunction. J Pediatr 1964;65:645–63.

52. Kornfield SJ, Kratz J, Diamond F et al. Shwachman–Diamond syndrome associated with hypogammaglobulinemia and growth hormone deficiency. J Allergy Clin Immunol 1995;96:247–50.

53. Smith OP, Hann IM, Chessells JM et al. Haematological abnormalities in Shwachman–Diamond syndrome. Br J Haematol 1996;94:279–84.

54. Aggett PJ, Thorn JM, Delves HT et al. Trace element malabsorption in exocrine pancreatic insufficiency. Monogr Paediatr 1979;10:8–11.

55. Kent A, Murphy GH, Milla P. Psychological characteristics of children with Shwachman syndrome. Arch Dis Child 1990;65:1349–52.

56. Mann NS, Mann SK. Enterokinase. Proc Soc Exp Biol Med 1994;206:114–8.

57. Green JR, Bender SW, Posselt HG et al. Primary intestinal enteropeptidase deficiency. J Pediatr Gastroenterol Nutr 1984;3:630–3.

58. Ligumsky M, Granot E, Branski D et al. Isolated lipase and colipase deficiency in two brothers. Gut 1990;31:1416–8.

In memory and honor of the late Dr H Shwachman of CHMC, Boston (died 1986)

chapter 16

Eating Disorders

Obesity is harmful to the body and makes it sluggish, disturbs its functions and hinders its movements.

The Medical Aphorisms of Moses Maimonides (1135–1204)

OBESITY

Obesity is defined as an excess of body weight over 20% of the ideal. The clinical estimate of body fat by skinfold thickness correlates well with physicochemical techniques. In most of the industrialized world, but particularly in the USA, the incidence of obesity and its severity have increased yearly in alarming proportions. Obese children need help, not only because of the adverse effects on their health, but also because they inevitably suffer much teasing and unhappiness. Even though an adverse social and psychological background can produce overeating and subsequently obesity, it is mandatory while establishing therapy or support to start the child on a diet. It is undeniable that unhappiness can cause obesity; and obesity, unhappiness. In addition, obesity in adulthood is no longer believed to be inevitable after a childhood problem with weight; furthermore, most overweight babies are not so by the age of 4 years.

ASSESSMENT OF BODY FATNESS

Clinical examination needs to include an assessment of pubertal development and anthropometry, which must be carefully evaluated. Body fatness can be assessed in a clinical setting with a skinfold caliper (Fig. 16.1), a tapemeasure, a stadiometer and weighing equipment; or, in a research setting, with techniques such as total body electrical conductivity (TOBEC), underwater weighing, dual energy X-ray absorptiometry (DEXA) and ^{40}K [1,2]. Centile charts for triceps skinfold thickness in boys and girls are available. Where values exceed the 97th centile, there is obesity. Weight in itself is a poor way to assess body fatness. Centile standards for height, weight, age and sex enable a diagnosis of obesity to be made; one criterion defines obesity as a weight exceeding the height-related weight by twice the standard deviation or more.

In adults, one indicator of obesity is the body mass index (BMI), which determines the body mass (weight/height^2 = body mass); however, this is less useful in children because of variation with age [3]. Childhood obesity could be defined as a BMI at or above the 85th percentile for age and sex, and obesity in adulthood as a mean BMI at or above 27.8 for men and 27.3 for women.

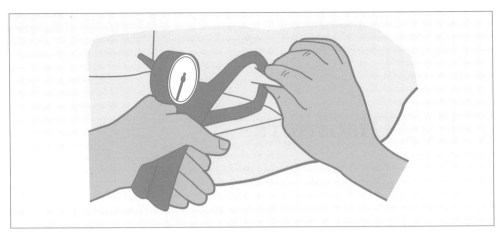

Figure 16.1 Measuring skinfold thickness with calipers.

Alternatively, body mass can be related to a theoretical child with height and weight upon the 50th centile and the measure then given a percentage value:

- 90% = underweight
- 90–110% = normal weight
- 110–120% = overweight
- >120% = obese

PREVALENCE OF OBESITY IN CHILDHOOD

Estimates indicate that as many as one-third of the population of the developed countries is overweight. As different definitions are used internationally to diagnose obesity, relevant comparisons are difficult.

Prevalence estimates of overweight among youth in the USA range from 11% to 24% [4] and the numbers have been increasing steadily. The prevalence of overweight and obesity has increased dramatically in African-American children. An analysis of secular trends suggested a clear upward tendency in body weight in children of 0.2 kg per year between 1973 and 1994 [5].

Prevalence data reveal an increase in childhood obesity throughout Europe but with marked variability relating to age, sex and demographic factors [6]. In Spain, the overall prevalence of overweight and very overweight were significantly higher in a 1995 survey compared with one performed in 1985 – 18% versus 12% (P<0.05) for overweight, and 7% versus 3% (P<0.05) for very overweight [7].

The prevalence of both overweight and obesity increased significantly in English and Scottish children between 1984 and 1994, although there had been no such change in the decade before 1984 [8]. Chinn and Rona [8] analyzed results from cross-sectional surveys carried out at schools in England and Scotland: 10,414 boys and 9737 girls in England, and

5385 boys and 5219 girls in Scotland, all aged 4 to 11 years, were assessed. From 1984 to 1994, the prevalence of overweight increased from 5.4% to 9.0% in English boys and from 6.4% to 10.0% in Scottish boys. In girls, the rate rose from 9.3% to 13.5% and from 10.4% to 15.8%, respectively. The prevalence of obesity increased correspondingly, reaching 1.7% (English boys), 2.1% (Scottish boys), 2.6% (English girls) and 3.2% (Scottish girls).

In a more recent series of cross-sectional studies of routinely collected data in the Wirral Health Authority, England, between 1989 and 1998, there was a highly significant increase in weight and body mass index in children under 4 years of age [9]. A total of 35,662 infants aged 1–3 months (representing 88% of live births) and 28,768 children aged 2.9–4.0 years were evaluated by health visitors. The proportion of overweight children rose from 14.7% to 23.6% (P<0.001) and that of obese children from 5.4% to 9.2% (P<0.001). There was also a very marked increase in the mean SD score for weight (0.05 to 0.29; P<0.001) and body mass index (–0.15 to 0.31; P<0.001). Infants showed a small but significantly increasing trend in mean SD score for weight (–0.17 to –0.05; P<0.005).

ETIOLOGY OF CHILDHOOD OBESITY

Children uncommonly have obesity secondary to a pathologic disease, but, if present, this must be identified (e.g. Prader–Willi or Laurence–Moon–Biedl syndrome). Prader–Willi syndrome is a multi-system disorder characterized by neonatal hypotonia and poor appetite, followed later by hyperphagia, morbid obesity, tantrums or oppositional behavior and mild-to-moderate mental retardation. Yet, up to 10% of affected adults have an IQ within the normal range. It occurs sporadically, either as a result of microdeletion of chromosome 15p (70%) or due to maternal disomy of chromosome 15 (30%) [10]. The voracious appetite in this syndrome can cause gross and unsightly obesity unless early attempts are made to curtail excessive eating.

Regardless of the presence of an underlying condition, obesity develops if there is a positive energy balance. Adipose tissue is formed in childhood with only a small positive energy balance. During the first year of life, the average rate of energy store in fat is 37 kcal/day (155 kJ/day), which progressively falls to 13 kcal/day (54 kJ/day).

Contrary to some professional subjective opinions, not all obese children eat excessively. Overweight children are less active than their leaner counterparts and this pattern of reduced physical activity is more important than excess eating. Such children are known in America to indulge in prolonged television viewing [11]. Observations in animals and adult men have shown that with reduced activity a corresponding decrease in food intake does not happen. Many factors are involved in the etiology of obesity, including behavioral problems, feeding patterns within the family, nature of feeding in the newborn period [12], attitude of parents and siblings to obesity and physical activity.

Childhood obesity increases the risk in adulthood, but how parental excess weight affects the chances of a child becoming an overweight adult is unknown. The risk of obesity in young adulthood associated with both obesity in childhood and in one or both parents has been investigated [13]. The findings indicated that in individuals who were obese during childhood, the likelihood of that problem in adulthood ranged from 8% for those aged 1 or 2 years without obese parents to 79% for those aged 10–14 years with at least one obese parent. Following adjustment for parental obesity, the odds ratio was 1.3 for obesity at 1 or 2 years of age up to 17.5 at 15–17 years of age. After adjustment for the child's obesity status, the odds ratio in adulthood associated with having at least one obese parent ranged from 2.2 at 15–17 years of age to 3.2 at 1 or 2 years of age. The authors concluded that obese children under 3 years of age without obese parents are at low risk from the problem in adulthood, but among older children it is an increasingly important predictor of adult obesity, regardless of whether the parents are overweight. Parental obesity more than doubles the risk of adult obesity among both obese and non-obese children under 10 years of age.

The most recent discoveries regarding obesity are related to the hormone leptin and the identification of certain genes in animal models. Leptin, comprising 167 amino acids, is mainly expressed in adipocytes, and its hypothalamic receptors are integral components of a complex physiologic system involved in the regulation of fuel stores and energy expenditure [14]. The discovery of leptin has constituted a great breakthrough in the understanding of body weight regulation and of the role of the fat tissue as an endocrine organ. Leptin precursors and the hormone itself are produced by placenta, fetal tissues, gastric mucosa and hepatic stellate cells. They can participate in many physiologic functions such as fetal growth, gut-derived satiety, immune or proinflammatory responses, reproduction, nutrient intestinal absorption, angiogenesis and lipolysis. Circulating concentrations of leptin exhibit pulsatility and circadian rhythmicity [15]. The levels of plasma leptin vary directly with the BMI and percentage body fat, and leptin contributes to the regulation of body weight [16–18].

Plasma leptin concentrations are also influenced by metabolic hormones, gender and body energy requirements. Defects in the leptin signaling pathway result in obesity in animal models. Only a few obese humans have been identified with mutations in the leptin or leptin receptor genes; however, most cases of obesity in humans are associated with high leptin levels. Thus, in humans, obesity may represent a state of leptin resistance.

Another area of development has been the molecular basis of body fat regulation. Identification of mutations in several genes in animal models of obesity and development of transgenic models has indicated the physiologic roles of many genes in the regulation of body fat distribution. In humans, mutations in a number of genes, including those for leptin and leptin receptors, have been described in patients with severe obesity [15]. Most of these obesity disorders exhibit a distinct phenotype with varying degrees of hypothalamic and pituitary dysfunction and a recessive inheritance. As the genes that mediate susceptibility to obesity may affect energy intake, as well as energy expenditure and/or the partitioning of calories between lean tissues and fat, the ability to define the gross metabolic basis for the obesity is very important in determining which genes are relevant to the phenotype [19]. Animal models of obesity have been studied intensively for clues to the relevant genes in humans because of the difficulties in defining and controlling the environment of humans. Over the past 40 years, a series of autosomal dominant (Yellow) and recessive (obese, diabetes, tubby, fat, fatty) obesity mutations have been described in mice and rats.

MANAGEMENT

Specialized obesity clinics have many advantages, particularly if they are located in schools. After the initial assessment by an experienced clinician, it is not essential that such a service be maintained at consultant or equivalent level. Dietary education and caloric restriction with an exercise program are the mainstay of treatment. Compliance can be poor; hence, the child and parent(s) must be highly motivated in initiating a program of nutritional re-education to justify the enterprise.

METHODS OF MANAGEMENT

Energy restriction

Whatever the cause(s) of obesity, there must be a reduction in the caloric intake. Serial measurements of height, weight and skinfold thickness need to be recorded. An integrated school-based program of behavior modifications, nutritional guidance and physical education over 10 weeks resulted in 60 (95%) of 63 obese children losing weight compared with three (21%) of the 14 controls. The average loss in this very successful study was 4.4 kg [20]. Similarly, a school-based behavioral weight-reduction program in New York among obese junior high school pupils resulted in 51% losing weight compared with 16% of the controls [21]. A slow weight loss is more beneficial in the long term if deceleration of linear growth and rapid regain is not to occur. Total fasting ('zero-calories regimen') is not recommended in growing individuals.

A ketogenic diet can be implemented in children whose weight is approximately 150–200% of their ideal body weight. This diet requires that the patient be closely supervised throughout the period, especially during the first 5 or 6 days of the regimen. A diet very low in carbohydrate and relatively high in fat is taken until the patient exhibits ketones in the urine. Ketosis decreases the appetite. A small amount of carbohydrate is then introduced in the diet. An example of such a diet for adolescents is as follows: daily intake of 650 to 725 kcal (962–1073 kJ), comprising 80–100 g of protein, 25 g of carbohydrate and 25 g of fat [22].

Protein-sparing modified fast

This is a hypocaloric, ketogenic regimen that provides 1.5–2 g of protein per kilogram target weight per day [23]. The patient's target weight is defined as approximately 20% above the ideal weight for height. This diet is designed to promote rapid weight loss. It is indicated for morbidly obese (≥150% of their ideal body weight), rapidly growing children and adolescents who have been unsuccessful with other diets and have developed complications from their obesity. It provides sufficient protein to keep the body from losing muscle mass but is very low in carbohydrates and fats. The diet is nutritionally inadequate and requires calcium, potassium, magnesium and multivitamin supplementation together with iron. It is not recommended that this schedule be continued for more than 4 months at a time [24]. The effects of this type of regimen on potassium, magnesium and calcium were evaluated and it was found that the vitamin- and mineral-supplemented diet allowed a positive calcium and potassium balance and improved the magnesium balance [25].

Physical exercise

Clinical studies have shown that regular exercise results in weight loss but, not surprisingly, when combined with dieting is even more effective. People tend to overestimate both the amount of exercise they perform and the calories spent in its performance.

Behavior therapy

This has produced promising results and should form part of a comprehensive therapeutic and educational program of management.

Anorectic drugs

These are effective but are not indicated in children because of the risk of side effects. Although studies using amphetamines have demonstrated an initial weight loss, later follow-up revealed that most patients were still obese. There are risks in both over-reliance on anorectics and their long-term use. Such problems have been described in adults using amphetamine-like appetite suppressants [26]. Mefenorex, an alternative therapy, is an indirect sympathomimetic amine that does not cause an amphetamine-like EEG profile (i.e. a significant decrease in slow delta waves and an increase in fast beta activities) [27].

Surgery

Some grossly obese adults have had bypass surgery, which induces malabsorption, to cause weight loss. Such patients must also reduce their food intake to avoid diarrhea. However, these procedures are not without undesirable sequelae and should not be carried out in children. Gastric stapling is another technique used in adults but not recommended for children.

Joint management

A multidisciplinary approach involving the support of parents, peers, nutritionist, pediatrician and behavioral therapist or clinical psychologist is the most advisable method of joint management. Without eliciting an attitude of high motivation, most endeavors will fail. A change in lifestyle is recommended in the useful and comprehensive guidelines issued by the Office of Health Information and Health Promotion (OHIHP – USA) in a publication entitled *Matrix for Action*. A WHO consultation report advises on both prevention and management [28].

DIETARY TREATMENT

Dietary history

The child and parents should be interviewed separately in an effort to determine the cause of previous failures, if any, of dieting. The child's age, degree of obesity, motivation and carer's support are important factors in selecting the dietary regimen to be recommended. Details of ethnic background, family structure, typical daily schedules and activities and interests provide useful information of the family lifestyle. Food-purchasing habits, methods of preparation, availability of money and frequency of eating outside the home enable the meal pattern to be ascertained. A 72-h recall, combined with noted frequency of consumption of individual items, can be a useful guide. The dietician ought to be aware of bizarre habits such as night feasting.

Principles of dietary treatment

The nutritional adequacy of any diet is of prime importance if growth is not to be jeopardized. Furthermore, treatment can provoke antagonistic psychological responses. The parents and the child need to be jointly involved in planning the dietary regimen. Such shared management encourages motivation and participation. Ideally, a target weight should be agreed at an early stage.

Parents should be told that fad and crash diets are potentially dangerous and must be avoided. The aim of the treatment is to correct faulty eating habits. In mild or moderate obesity it is recommended that the intake be modified to keep weight stable and allow for catch-up growth, whereas in severe obesity the purpose is to induce a negative energy balance and slow loss of body weight. Very-low-energy diets need careful supervision.

Infants

Dietary restriction is not recommended for infants under 18 months old. Excessive weight gain can be controlled by correcting inappropriate feeding practices. For example, bottlefed infants may be force-fed the residual volume of a feed to fulfill the parent's desire for an empty bottle: a smaller feed may be all the infant requires. The use of low-fat milks is not recommended until age 2 years. Parents of fat infants may be in the habit of unnecessarily encouraging the child to empty the bowl or jar. Food is frequently used as a reward; also, the infant's cries may be misinterpreted as hunger. If physical activity is confined to a chair or playpen and the child force-fed in any way, the self-regulating mechanism for weight control is overruled.

Childhood

Parents of children under 5 years old need general advice to avoid a high intake of fat and sugar. This includes removal of visible fat, use of butter or margarine in moderation and replacement of frying with other methods of cooking. A policy to limit potato-chips, French fries, candy and chocolate needs to be carefully planned to avoid feelings of deprivation and isolation from peers. Carers need to be aware that eating patterns established during the formative years lay the foundation for later life.

Children over 5 years of age can increasingly participate in the management of their eating habits. Foods taken in excess must be identified. It is unrealistic to expect total avoidance, and both parents and child need to learn how to include these foods occasionally. Smaller portions, no second helpings and low-calorie brands of items (e.g. sugar-free drinks) may be sufficient to control weight gain. Any modification must ensure variety and satiety and be based on the existing family diet.

In cases of moderate obesity the child needs to grow into his or her present weight, whereas in more severe cases the aim is to achieve a slow loss, avoiding harmful fluctuations. As one pound of excess body weight represents 3500 kcal (14.7 MJ) – i.e. 7700 kcal (32.3 MJ) for 1 kg – a daily reduction of 500 kcal (2 MJ) is needed to lose one pound (450 g) of weight per week. An average weight loss over a month shows a realistic trend. Weighing easily becomes an obsessive habit, and when no weight loss is observed, disappointment, if not negativism and disinterest, ensue.

A reducing diet must provide 60% of the energy requirements for the child's age. A daily intake of between 800 and 1200 kcal (3.4–5.1 MJ) is generally advised and most children lose weight on 1000 kcal (4.2 MJ). Adolescents will need higher caloric levels to achieve adequate nutrition, and may require 1500 kcal (especially boys). If the nutritional adequacy of the diet is in doubt, supplements may be needed. Parents need to know of the unrestricted foods and of items to use with caution, as well as the interchangeable isocaloric portions (Appendices VI.1 and VI.6). The skilled help of a dietitian is invaluable in aiding parents to use this information to develop an acceptable eating pattern. Once initial weight has leveled out, increased exercise is recommended to balance the lowered metabolic rate.

Adolescents

A long-standing history of childhood obesity and associated psychological difficulties is not uncommon. It is important not to pressurize this group to lose weight, particularly in early adolescence when motivation is less evident. Emphasizing the child's failure to lose weight can result in poor self-esteem. Psychological support and behavioral modification techniques may be valuable.

At each consultation, there should be an opportunity to discuss feelings and experiences and plan coping strategies for dealing with identifiable problems. A food diary can provide useful insights into eating behavior and associated emotions. Non-diet-related assignments given between visits encourage participation and help to keep the issue of food and weight in perspective. Planned activities and an exercise program should be encouraged. Endeavors to counteract boredom should be emphasized, particularly during the school holidays, because long periods of unstructured time provide ample opportunities for eating and inactivity.

In cases of severe obesity, a protein-sparing modified fast may be useful as part of a supervised program. However, there is the risk of inducing eating disorders such as 'bingeing' when advocating strict dietary measures.

In-patient treatment is used as a last resort to show both child and parent that weight loss can be achieved. However, facilities for intensive education are rarely available and weight is often regained after discharge from hospital. Group therapy is not as widely used with children as with adults. Successful treatment of obesity requires a prolonged commitment by the whole family. Compliance consists of implementing dietary knowledge over considerable time, and long-term positive support is essential in maintaining motivation. There is a need for programs that encourage positive attitudes and awareness of self-image and an easier relationship with food and body weight. In addition, health professionals must understand more of the psychological dynamics of food choice, eating behavior, self-image and weight control.

The limited information currently available from studies in adult patients suggests that antidepressant treatment may be associated with a reduction in binge frequency in obese patients with this eating disorder, but does not lead to weight reduction [29].

ANOREXIA NERVOSA AND BULIMIA NERVOSA

Whosoever fasts for the sake of self-affliction is termed a sinner.

Talmud, Ta'anit 11a The Babylonian Mar Samuel

(circa 165–257)

Anorexia nervosa is a very serious disorder seen predominantly in teenage girls and young women. However, cases may present as young as 7 years of age. The female-to-male ratio in one UK study was 4:1 [30], but in the USA only 5–10% of cases are male. It was described with its present terminology in 1873 in the French medical literature by Ernest C. Laségue under the title 'anorexia hysterique', and in the same year Sir William Gull in England used the description 'anorexia nervosa'. However, prior to 1873, sporadic case reports of what was known as 'apepsia hysterica' appeared in publications such as the *British Medical Journal* [31].

Anorexics who have reached reproductive age frequently have amenorrhea. The morbid fear of obesity is such that the mean weight loss, when calculated by the norm for height and age, can be as high as 32% [32]. In the UK, given a prevalence of one percent amongst women aged 15–29 years, it is estimated there are at least 70,000 cases. National incidence rates vary widely, from 0.08 per 100,000 in Sweden to 8.1 per 100,000 in Holland [33,34]. There is evidence suggesting the incidence in the USA is increasing significantly. Jones et al. [35] found cases in Monroe County, NY, had nearly doubled from 0.35 per 100,000 (1960–1969) to 0.64 per 100,000 (1970–1976); however, Lucas et al. [36] calculated that the overall age-adjusted incidence rate per 100,000 person-years was 14.6 for females.

In a study of 30 children who were followed up over a 7-year period, poor prognostic factors included early age at onset (less than 11 years), depression during the illness, disturbed family life, and one-parent families and families in which one or both parents had been married before [37]. The outcome was good in only 60%. Another small study, however, indicated that the age of onset had no prognostic significance [38]. One group of workers found that late onset was associated with poor outcome [39]. Many of the girls have been described as 'overachievers' [40]. A Canadian study revealed both males and females experience a similar psychosocial morbidity [41].

Numerous endocrine, gastrointestinal peptide [42] and hypothalamic anomalies accompany anorexia nervosa, including abnormal thyroid function. Some may be adaptive phenomena secondary to the malnutrition. Many investigators have reported abnormal gonadotropins and there is also a delayed response to thyrotropin-releasing hormone. The basal plasma cortisol level can be elevated and a loss of the diurnal variation occurs.

Bulimia means 'ox-hunger' and is also known as 'binge-eating'. It was described by Russell [43] as an "ominous variant of anorexia nervosa". This obsessive–compulsive disorder [44] is characterized by episodic overeating that is followed by self-induced vomiting, purgation or periodic starvation in an endeavor to avoid weight gain. In common with anorexia nervosa, to which it is related, the patients are mainly young women who have a fear of obesity – indeed, a history of obesity and anorexia is seen in almost 50% of cases. There may be a switch from bulimia nervosa to anorexia nervosa or the features of both might coexist (Fig. 16.2).

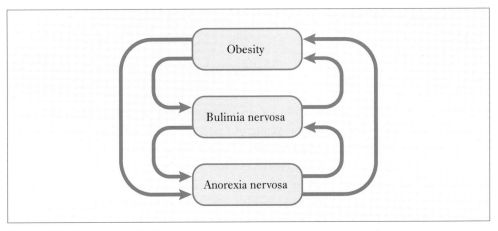

Figure 16.2 Interrelationship between anorexia nervosa, bulimia nervosa and obesity.

Bulimia nervosa has been reported most frequently in whites living in Western Europe, North America and Australasia, with few cases among non-whites. However, a high prevalence has been observed among Asian schoolgirls in Bradford, England [45]. Depression, suicidal ideas, shoplifting, alcoholism and drug abuse are some of the features of this psychological disease. Bulimic episodes are associated with distress and anger.

DIAGNOSIS

The diagnosis of anorexia nervosa is readily suspected. Any young girl, especially if from a middle-class family, with drastic weight loss from starvation and self-induced vomiting and/or diarrhea and obsessed with food needs to be regarded as a case. Often, a case history may include features such as an acrimonious parental divorce, alcoholic parents, physical/sexual abuse, perfectionism and obsessionality. In the UK, there appears to be an excess presence of the disorder among young ballerinas and professional dancers. In Canada, 7.6% of professional ballet students fulfill the diagnostic criteria for anorexia nervosa [46]. Crohn's disease can coexist with anorexia nervosa. More commonly, however, that form of inflammatory bowel disease is missed as a diagnosis but erroneously labeled as anorexia nervosa. Restlessness and insomnia with early wakening may result in the false diagnosis of severe depression. Before symptoms are so overt, the carers may observe the following tell-tale features: complaints of abdominal pain or nausea whenever eating; cutting food into very small pieces; paying exaggerated attention to what is eaten; calculating calories, etc.

The most frequently used criteria for the diagnosis of anorexia nervosa are those of the American Psychiatric Association's *Diagnostic and Statistical Manual for Mental Disorders*, fourth edition (DSM-IV) [47], presented in Tables 16.1 and 16.2. Although the DSM-IV version suggests such, it does not require a minimum body weight for a diagnosis. It has been shown that there is no point in separating patients into different groups based upon the amount of weight loss. The DSM-IV criteria also limit the amenorrhea requirement of previous criteria to postmenarchal females. What is important for the diagnosis is that weight and shape are central themes to the subject's self-evaluation and that there is denial of the seriousness of the low weight. DSM-IV separates anorexia nervosa into two subtypes: one group is for those who strictly limit food intake, and the other is confined to patients who binge and purge [48–52].

The DSM-IV criteria for bulimia nervosa are presented in Table 16.3. The amount of food characterizing a 'binge' is specified as being more than that which most people would consume, given the same period of time and circumstances. In addition, to comply with the definition, binge eating (as in DSM-III-R) as well as the inappropriate compensatory behavior must occur at least twice a week, and last for 3 months.

DIFFERENTIAL DIAGNOSIS

Differential diagnosis between anorexia nervosa and bulimia nervosa is difficult, as the disorders share some common features. Williamson [53] reported that both groups are similar in their body image distortion and anxiety after eating, but, while anorexics are 15% or more below normal weight, bulimics are within 10% of normal weight. Anorexics only occasionally engage in binge eating, but bulimics do so frequently. Furthermore, anorexics typically fast and avoid forbidden food, whereas bulimics binge on banned food and purge to control weight (Table 16.4). There are three observable signs that should alert the clinician to the possibility of bulimia nervosa [54]:

- Dental enamel erosion

- Lesions on the skin over dorsum of the hand

- Hypertrophy of the salivary glands

Further differential diagnoses include inflammatory bowel disease (particularly Crohn's), pancreatitis, superior mesenteric artery syndrome, hyperthyroidism, Addison's disease, infections and increased intracranial pressure.

MANAGEMENT

The essential need is to save the patient's life and correct the malnutrition. Delayed gastric emptying complicates food aversion by giving a sensation of early satiety and 'fullness' long after a meal has been ingested or delivered by nasogastric tube as a bolus. Persons with a weight loss below 75% of the ideal weight for height need hospital admission; those with drastic weight loss (35–40% below their usual weight), cardiac arrhythmias or those under metabolic stress justify enteric infusions of nutrients. This technique may achieve an impressive, albeit transient, response. If admitted to hospital, close surveillance is essential to deter illicit physical activity and the disposal of food. Outmaneuvering of the nursing and medical staff is common and patients often undertake brisk walks through the wards until confined to bed. The anorexic may devise devious modes of exercise when restricted to his or her room. Such initiatives may include repetitive opening and closing of a window or illicit knee-bending exercises. The mortality rate is as high as 10% in some series of hospitalized patients. Suicide is a common cause of death. The mortality in one group of 94 revealed a rate of 18% over 33 years [55].

- Refusal to maintain body weight at or above a minimally normal weight for age and height (e.g. weight loss leading to maintenance of body weight less than 85% of that expected, or failure to make expected weight gain during periods of growth, leading to body weight less than 85% of that expected)

- Intense fear of gaining weight or becoming fat, even though underweight

- Disturbance in the way in which one's body weight or shape is experienced, undue influence of body weight or shape on self-evaluation, or denial of the seriousness of the current low body weight

- In postmenarchal females, amenorrhea, i.e. the absence of at least three consecutive menstrual cycles (a woman is considered to have amenorrhea if her periods occur only following hormone, e.g. estrogen, administration)

Specify type:

Restricting type: during the current episode of anorexia nervosa, the person has not regularly engaged in binge-eating or purging behavior (i.e. self-induced vomiting or the misuse of laxatives, diuretics or enemas)

Binge-eating/purging type: during the current episode of anorexia nervosa, the person has regularly engaged in binge-eating or purging behavior (i.e. self-induced vomiting or the misuse of laxatives, diuretics or enemas)

Table 16.1 DSM-IV criteria for anorexia nervosa.

- Body weight is maintained at least 15% below that expected, or body mass index (BMI) is 17.5 or less; prepubertal patients may fail to make expected weight gains

- The weight loss is self-induced by avoidance of fattening foods and by the use of self-induced purging, excessive exercise, appetite suppressants and/or diuretics

- There is body image distortion whereby a dread of fatness persists as an intrusive overvalued idea, and the patients impose a low weight threshold on themselves

- An endocrine disorder involving the hypothalamic–pituitary–gonadal axis is present, manifested in the female as amenorrhea and in the male as loss of sexual interest and potency

- If onset is prepubertal, the sequence of pubertal events is delayed or even arrested; in girls, breasts do not develop and there is amenorrhea; in boys, the genitals remain juvenile

Table 16.2 Diagnostic guidelines for anorexia nervosa.

NUTRITIONAL MANAGEMENT

Enteral and parenteral feeding

Parenteral infusions are only justifiable as a life-saving measure. Enteral nutrition delivered through a nasogastric tube as a bolus or as a constant infusion is the preferred way to administer calories to patients unwilling to do so by mouth. Any regimen should have as its main aim the correction of fluid and electrolyte disturbances; the replacement of body tissue is a long-term objective best met by voluntary feeding.

In any state of chronic malnutrition, a deficiency of sodium and potassium exists. The potassium deficits should be repleted over several days. If correction is too rapid, there will

- Recurrent episodes of binge eating – an episode of binge eating is characterized by both of the following:

  (i)   eating, in a discrete period of time (e.g. within any 2-h period), an amount of food that is definitely larger than most people would eat during a similar period of time and under similar circumstances

  (ii)   a sense of lack of control regarding what or how much one is eating

- Recurrent inappropriate compensatory behavior in order to prevent weight gain – e.g. self-induced vomiting, misuse of laxatives, diuretics, enemas or other medications, fasting, or excessive exercise

- The binge-eating and inappropriate compensatory behaviors both occur, on average, at least twice a week for at least 3 months

- Self-evaluation is unduly influenced by body shape and weight

- The disturbance does not occur exclusively during episodes of anorexia nervosa

Specify type:

Purging type: during the current episode of bulimia nervosa, the person has regularly engaged in self-induced vomiting or the misuse of laxatives, diuretics or enemas

Non-purging type: during the current episode of bulimia nervosa, the person has used other inappropriate compensatory behaviors, such as fasting or excessive exercise, but has not regularly engaged in self-induced vomiting or the misuse of laxatives, diuretics or enemas

Table 16.3 Criteria for bulimia nervosa.

	Anorexia	**Bulimia**
Age of onset	Early or late adolescence	Early or late adolescence
Percentage below normal weight	≤ 15%	≥ 10%
Binge eating	Occasional	Frequently
Behavior	Fast and avoid forbidden foods	Binge on forbidden foods

Table 16.4 Characteristics of anorexia and bulimia nervosa.

be severe metabolic consequences. When protein deficiency is marked, an infusion of plasma may be used as a short-term replacement. Whatever enteral preparation is chosen, it should be introduced slowly, giving no more than half-strength or 50% of the estimated volume of requirements in the first 24 h. An adult preparation is usually suitable (see Appendix III.1).

Continuous infusion is likely to cause less distress than bolus feeding; introduction of enteral feeds can induce nausea and a bloated sensation. Supervision by nursing staff (often on a one-to-one basis) is vital at all times, because infusions can be disconnected and enteral fluids disposed of by the anorexic.

Oral feeding

When planning a scheme for nutritional rehabilitation it is essential that all members of the team – psychiatrist, pediatrician or adolescent medicine specialist, nursing staff and dietitian – are fully involved. Adolescents with anorexia are notoriously manipulative and quickly perceive which staff members are unsure about procedures. The full nutritional requirements, taking height and age into consideration, should be calculated and a realistic 'target weight' set. The complete energy intake may not be achieved immediately, but, with a planned series of increments, should be reached over 5–7 days.

The regimen should be based on normal meals that are appropriate for age. Too much choice is to be avoided, because this facilitates manipulation. A long list of dislikes must be discouraged, as such items may well include bread and potato, which are regarded as fattening. Ideally, all portions should be weighed to avoid conflict about daily variations of quantity. If this is not possible, portion sizes should be clearly stated in handy measures such as tablespoons, slices, number of cookies, etc. and displayed so that both food-service staff and patients can see them. Rules about mealtimes and exactly what may be uneaten must be established at an early stage and this strategy then firmly enforced. If the patient is very underweight, a complete nutritional supplement should be administered. Unfortunately, a dogmatic, inflexible attitude is justified in view of the bleak outlook. A schedule that is acceptable to the patient needs to be negotiated and it may be useful to draw up a 'contract' specifying what has been agreed upon about eating and levels of physical activity. This protocol can be signed by the patient and care staff. Pleasurable activities, for example watching television or being allowed outside the ward area, are used to encourage good behavior, and bed rest or restriction of visitors is imposed if compliance is poor. All members of the caring team must liaise frequently and be fully in agreement regarding decisions and procedures to be followed in any circumstance.

PSYCHOTHERAPY AND PHARMACOTHERAPY

Research on the treatment of eating disorders has focused primarily on cognitive-behavioral therapy [56] and, more recently, on interpersonal psychotherapy [57]. Numerous studies have shown that cognitive-behavioral therapy is helpful in reducing symptoms of bulimia nervosa and binge-eating disorder. Antidepressant medications are also useful, but are less likely to result in remission of symptoms than is cognitive-behavioral therapy. The results from comparison studies are inconsistent, with modest evidence that combining antidepressant medication and psychotherapy produces greater improvement in bulimic symptoms. Limited research has been conducted on the treatment of anorexia nervosa, although preliminary studies suggest that psychotherapy and fluoxetine may be helpful in preventing relapse after weight restoration.

There is now compelling evidence from double-blind, placebo-controlled studies that antidepressant medication is useful in the treatment of bulimia nervosa [29]. What is less clear is which patients are most likely to benefit from such medication and how best to sequence the various therapeutic interventions available. Statistically significant effects concerning the reduction of bulimic or depressive symptoms in bulimia nervosa have been demonstrated for tricyclic antidepressants (imipramine, desipramine), serotonergic agents (fluoxetine, d-fenfluramine), non-selective monoamine oxidase inhibitors (isocarboxazide, phenelzine) and trazodone. The utility of antidepressant medications in bulimia nervosa has led to their evaluation in binge-eating disorder. Additional studies of the use of medication in the treatment of binge-eating disorder and of the role of pharmacotherapy in the treatment of bulimia nervosa are needed.

PROGNOSIS

One of several studies directed to assess the course and outcome of anorexia and bulimia nervosa indicated that, during a median follow-up of 90 months, the full recovery rate of women with bulimia was 74% while that for women with anorexia was 33% [58]. Intake diagnosis of anorexia was the strongest predictor of worse outcome. No predictors of recovery emerged among bulimic subjects. Eighty-three percent of women with anorexia and 99% of those with bulimia achieved partial recovery. Approximately one-third of women with either disorder relapsed after full recovery. The authors concluded that the course of anorexia is characterized by high rates of partial recovery and low rates of full recovery, in comparison with bulimia, where there are higher rates of both partial and full recovery.

In another study, the long-term course of severe anorexia nervosa was examined with respect to recovery, relapse and predictors of outcome [59]. Patients were assessed over 10–15 years from the time of their index admission. Nearly 30% of patients had relapses following hospital discharge, prior to clinical recovery. However, most patients were weight recovered and menstruating regularly by the end of follow-up, with nearly 76% of the cohort meeting criteria for full recovery. Relapse after recovery was relatively uncommon. The time to recovery, however, was protracted, ranging from 57 to 79 months. Among restrictors at intake, nearly 30% developed binge eating, occurring within 5 years of intake. There were no deaths in the cohort.

Another group of workers reviewed 88 studies that had conducted follow-up assessments with bulimic subjects at least 6 months after presentation [60]. The crude mortality rate due to all causes of death for subjects with bulimia nervosa in these studies was 0.3% (seven deaths among 2194 subjects); however, ascertainment rates and follow-up periods were small and likely to produce underestimation. At 5–10 years following presentation, approximately 50% of women initially diagnosed with bulimia nervosa had fully recovered, while nearly 20% continued to meet full criteria for the disorder. Approximately 30% of women experienced relapse into bulimic symptoms. The risk of relapse appeared to decline 4 years after presentation. This study reconfirmed that there are few prognostic factors consistently identified, but certain personality traits, such as impulsivity, may contribute to poorer outcome.

FEEDING DISORDERS IN INFANTS AND YOUNG CHILDREN

Feeding difficulties and anorexia in children younger than 4 years of age are a relatively frequent cause for consulting with the general pediatrician. The child who will not eat what and when the parents wish him or her to needs to be distinguished from the child who will not eat anything at anytime. The first kind does not appear to be undernourished; indeed, sometimes they are overweight. Anemia, however, may occur. The child who is truly anorectic has poor weight gain and looks undernourished, even stunted.

Frequently, parents of children who do not eat at mealtimes complacently witness them consuming juices, crackers, potato-chips or candy even during the consultation. Often, in this phase of junk eating, the pediatrician will be told that the infant or child 'never eats' because that is how the carer(s) perceives the situation. Such events need to be clearly explained to the parents, and feeding norms set: the child should be in an infant seat and not running all over the house causing pandemonium while eating; the carer should prepare only one or two types of food and not a whole series of options and bribes. The child needs to receive positive reinforcement if he or she eats but should not be punished if he or she does not; milk should be offered at the end of the meal and not at the beginning. No compensatory food or snacks ought to be given between meals because the child did not have an appropriate earlier intake. Mealtimes should not be a power struggle. Even a young non-verbal infant can wield considerable emotional control by rejecting the offerings from the parents. Obviously, no attempts must ever be made to force-feed consequent to maternal distress when a child refuses to eat. This practice is not uncommon among certain ethnic communities. These children may benefit from behavioral modification therapy and dietary supplements.

REFERENCES

1. Butte N, Heinz C, Hopkinson J et al. Fat mass in infants and toddlers: comparability of total body water, total body potassium, total body electrical conductivity, and dual-energy X-ray absorptiometry. J Pediatr Gastroenterol Nutr 1999;29:184–9.

2. Ellis KJ. Measuring body fatness in children and young adults: comparison of bioelectric impedance analysis, total body electrical conductivity, and dual-energy X-ray absorptiometry. Int J Obes Relat Metab Disord 1996;20:866–73 .

3. Dietz WH, Bellizzi MC. Introduction: the use of body mass index to assess obesity in children. Am J Clin Nutr 1999;70:123S–5S.

4. Troiano RP, Flegal KM. Overweight prevalence among youth in the United States: why so many different numbers? Int J Obes Relat Metab Disord 1999;23:S22–7.

5. Goran MI. Metabolic precursors and effects of obesity in children: a decade of progress, 1990–1999. Am J Clin Nutr 2001;73:158–71.

6. Livingstone MB. Childhood obesity in Europe: a growing concern. Public Health Nutr 2001;4:109–16.

7. Rios M, Fluiters E, Perez Mendez LF et al. Prevalence of childhood overweight in Northwestern Spain: a comparative study of two periods with a ten year interval. Int J Obes Relat Metab Disord 1999;23:1095–8.

8. Chinn S, Rona RJ. Prevalence and trends in overweight and obesity in three cross sectional studies of British children, 1974–94. BMJ 2001;322:24–6.

9. Bundred P, Kitchiner D, Buchan I. Prevalence of overweight and obese children between 1989 and 1998: population based series of cross sectional studies. BMJ 2001;322:326–8.

10. Couper R. Prader-Willi syndrome. J Paediatr Child Health 1999;35:331–4.

11. Gortmaker SL, Must A, Sobol AM et al. Television viewing as a cause of increasing obesity among children in the United States, 1986–1990. Arch Pediatr Adolesc Med 1996;150:356–62.

12. Butte NF. The role of breastfeeding in obesity. Pediatr Clin North Am 2001;48:189–98.

13. Whitaker RC, Wright JA, Pepe MS et al. Predicting obesity in young adulthood from childhood and parental obesity. N Engl J Med 1997;337:869–73.

14. Prolo P, Wong ML, Licinio J. Leptin. Int J Biochem Cell Biol 1998;30:1285–90.

15. Chen D, Garg A. Monogenic disorders of obesity and body fat distribution. J Lipid Res 1999;40:1735–46.

16. Ellis KJ, Nicolson M. Leptin levels and body fatness in children: effects of gender, ethnicity, and sexual development. Pediatr Res 1997;42:484–8.

17. Argente J, Barrios V, Chowen JA et al. Leptin plasma levels in healthy Spanish children and adolescents, children with obesity, and adolescents with anorexia nervosa and bulimia nervosa. J Pediatr 1997;131:833–8.

18. Lindgren AC, Marcus C, Skwirut C et al. Increased leptin messenger RNA and serum leptin levels in children with Prader-Willi syndrome and nonsyndromal obesity. Pediatr Res 1997;42:593–6.

19. Leibel RL. Single gene obesities in rodents: possible relevance to human obesity. J Nutr 1997;127:1908S.

20. Brownell KD, Kaye FS. A school-based behavior modification, nutrition education, and physical activity program for obese children. Am J Clin Nutr 1982;35:277–83.

21. Botvin GJ, Cantlon A, Carter BJ et al. Reducing adolescent obesity through a school health program. J Pediatr 1979;95:1060–3.

22. Willi SM, Oexmann MJ, Wright NM et al. The effects of a high-protein, low-fat, ketogenic diet on adolescents with morbid obesity: body composition, blood chemistries, and sleep abnormalities. Pediatrics 1998;101:61–7.

23. Yang SP, Martin LJ, Schneider G. Weight reduction utilizing a protein-sparing modified fast. J Am Diet Assoc 1980;76:343–6.

24. Figueroa-Colon R, von Almen TK, Franklin FA et al. Comparison of two hypocaloric diets in obese children. Am J Dis Child 1993;147:160–6.

25. Stallings VA, Archibald EH, Pencharz PB. Potassium, magnesium, and calcium balance in obese adolescents on a protein-sparing modified fast. Am J Clin Nutr 1988;47:220–4.

26. de-Lima MS, Beria JU, Tomasi E et al. Use of amphetamine-like appetite suppressants: a cross-sectional survey in southern Brazil. Subst Use Misuse 1998;33:1711–9.

27. Patat A, Cerclé M, Trocherie S et al. Lack of amphetamine-like effects after administration of mefenorex in normal young subjects. Hum Psychopharmacol 1996;11:321–35.

28. Report of a WHO consultation on obesity: preventing and managing the global epidemic. Geneva: WHO, 1997.

29. Walsh BT, Devlin MJ. Pharmacotherapy of bulimia nervosa and binge eating disorder. Addict Behav 1995;20:757–64.

30. Lask B, Bryant-Waugh R. Childhood onset anorexia nervosa. In: Recent Advances in Paediatrics, No. 8. Edinburgh: Churchill Livingstone, 1986.

31. Anon. Apepsia hysterica. Br Med J 1870;i:39.

32. Casper RC, Offer D, Ostrov E. The self-image of adolescents with acute anorexia nervosa. J Pediatr 1981;98:656–61.

33. Hoek HW. The incidence and prevalence of anorexia nervosa and bulimia nervosa in primary care. Psychol Med 1991;21:455–60.

34. Hoek HW, Maiwald M, Bartelds A et al. The incidence of eating disorders and the influence of urbanization. Fifth International Conference on Eating Disorders, New York, USA, 1992 (Abstr. 163).

35. Jones DJ, Fox MM, Babigian HM et al. Epidemiology of anorexia nervosa in Monroe County, New York, 1960–1976. Psycho Som Med 1980;42:551–8.

36. Lucas AR, Beard CM, O'Fallon WM et al. 50-year trends in the incidence of anorexia nervosa in Rochester, Minn: a population-based study. Am J Psychiatry 1991;148:917–22.

37. Bryant-Waugh R, Knibbs J, Fosson A et al. Long term follow up of patients with early onset anorexia nervosa. Arch Dis Child 1988;63:5–9.

38. Hawley RM. The outcome of anorexia nervosa in younger subjects. Br J Psychiatry 1985;146:657–60.

39. Ratnasuriya RH, Eisler I, Szmukler GI et al. Anorexia nervosa: outcome and prognostic factors after 20 years. Br J Psychiatry 1991;158:495–502.

40. Warren MP, Vande Wiele RL. Clinical and metabolic features of anorexia nervosa. Am J Obstet Gynecol 1973;117:435–49.

41. Woodside DB, Garfinkel PE, Lin E et al. Comparisons of men with full or partial eating disorders, men without eating disorders, and women with eating disorders in the community. Am J Psychiatry 2001;158:570–4.

42. Baranowska B, Radzikowska M, Wasilewska-Dziubinska E et al. Disturbed release of gastrointestinal peptides in anorexia nervosa and in obesity. Diabetes Obes Metab 2000;2:99–103.

43. Russell G. Bulimia nervosa: an ominous variant of anorexia nervosa. Psychol Med 1979;9:429–48.

44. Bellodi L, Cavallini MC, Bertelli S et al. Morbidity risk for obsessive-compulsive spectrum disorders in first-degree relatives of patients with eating disorders. Am J Psychiatry 2001;158:563–9.

45. Mumford DB, Whitehouse AM. Increased prevalence of bulimia nervosa among Asian schoolgirls. BMJ 1988;297:718.

46. Garner DM, Garfinkel PE. Socio-cultural factors in the development of anorexia nervosa. Psychol Med 1980;10:647–56.

47. American Psychiatric Association. Diagnostic and Statistical Manual for Mental Disorders (DSM-IV), 4th ed. Washington, DC: American Psychiatric Association, 1994.

48. Casper RC, Eckert ED, Halmi KA et al. Bulimia. Its incidence and clinical importance in patients with anorexia nervosa. Arch Gen Psychiatry 1980;37:1030–5.

49. Garfinkel PE, Moldofsky H, Garner DM. The heterogeneity of anorexia nervosa. Arch Gen Psychiatry 1980;37:1036–40.

50. Strober M. The significance of bulimia in juvenile anorexia nervosa: an exploration of possible etiological factors. Int J Eat Disord 1981;1:28–93.

51. Strober M, Salkin B, Burroughs J et al. Validity of the bulimia-restricter distinction in anorexia nervosa. Parental personality characteristics and family psychiatric morbidity. J Nerv Ment Dis 1982;170:345–51.

52. West R. Eating Disord rs: Anorexia Nervosa and Bulimia Nervosa. London: Office of Health Economics, 1994.

53. Williamson DA. Assessment of Eating Disorders: Obesity, Anorexia, and Bulimia Nervosa. NY: Pergamon Press, 1990.

54. Mitchell JE, Pomeroy C, Colon E. Medical complications in bulimia nervosa. In: Fichter M (ed). Bulimia Nervosa: Basic Research, Diagnosis, and Therapy. New York: Wiley, 1990:71–83.

55. Theander S. Anorexia nervosa. A psychiatric investigation of 94 female patients. Acta Psychiatr Scand Suppl 1970;214:1–194.

56. Fernandez-Aranda F, Bel M, Jimenez S et al. Outpatient group therapy for anorexia nervosa: a preliminary study. Eat Weight Disord 1998;3:1–6.

57. Peterson CB, Mitchell JE. Psychosocial and pharmacological treatment of eating disorders: a review of research findings. J Clin Psychol 1999;55:685–97.

58. Herzog DB, Dorer DJ, Keel PK et al. Recovery and relapse in anorexia and bulimia nervosa: a 7.5-year follow-up study. J Am Acad Child Adolesc Psychiatry 1999;38:829–37.

59. Strober M, Freeman R, Morrell W. The long-term course of severe anorexia nervosa in adolescents: survival analysis of recovery, relapse, and outcome predictors over 10–15 years in a prospective study. Int J Eat Disord 1997;22:339–60.

60. Keel PK, Mitchell JE. Outcome in bulimia nervosa. Am J Psychiatry 1997;154:313–21.

Food Intolerance and Aversion

chapter **17**

'Food intolerance' is used to describe the condition in which an individual experiences adverse and reproducible manifestations following the intake of a particular food or food ingredient, whereas 'aversion' is taken as meaning psychological intolerance or food avoidance. Definitions are by no means well accepted by all authors. It has been suggested that the term 'allergy' be applied only to those with immediate allergic responses to food and with the presence of specific Immunoglobulin E (IgE) antibodies [1]. Among the food allergies, we include the reactions mediated by IgE (hypersensitivity or immediate-type allergy), as well as those produced by any other known immunological mechanism (reactions not mediated by IgE). Mast cells, basophils, eosinophils, macrophages and platelets can all be activated by IgE antibodies, causing the release of preformed or instant mediators. The subject of food intolerance has been complicated by disagreement regarding the diagnostic criteria, and by the fact that laboratory and skin tests are seldom helpful in corroborating a suspected diagnosis [2]. The reliability of skin testing, particularly in those under 1 year of age, has been questioned in the USA [3]. Furthermore, symptoms can be diverse and change within the same patient from one antigen exposure to the next. Also, parents and many pediatricians tend to either overdiagnose this entity or minimize its relevance. The clinical manifestations of food intolerance are listed in Table 17.1 [4–6].

FOOD AVERSION

Food aversion, in contrast to intolerance, is the result of either psychological intolerance or food avoidance. This problem may be seen as early as infancy, particularly in those who have had a complicated neonatal illness such as prematurity, bronchopulmonary dysplasia, necrotizing enterocolitis and/or severe heart disease. It can also be observed in toddlers who are described as 'picky eaters', as well as in older children and adults. In many cases, the child or adolescent will describe symptoms that occur following the intake of the foods to which they have an aversion. The causative association is not always apparent in that abdominal pain or nausea may follow a spoonful of a specific brand of yogurt yet not after a glass of milk.

FOOD INTOLERANCE

INCIDENCE

Approximately 5% of children under the age of 3 years experience food allergic disorders [4], although an incidence as high as 8% has been reported [7]. In 75% of cases, symptoms occur

Symptom	%
Vomiting	47
Diarrhea	41
Crying/colic	35
Failure to thrive	31
Eczema	22
Abdominal pain	19
Wheeze	19
Urticaria	18
Other rashes	13
Mood alteration	12
Angioneurotic edema	10
Flatulence	10
Abdominal distension	7
Steatorrhea	3

Table 17.1 Intestinal and extraintestinal manifestations of food intolerance in a study group of 68 children. Adapted from [6].

in the first 2 months of life. In a prospective and descriptive study by Rance et al. [8], a family history of atopic disease was found in 70.5% of 554 pediatric patients with food allergies. The main symptoms were atopic dermatitis (50.5% of patients), followed by urticaria and angioedema (30%). Asthma was present in 8.6% of patients and anaphylaxis in 4.5%.

ETIOLOGY

Food intolerance is a reaction that can be caused by:

1. Allergic reactions, which implies an unpleasant and immediate response to food(s). Such a mechanism may be via IgE antibody formation, a T cell-mediated reaction or the systemic formation of antigen–antibody complexes [9].

2. Enzyme deficiency, e.g. lactose intolerance due to hypolactasia (see p. 109) and fructose avoidance, as observed in patients with congenital fructose intolerance due to the deficiency of fructose-1-phosphate aldolase.

3. Pharmacologic factors, e.g. tyramine. There is a high concentration of tyramine in fermented cheese and this can elevate blood pressure and produce symptoms. Caffeine in coffee and tea can, in the hypersensitive, cause symptoms such as anxiety and tachycardia.

4. Toxic effect. Naturally occurring toxins occur in many foods, such as lectins in raw beans and hemagglutinins in soya; however, these heat-labile toxins are destroyed when cooked.

If particular foods, such as mushrooms and cereal grains, are stored, they can become contaminated with moulds and produce mycotoxins.

5. Other intolerances:

(i) Tartrazine, an azo dye, is a common coloring substance contained in many foods, soft drinks and pharmaceutical products. Its mechanism of action may be mediated by IgE antibodies. In a double-blind, placebo-controlled, repeated-measure study in Melbourne, Australia [10], it was demonstrated that tartrazine was responsible for irritability, restlessness and sleep disturbances in some children. Moreover, the investigators noted a dose-related response effect. Benzoates or sulfur dioxide preservatives and butylated hydroxyanisole or butylated hydroxytoluene antioxidants may cause urticaria and asthma. Manifestations of symptoms due to food additives include urticaria, asthma, migraine and rhinitis.

(ii) Acetylsalicylic acid (ASA), present in some vegetables and a variety of fruits and plants, can cause a range of symptoms in sensitive patients, including asthma, urticaria and rhinitis. Synthetic salicylates are found as flavoring products (see Appendix IV.40) and occur in high concentrations in curry powder and paprika.

PATHOGENESIS

We will refer exclusively to sensitivity to dietary protein. A genetic predisposition may well play an important part in the development of an adverse food reaction, as evidenced by HLA haplotyping [11] (Fig. 17.1). However, a key determinant is the integrity of the small-bowel mucosa to macromolecules. The permeability of the gastrointestinal tract to structures that can behave as allergens is believed to be a major factor in the pathogenesis of antigenic food reactions. Facilitated intestinal uptake of dietary antigens in severe or chronic diarrhea might be associated with subsequent allergy [12]. The intactness of the bowel mucosa is maintained in part by secretory IgA and the glycocalyx (a glycoprotein that coats the bowel enterocytes), as well as by the mucosa-associated lymph tissues (MALTs) [13]. Alteration to this protective barrier will enable the uptake of undigested macromolecules and increase the risk of a subsequent allergic reaction. It has been suggested that following a food challenge there is deposition of immune complexes in different target organs and sites, which can result in migraine, arthralgia or eczema. Antigen-specific protection is related to oral or parenteral immunization as well as the secretory immunoglobulins IgA and IgM. The absorbed antigens are presented to the gut-associated lymphoid tissue (GALT) of the lamina propria. GALT is an important component of the immune system and it gathers information from an antigen-filled tube, the gut. It is comprised of nodular lymphoid tissues (Peyer's patches and mesenteric lymph nodes), the mucosal phagocytes and lymphoid cells as well as lymph nodes. It is the specialized M cell on the membrane of the enterocyte (Fig. 17.2) that facilitates access of an antigen to the intestinal lymphoid tissue. These cells thus act as a gateway between the mucosal surface and the follicles in Peyer's patches of the foregut. M cells have scant villi with a deficient glycocalyx; these features together with absent lysosomes suggest that M cells are especially adapted for active vesicular transport of antigens [14].

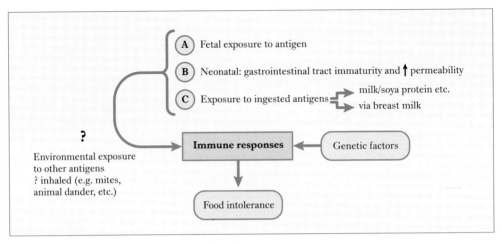

Figure 17.1 Possible pathways of food intolerance.

Mast-cell triggering and tryptase

The role of mast cells in mediating immediate-type hypersensitivity reactions is well established but their involvement in chronic inflammation and immune responses is only now becoming better understood. These cells, in common with basophils, express the high-affinity Fc receptor for IgE, but these two leukocytes are very distinct in their development. Activation of mast cells in the bowel can be evaluated by an assay for the serine protease tryptase: this will convey information about intestinal mucosal integrity and permeability [15]. It is known that mast cells that have been sensitized with IgE antibody and exposed to an antigen will be triggered to cause degranulation of the cell and release of mediators. Also, an IgG subclass can induce mast cell secretion. Mast cells synthesize and release large amounts of active proteinases, including tryptase and chymase. In addition, mast cells are able to produce a variety of cytokines such as interleukin (IL)-4, IL-5, IL-6, tumor necrosis factor (TNF)-α and interferon (IFN)-γ [16]. Mature tryptase and chymase are packaged and released together. One possible role for chymase is potentiation of histamine-induced vascular permeability [17]. Until recently, evaluation of mast cell activity has been dependent upon biopsy specimens from the small-bowel mucosa, but current and sophisticated developments in immunocytochemistry now allow access to non-invasive options.

Although protein hypersensitivity may follow an episode of gastroenteritis, in most cases a preceding event cannot be identified [18]. Each type of food contains substances that have the capacity to act as allergens: some are characteristic of that particular food, others can be shared with species of the same family or a closely related one (e.g. fish, legumes), while yet others may be present even in families that are phylogenetically distant. The last of these usually correspond to proteins with a similar function (profilins, tropomyosins, seralbumins, etc.). Some of these allergens are so ubiquitous they are known as panallergens [19]. These panallergens can be implicated in the sensitization to multiple allergens, as observed in many patients. These allergens may be limited to food, or act as pneumoallergens also.

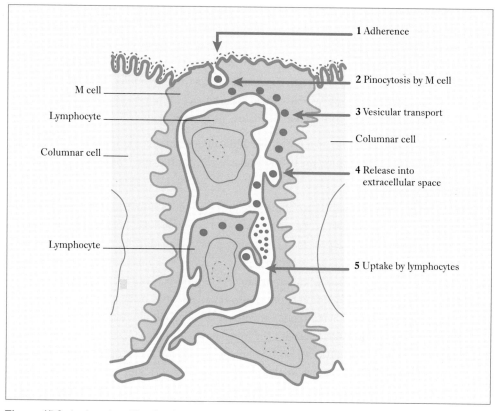

Figure 17.2 Antigen handling by the small intestine.

DIAGNOSIS

Proper diagnosis can be established through a careful history and examination, tests for IgE antibodies specific for food antigens, a favorable response to an allergen elimination diet and, if necessary, blinded and controlled antigen challenge (see p. 304).

In North America and Canada, it is common clinical practice to use skin testing. Parameters for this option, which is not without risk [20], have been published [21].

TREATMENT

Dietary management of adverse reactions to foods

Almost every food consumed by man has been cited as an allergen in the literature. Many food dyes, which have a low molecular weight and are not allergens in themselves, act as haptens and become allergenic if linked to a larger protein molecule. Some substances may undergo transformation to allergens only after they have been through the digestive process. Cooking or food processing can also affect allergenicity: a hard-boiled egg is less allergenic than a raw one. Certain combinations of foods may be allergenic while failing to give rise to symptoms when eaten separately. Allergy to one food is likely to produce cross-reactions with biologically related compounds [22]: if eggs are not tolerated, then chicken should be suspected until proved otherwise; similarly, beef and veal in milk protein allergy, and broad beans, peas, and lentils where peanuts are known to be allergenic [23]. The allergenicity of some items may be dose related: one strawberry may be tolerated while a plateful will produce urticaria. Nevertheless, from this morass of facts it is usually possible to select items that are likely offenders. Certain foods are linked with particular symptoms and this may be of help when deciding which should be avoided (Table 17.2) [24]. However, the symptoms may change with subsequent exposure, as with peanuts [25,26].

The most common food allergens reported are milk, cheese and dairy products, egg, fish and shellfish, chocolate, citrus fruits, meat (particularly pork), nuts and wheat.

Elimination diets [27]

A careful diet history in relation to clinical features is most important: if symptoms are continuous, the culprit is likely to be something that is taken daily; occasionally, a reaction occurs within hours of eating a food, and the cause is readily identified. Those with intermittent symptoms should keep a food diary including every item eaten or drunk, with brand names of processed food where applicable. A careful scrutiny of foods ingested 48 h prior to the development of symptoms, preferably on at least two occasions, should result in a 'short list' of offenders. These foods, and those biologically related to them, are then removed from the diet for 4–6 weeks with the intake/symptom record being continued. After this time, the offending item(s) should be given, ideally in a disguised form, to see if symptoms reappear. Failure to test in this objective way may result in many foods being wrongly branded as allergens and the child being condemned to a more restricted diet than is necessary. If a full diet history fails to give any clues, it is worthwhile excluding the most common allergens, according to symptoms, for 4–6 weeks before embarking on a full elimination diet. It is important that all traces of allergens are removed; thus, manufactured products, which may contain hidden ingredients, should be completely avoided.

A full elimination diet should only be proposed as a last resort, because this is a major undertaking for all concerned. A suggested protocol for an elimination diet is given in Appendix IV.39.

COW AND SOY MILK PROTEIN INTOLERANCE

Because the pathogenesis and symptoms of cow milk protein intolerance [CMPI; cow milk protein-sensitive enteropathy/cow milk allergy (CMA)] and those of soy milk protein intolerance are similar, we will describe them as a single entity and refer to them as dietary protein intolerance (DPI).

DPI can be preceded by an episode of acute enteritis [28] or present suddenly without any overt predisposing conditions. It is postulated that the mechanism is an allergic one, and a personal and family history of atopy is often present. There are more than 20 protein fractions in cow milk: β-lactoglobulin (not present in human milk) is the most common culprit, but α-lactalbumin, casein and bovine serum albumin can also cause enteropathy. Some of the milk antigens can cross-react with those found in goat milk. Use of this

Food	%
Egg	58.0
Soy milk	47.0
Orange	35.0
Peanuts	34.0
Casein hydrolysate	22.0
Banana	18.0
Wheat	16.0
Beef	14.5
Fish	13.0
Tomato	12.0
Strawberry	11.0
Chicken	9.0
Pear	8.0
Lamb	7.0
Apple	5.0

Table 17.2 Percentage of children with cow milk allergy showing an adverse reaction to individual foods. Adapted from [24].

non-bovine source of nutrition may sometimes be of help, but is not without risks – unless supplemented, goat milk is deficient in folate and vitamin B_{12}, and, in many communities, it may not have been pasteurized.

DIETARY MILK PROTEIN (AND MATERNAL MILK PROTEIN) INDUCED ENTEROPATHY [29]

Gastrointestinal symptoms may mimic a prolonged gastroenteritis and can include vomiting and loose mucusy stools containing macroscopic or microscopic blood. Failure to thrive may be the presenting feature. In some instances, it can follow an episode of acute gastroenteritis in which symptoms fail to resolve in the usual 5–7 days (post-enteritis syndrome). Furthermore, hypoproteinemia may arise as a result of a protein-losing enteropathy. Secondary carbohydrate intolerance may occur as a consequence of the blunting of the villi and depletion of the brush-border disaccharidases.

Whenever CMPI is suspected and a switch is made to soy milk, there is the possibility that an allergic reaction will recur. As many as 25% of children intolerant to cow milk react adversely to soy proteins. Ament and Rubin [30] described an intolerance to soy protein that caused flattening of the small-bowel villi which was morphologically indistinguishable from celiac disease. Moreover, the villi became atrophied as early as 24 h after soy challenge. The lesion was reversible within 4 days following removal of the offending soy protein.

DIETARY MILK PROTEIN (AND MATERNAL MILK PROTEIN) INDUCED COLITIS [31]

Protein-induced colitis is characterized by blood and mucus in the stools, with or without diarrhea. Proctoscopy or colonoscopy will reveal a friable mucosa that bleeds or a zone of hyperemia around blood vessels. Biopsy may demonstrate changes of an acute colitis with crypt distortion or abscesses, depletion of mucus from rectal glands and inflammatory changes within the lamina propria. In food-sensitive colitis, eosinophilia, as well as IgE-bearing mononuclear cells, are often found in the biopsy material.

Proctocolitis can also be observed in infants who are exclusively breastfed. Protein-sensitive colitis is the most common cause of rectal bleeding in infants. The diagnosis can be substantiated if withdrawal of the offending allergen leads to remission of symptoms. The prognosis is excellent. If the child has diarrhea, stools should be cultured for bacteria to exclude an infectious cause of colitis. In the preterm and newborn infant, necrotizing enterocolitis needs to be ruled out.

OTHER GASTROINTESTINAL SYMPTOMS ATTRIBUTED TO DPI

In young children, protein hypersensitivity may also manifest as

- Colic

- Esophagitis

- Chronic constipation [32]

Colic

Although the etiology of colic is multifactorial, one of the few identifiable causes in infants is intolerance to cow milk protein [33]. In a study by Jakobsson et al. [34], CMPI from formula or transmitted through maternal milk was clearly demonstrated.

Esophagitis

The histologic appearance of esophageal eosinophils has been correlated with esophagitis and gastroesophageal reflux disease in children. It has been suggested that esophageal eosinophilia that persists despite traditional antireflux therapy might depict allergic esophagitis rather than treatment failure. In a study by Kelly et al. [35], 10 infants with long-standing symptoms of gastroesophageal reflux despite standard antireflux measures, responded to semi-elemental or elemental diets. However, in some cases, a brief course of corticosteroids may be necessary [36].

OTHER DIETARY PROTEINS

Small-intestinal enteropathies associated with egg, fish, chicken and rice in infants have been described [37].

DIAGNOSIS

At present, there is no widespread agreement concerning the criteria for diagnosing DPI [38]. Despite the large number of publications describing different *in vivo* and *in vitro* tests to diagnose this entity, the response to a blinded challenge with the suspected offending protein remains the gold-standard method.

In 1963, Goldman established the criteria for the diagnosis of protein hypersensitivity: symptoms must subside following dietary elimination of milk and become exacerbated within 48 h of its reintroduction (three challenges in all) [39]. Extreme caution is required upon challenging an infant, because an anaphylactic-type reaction may occur. Shock and, rarely, death have followed milk ingestion in this situation. Therefore, nursing and medical staff should be on site in a well-equipped facility when vulnerable infants are challenged with milk. In an obese infant, and in other situations where venous access might be difficult in an emergency situation, it is prudent to have an intravenous line in position prior to the challenge.

Investigations

Skin tests

Skin (prick) tests ('immediate') and the radioallergosorbent test (RAST) produce false-positives as well as false-negatives and fail to identify problems not due to IgE, i.e. reactions that occur after some hours [40]. Although the positive predictive value of a prick test is lower than 50%, a negative skin test in those older than 12 months of age practically excludes the possibility that the patient will develop symptoms in a challenge unless the reaction in question is not mediated by IgE.

Rance and colleagues [41] investigated the associations between results obtained with prick tests using commercial extracts and fresh foods, for four foods, in 430 children with suspected food allergy. For cow milk, wheal diameters at 15 min were larger with commercial extracts, but the difference was not significant. Conversely, skin responses were significantly larger with fresh foods for the other ingested allergens. Skin prick tests were positive in 40% of cases with commercial extracts and in 81.3% with fresh foods. The overall concordance between a positive prick test and a positive labial and/or oral challenge was 58.8% with commercial extracts and 91.7% with fresh foods. The authors concluded that fresh foods may be more effective for detecting the sensitivity to food allergens and should be used for primary testing for egg, peanut and cow milk sensitivity.

Majamaa et al. [42] evaluated the relevance of skin tests and the concentration of specific IgE antibodies correlating with oral cow milk challenge in 143 infants aged under 2 years with suspected CMA. Seventy-two (50%) of the challenges were positive. Of the positive reactions, 22 involved immediate-type reactions; in 50 patients, delayed-onset reactions of eczematous or gastrointestinal type occurred. Of the infants with challenge-proven CMA, 26% showed elevated IgE concentrations to cow milk, 14% had a positive skin prick test and 44% had a positive patch test for cow milk. In most patients with a positive patch test, the prick test for cow milk was negative.

Small-bowel biopsy

If the small intestine is affected, small-bowel biopsy will show a patchy enteropathy, with mostly a chronic, non-specific inflammatory infiltrate that consists of lymphocytes and plasmocytes as well as eosinophils [43]. The histopathology can resemble celiac disease in relapse. Also, the lamina propria may be infiltrated with eosinophils and/or have an increase in IgE plasma cells. The mucosa improves when the offending protein(s) is removed from the diet.

Proctoscopy/sigmoidoscopy

This test is only indicated if the diagnosis is not clear. The mucosa may be friable, hemorrhagic and with abundant mucus. Histopathology will demonstrate acute and chronic inflammatory infiltrates, with a predominance of lymphocytes and plasmocytes and an increased number of eosinophils [44]. There may also be hyperplasia of goblet mucus cells. HLA-DR antigens are not normally expressed on the mucosal lining cells but have been reported in food-sensitive colitis, although this is not exclusive to this entity (Figs 17.3 and 17.4).

Other tests

Other laboratory tests are not generally necessary, but findings may include:

- Eosinophilia ($>450/mm^3$)

- Elevated total IgE

- Low IgA and reduced C3

- Blood – investigate iron-deficiency anemia if the history reflects abundant and/or prolonged bleeding

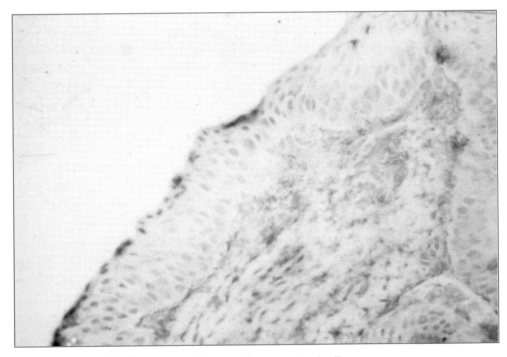

Figure 17.3 HLA-DR (immunoperoxidase stain) – normal anal cell appearance.

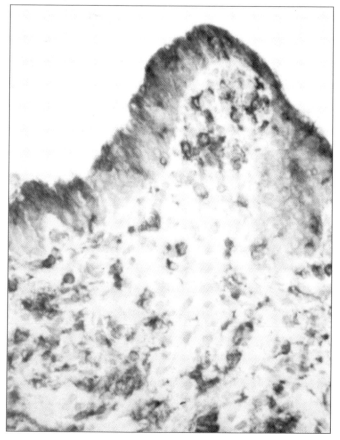

Figure 17.4 HLA-DR positive stain in food-sensitive colitis in anal cells – note increased darkly stained cells. (By kind permission of Dr I Lampert.)

- Stools – presence of Charcot–Leyden crystals (eosinophils); in addition, a useful clue to the diagnosis of protein-sensitive colitis is the presence of occult or gross blood and/or mucus in the stools in an infant who is otherwise healthy and whose stools are neither hard nor extremely watery

Differential diagnosis

In patients with diarrhea, the following conditions need to be excluded:

- Lactose malabsorption

- Celiac disease

- Giardiasis

- Irritable bowel syndrome (toddler diarrhea)

- Enteritis – infectious, autoimmune, inflammatory bowel disease, intractable diarrhea

- Intestinal lymphangiectasia

- Immunodeficiency syndrome

The difficulty is that lactose malabsorption can coexist with DPI, as can transient gluten intolerance. Once the intestinal mucosa heals, lactose will be tolerated and, later, milk proteins.

In patients with diarrhea and blood and/or mucus in the stool, the differential diagnosis should include:

- Necrotizing enterocolitis, particularly in the first few weeks of life
- Infectious colitis – *Campylobacter jejunii*, ameba, *Clostridium difficile*
- Inflammatory bowel disease – Crohn's disease or ulcerative colitis
- Food-sensitive colitis, especially in the early weeks of life or when breast milk is switched for formula

DIETARY MANAGEMENT

In the exclusively breastfed infant, intolerance is not to maternal milk protein but to proteins from the mother's diet and present in her milk. If an elimination diet in the mother does not resolve the problem and the infant is clinically well and growing with normal rectal biopsy findings, reassurance may be all that is required. In the formula-fed infant, identifying the suspected allergen is the easiest of all situations, and the problem can frequently be resolved with a switch to a hydrolyzed milk protein.

The nutritional requirements of children with DPI may be increased because of pre-existing undernutrition. If so, a higher energy intake can be achieved by one or more of the following:

- Concentrating the formula powder
- Adding carbohydrate such as glucose polymers to the formula
- Adding fat to the formula

Details are described in the section dealing with high-energy feeds in Appendix III.

Formula alternatives

Alternatives to cow milk fall into three broad categories:

- Hydrolyzed milk protein
- Milk of another species (e.g. human, goat or sheep) – goat and sheep milk are not routinely recommended because of the risk of cross-reactivity, and human milk only if the mother is capable of, or wants to re-establish, lactation
- Feeds based on soy milk – rarely effective as a substitute for true casein hypersensitivity (cross-reactivity risk)

Milk protein hydrolysates

Cow milk protein products that have undergone enzymatic hydrolysis into their constituent peptides and amino acids are frequently used in the treatment of DPI. These milks are generally lactose-free, with glucose polymers added as the carbohydrate. A small proportion of infants have been reported to react to these special milks. This might be attributable to vat contamination with whole-milk proteins during manufacture. Care must be taken to ensure that the product used is suitable for infants and contains adequate vitamin and mineral supplementation. For extreme cases of hypersensitivity, products containing small peptides have been developed. Special products designed for use as an infant formula and which contain adequate vitamin and mineral supplementation include:

- Alfaré (Nestlé Nutritionals) – not available in the USA

- Alimentum (Ross Laboratories) – available in the USA and UK

- Nutramigen (Mead Johnson) – available in the USA and UK

- Pregestimil (Mead Johnson) – available in the USA and UK

- Pepdite (for infants aged <1 year) and Pepdite 1+ (for those aged >1 year; SHS International) – Pepdite is not available in the USA; Pepdite 1+ is available in the USA and UK

Further details of these products are found in Appendix IV.6.

It needs to be remembered that infants ingesting any of the above are likely to have seedy, non-formed stools.

Human milk

Where lactation in the mother has not entirely ceased, continuation of breastfeeding can be encouraged. Pasteurized and banked human milk has been used for very sick infants in hospital as a temporary measure. (HIV is readily destroyed by pasteurization.) In some communities, for personal as well as cultural reasons, mothers will not permit their infants to receive human milk from unrelated donors. A supplement of iron and vitamins A, B group $(B_1, B_2, B_3$ and $B_6)$, C and D should be given with breast milk. In addition, unless the mother excludes cow milk protein and/or other potential allergens from her diet, reactions can be caused via breast milk.

Goat milk

This is sometimes tolerated by infants allergic to cow milk protein. However, a number of the proteins of cow and goat milk do cross-react and many infants show symptoms when challenged with this milk. Furthermore, folate deficiency, a potential cause of megaloblastic anemia, may develop, because, unless supplemented by the manufacturer, goat milk contains only 6.5 μg/l of folate compared with 42 μg/l in cow milk. Goat milk may also be deficient in vitamin B_{12} [45].

Vegetable proteins

The most common vegetable-based milk substitutes contain soy, which has a high biological value and a bland taste. These preparations are free of lactose and would therefore be suitable for lactose-intolerant infants. Although some adverse reactions have been noted in milk-intolerant infants fed with soy formula these have mainly occurred with products based on soy flour; most modern infant formulas contain a soy protein isolate, which is less likely to give rise to problems.

Care must be taken to choose a product specifically designated for pediatric use. Products intended for adult vegans are generally not nutritionally adequate; the methionine content is low and vitamins and minerals may not be added.

Soy protein isolates that are suitable for infants include:

- Isomil – available in the USA (Ross) and UK (Abbott Nutrition)

- Prosobee (Mead Johnson) – available in the USA and UK

- Nursoy (Nestlé) – not available in UK, available as Carnation Alsoy in USA

- Wysoy (Wyeth; UK) – not available in the USA

Further details of these products are found in Appendix IV.3.

Chemically defined diets

Chemically defined diets are based on synthetic amino acid mixtures with a source of fat and carbohydrate, and are theoretically the least likely product to cause allergy. However, they have several disadvantages, such as low palatability and high osmolality, which are more fully discussed in the section in Appendix IV.20. Suitable feeds of this type are:

- Neocate Infant formula, for infants aged <1 year, and Neocate 1+ for infants over one year. Neocate Advance (UK) or Neocate Junior (USA) for older children (SHS)

- Vivonex Pediatric (Novartis Nutrition; USA)

- Tolerex (Novartis Nutrition; USA)

Reintroduction of cow or soy milk

Where milk protein is to be reintroduced after a period on a milk-free diet, care should be taken to minimize the risk of an anaphylactic reaction developing. This acute reaction has been seen in infants who exhibited only fairly minor symptoms while receiving cow or soy milk on previous occasions. Ideally, prior to a milk challenge in a patient with an enteropathy, a small-bowel biopsy should show a normal healed mucosa. If the mucosa still reveals features of DPI, postpone the challenge. However, a normal mucosal pattern does not exempt the child from the risk of an adverse reaction to a milk challenge. Also, lactose absorption should be proven either by a lactose breath hydrogen test (see p. 166) or by demonstrating clinical tolerance following gradual reintroduction of the carbohydrate and stool monitoring for carbohydrate and pH (see p. 107). In addition, milk should be applied topically to the skin as a scratch test. A severe cutaneous reaction would suggest persistence of milk intolerance, but the absence of a skin response does not nullify the risk of

Day 1	5, 10, 20, 30 and 60 ml at 30-min intervals
Day 2	120 ml as a single morning dose
Day 3	240 ml as a single morning dose
Day 4	normal intake

Table 17.3 Procedure to perform milk challenge. Adapted from [46].

anaphylaxis. An intravenous drip should be *in situ* and observations maintained for about 12 h following the provocation. The patient must have immediate access to resuscitation facilities. The patient should not be exposed to this potentially hazardous procedure without the presence of trained personnel and equipment for treating systemic anaphylaxis.

The procedure for performing the challenge is outlined in Table 17.3 [46].

Milk-protein-free diet for older infants and children

In children over the age of 1 year, milk or a milk substitute is not an essential ingredient in the diet: provided that an adequate intake of protein, energy and calcium is achieved, the fluid intake can consist of non-milk-containing beverages.

Very small amounts of cow milk protein may provoke an allergic response; hence, for the diet to prove effective, all traces of bovine protein must be eliminated. Dairy products such as cheese, yogurt, ice cream, cream and butter are obvious sources of milk protein; however, in reality, many manufactured foodstuffs contain one or more types of milk protein. In countries where food legislation demands that the ingredients be shown on the packaging of processed foods, parents can be instructed to read the labels and omit any items that contain milk (often labeled as 'casein' or 'whey' products). Where such information is not available, all processed food should be avoided.

Soy protein intolerance

If soy protein intolerance is still present when solid food is to be introduced into the diet, care must be taken to exclude this protein. Soy flour is added to many processed foods, and any foods that are stated to contain soy, hydrolyzed protein or textured vegetable protein should be avoided. If exact ingredient information is not available, all processed foods likely to contain soy should be excluded. 'Made-up' meat dishes eaten in a restaurant, or from a hospital or school kitchen, are also likely to contain soy.

PROGNOSIS

In broad terms, the prognosis for the gastrointestinal manifestations of protein hypersensitivity is good. There is general agreement that chronic diarrhea due to CMA resolves with a cow milk-free diet, and that tolerance to cow milk is achieved by the age of 2 years. Businco et al. [47] followed, for 4—10 years, 37 infants with chronic diarrhea who, at onset of symptoms, had RAST and/or skin tests positive to cow milk. After the diarrhea subsided, reintroduction of cow milk was attempted at 6-month intervals. In 25 (68%) of these children, symptoms subsided at a median age of 2 years; however, the remaining 12 children (32%) did not tolerate cow milk at a median age of 6 years. In addition, during the follow-up period, 27 (73%) of the children suffered from other atopic manifestations, due either to CMA or to inhalant allergy.

Prediction of which patients will achieve tolerance and the time of resolution are speculative. Hill et al. [48] studied 98 children (median age 24 months) with CMA over a median period of 2 years to see whether acquisition of clinical tolerance to cow milk was associated with changes in levels of IgG and IgE anti-cow milk antibodies, and skin test reactivity to a cow milk extract.

Two groups of patients were examined. The first (n = 69) were IgE-sensitized and responded rapidly to small volumes of cow milk with one or more of the following: urticaria, exacerbations of eczema, wheeze and vomiting. The second (n = 29), a late-reacting group, demonstrated coughing, diarrhea and eczematoid rashes, alone or in combination, which developed more than 20 h after commencing normal volumes of cow milk. Significant immunological changes were confined to the first group. Of these, there were 15 children who achieved clinical tolerance to cow milk and they showed a significant fall in the levels of skin test reactivity to cow milk over the study period. In addition, these children had lower serum IgE antibodies to cow milk proteins, both at the outset and the final follow-up, compared with the patients whose allergy persisted. No consistent change in the IgG antibody responses to cow milk proteins was seen in either group of patients over the study period. The findings suggest that patients with immediate-type hypersensitivity to cow milk proteins whose disease persists for more than 2 years have a more severe dysregulation of IgE synthesis to cow milk proteins from the outset.

Similarly, James and Sampson [49] undertook a study to determine whether cow milk-specific antibody responses correlate with the development of clinical tolerance. Double-blind, placebo-controlled food challenges were performed annually in 29 children with CMA. Clinical reactivity was lost in 11 (38%) of the patients. The median age for all patients at the time of diagnosis by these food challenges was 3 years; more than 80% of patients in each group had atopic dermatitis as part of their presenting symptoms. Casein-specific and β-lactoglobulin-specific IgE, IgG, IgG1 and IgG4 antibody concentrations were analyzed in all patients at regular intervals. In the patients becoming clinically tolerant to cow milk, the IgE-specific antibody concentrations and IgE/IgG-specific ratios for both milk proteins were lower initially and decreased significantly with time, in comparison with those in the group who retained clinical sensitivity. The concentrations of IgG1- and IgG4-specific antibody to casein and the IgE/IgG1 and IgE/IgG4 ratios for both casein and β-lactoglobulin were significantly less in the patients losing clinical reactivity. No differences in the IgG-specific concentrations were observed in either group at any of the evaluation times. The authors concluded that monitoring similar casein-specific and β-lactoglobulin-specific IgE concentrations and IgE/IgG ratios may help predict which patients will ultimately lose their clinical reactivity to cow milk.

MIGRAINE AND FOOD INTOLERANCE

Migraine is a very contentious subject, in terms of both diagnostic criteria and management. The manifestations in children are quite dissimilar to those seen in adults, and in the latter, classic migraine is readily identified. Furthermore, gastrointestinal features are more prominent in children and neurological complications less evident.

DIAGNOSTIC AIDS AND RESEARCH PROCEDURES

The following tests should be carried out:

- Skin testing to foods

- Total IgE (see below)

- RAST to specific foods (see below)

Food allergens and RAST

Dependence on the results of RAST has been questioned because it is said by some authorities to be a semi-quantitative test [50] and others have rarely found positive RAST results to food samples in migraine patients. Normal IgE levels and negative RAST results have been reported in children with abdominal migraine. This suggests that the pathogenesis, if immunological, is not reaginic.

REFERENCES

1. Lessof MH. The diagnosis of food intolerance. Clin Exp Allergy 1995; 25(Suppl. 1):14–5.

2. David TJ. Patch tests. In: Food and Food Additive Intolerance in Childhood. Oxford: Blackwell Scientific, 1993:254–60.

3. Guerin B, Watson RD. Skin tests. Clin Rev Allergy 1988;6:211–27.

4. Sampson HA. Food allergy. JAMA 1997;278:1888–94.

5. Sampson HA. Clinical manifestations of adverse food reactions. Pediatr Allergy Immunol 1995;6 (Suppl. 8):29–37.

6. Minford AM, MacDonald A, Littlewood JM. Food intolerance and food allergy in children: a review of 68 cases. Arch Dis Child 1982;57:742–7.

7. Pearl ER. Food allergy. Lippincotts Prim Care Pract 1997;1:154–67.

8. Rance F, Kanny G, Dutau G, et al. Food hypersensitivity in children: clinical aspects and distribution of allergens. Pediatr Allergy Immunol 1999;10:33–8.

9. Sampson HA, Burks AW. Mechanisms of food allergy. Annu Rev Nutr 1996;16:161–77.

10. Rowe KS, Rowe KJ. Synthetic food coloring and behavior: a dose response effect in a double-blind, placebo-controlled, repeated-measures study. J Pediatr 1994;125:691–8.

11. Zwollo P, Ehrlich-Kautzky E, Sharf SJ, et al. Sequencing of HLA-D in responders and nonresponders to short ragweed allergen, Amb a V. Immunogenetics 1991;33:141–51.

12. Sanderson IR, Walker WA. Uptake and transport of macromolecules by the intestine: possible role in clinical disorders (an update). Gastroenterology 1993;104:622–39.

13. Mowat AM, Viney JL. The anatomical basis of intestinal immunity. Immunol Rev 1997;156:145–66.

14. Savidge TC. The life and times of an intestinal M cell. Trends Microbiol 1996;4:301–6.

15. Bacci S, Faussone-Pellegrini S, Mayer B, et al. Distribution of mast cells in human ileocecal region. Dig Dis Sci 1995;40:357–65.

16. Harvima IT, Horsmanheimo L, Naukkarinen A, et al. Mast cell proteinases and cytokines in skin inflammation. Arch Dermatol Res 1994;287:61–7.

17. Caughey GH. The structure and airway biology of mast cell proteinases. Am J Respir Cell Mol Biol 1991;4:387–94.

18. Walker-Smith JA. Cow milk-sensitive enteropathy: predisposing factors and treatment. J Pediatr 1992;121:S111–5.

19. Martin Esteban M, Pascual CY. Food allergies in Spain: causal allergens and diagnostic strategies. Pediatr Pulmonol Suppl 1999;18:154–6.

20. Zacharisen MC. Allergy skin testing infants: a safe or risky procedure? Ann Allergy Asthma Immunol 2000;85:429–30.

21. American Academy of Allergy and Immunology. Allergen skin testing. J Allergy Clin Immunol 1993;92:636–7.

22. Reese G, Lehrer SB. Food allergen cross-reactivity and clinical significance. Ann Allergy Asthma Immunol 2000;85:431–3.

23. Hill DJ, Heine RG, Hosking CS. Management of peanut and nut allergies. Lancet 2001;357:87–8.

24. Bishop JM, Hill DJ, Hosking CS. Natural history of cow milk allergy: clinical outcome. J Pediatr 1990;116:862–7.

25. Vander Leek TK, Liu AH, Stefanski K, et al. The natural history of peanut allergy in young children and its association with serum peanut-specific IgE. J Pediatr 2000;137:749–55.

26. Sampson HA. What should we be doing for children with peanut allergy? J Pediatr 2000;137:741.

27. Høst A, Koletzko B, Dreborg S, et al. Dietary products used in infants for treatment and prevention of food allergy. Arch Dis Child 1999;81:80–4.

28. Firer MA, Hosking CS, Hill DJ. Possible role for rotavirus in the development of cows' milk enteropathy in infants. Clin Allergy 1988;18:53–61.

29. Barnard J. Gastrointestinal disorders due to cow's milk consumption. Pediatr Ann 1997;26:244–50.

30. Ament ME, Rubin CE. Soy protein – another cause of the flat intestinal lesion. Gastroenterology 1972;62:227–34.

31. Halpin TC, Byrne WJ, Ament ME. Colitis, persistent diarrhea, and soy protein intolerance. J Pediatr 1977;91:404–7.

32. Iacono G, Cavataio F, Montalto G, et al. Intolerance of cow's milk and chronic constipation in children. N Engl J Med 1998;339:1100–4.

33. Lucassen PL, Assendelft WJ, Gubbels JW, et al. Infantile colic: crying time reduction with a whey hydrolysate: a double-blind, randomized, placebo-controlled trial. Pediatrics 2000;106:1349–54.

34. Jakobsson I, Lindberg T, Benediktsson B, et al. Dietary bovine beta-lactoglobulin is transferred to human milk. Acta Paediatr Scand 1985;74:342–5.

35. Kelly KJ, Lazenby AJ, Rowe PC, et al. Eosinophilic esophagitis attributed to gastroesophageal reflux: improvement with an amino acid-based formula. Gastroenterology 1995;109:1503–12.

36. Liacouras CA, Wenner WJ, Brown K, et al. Primary eosinophilic esophagitis in children: successful treatment with oral corticosteroids. J Pediatr Gastroenterol Nutr 1998;26:380–5.

37. Burks AW, Sampson H. Food allergies in children. Curr Probl Pediatr 1993;23:230–52.

38. Walker-Smith JA. Diagnostic criteria for gastrointestinal food allergy in childhood. Clin Exp Allergy 1995;25(Suppl. 1):20–2.

39. Goldman AS, Anderson DW, Sellers WA, et al. Milk allergy. I. Oral challenge with milk and isolated milk proteins in allergic children. Pediatrics 1963;32:425–43.

40. Eigenmann PA, Sampson HA. Interpreting skin prick tests in the evaluation of food allergy in children. Pediatr Allergy Immunol 1998;9:186–91.

41. Rance F, Juchet A, Bremont F, et al. Correlations between skin prick tests using commercial extracts and fresh foods, specific IgE, and food challenges. Allergy 1997;52:1031–5.

42. Majamaa H, Moisio P, Holm K, et al. Cow's milk allergy: diagnostic accuracy of skin prick and patch tests and specific IgE. Allergy 1999;54:346–51.

43. Manuel PD, Walker-Smith JA, France NE. Patchy enteropathy in childhood. Gut 1979;20:211–5.

44. Walker-Smith JA. Milk intolerance in children. Clin Allergy 1986;16:183–90.

45. Paul A, Southgate DAT. The Composition of Foods. Fourth revised and extended edition of MRC Special Report No. 297. London: HMSO, 1978.

46. Hill DJ, Firer MA, Shelton MJ, et al. Manifestations of milk allergy in infancy: clinical and immunologic findings. J Pediatr 1986;109:270–6.

47. Businco L, Benincori N, Cantani A, et al. Chronic diarrhea due to cow's milk allergy. A 4- to 10-year follow-up study. Ann Allergy 1985;55:844–7.

48. Hill DJ, Firer MA, Ball G, et al. Natural history of cows' milk allergy in children: immunological outcome over 2 years. Clin Exp Allergy 1993;23:124–31.

49. James JM, Sampson HA. Immunologic changes associated with the development of tolerance in children with cow milk allergy. J Pediatr 1992;121:371–7.

50. Speight JW, Atkinson P. Food allergy in migraine. Lancet 1980;2:532.

NUTRIENT REQUIREMENTS AND HEIGHT/WEIGHT DATA

UK DATA

USA DATA

I.1 RECOMMENDATIONS FOR ENERGY INTAKE

Estimated average intake					
Age	**UK**[1]		**Age**	**USA**[2]	
	kcal/kg/day	**kJ/kg/day**		**kcal/kg/day**	**kJ/kg/day**
1 month	115	480	0–6 months	108	450
3 months	100	420	6–12 months	98	410
6–36 months	95	400	1–3 years	102	425
Males:			4–6 years	90	375
3 years	97	405	7–10 years	70	290
4 years	94	395	*Males:*		
5 years	88	370	11–14 years	55	230
6 years	84	350	15–18 years	45	190
7 years	78	325	*Females:*		
Females:			11–14 years	47	195
3 years	92	385	15–18 years	40	170
4 years	87	365			
5 years	82	345			
6 years	71	320			
7 years	66	295			

	kcal/day	**MJ/day**
Males:		
7–10 years	1970	8.24
11–14 years	2200	9.27
15–18 years	2755	11.51
Females:		
7–10 years	1740	7.28
11–14 years	1845	7.92
15–18 years	2110	8.33

[1]From Dietary Reference Values for Food Energy and Nutrients for the United Kingdom. Department of Health Report on Health and Social Subjects No. 41. London: HMSO, 1991. Estimated Average Requirement.
[2]United States Recommended Daily Intakes 1989.

I.2 RECOMMENDATIONS FOR PROTEIN INTAKE

Age	UK[1]	Age	USA[2]
	g/kg/day		**g/kg/day**
0–3 months	2.10	0–6 months	2.16
4–6 months	1.65	6–12 months	1.55
7–9 months	1.55	1–3 years	1.23
10–12 months	1.54	4–6 years	1.20
1–3 years	1.16	7–10 years	1.00
4–6 years	1.11		
7–10 years	1.00		
	g/day		**g/day**
Males:		*Males:*	
11–14 years	42.10	11–14 years	45.00
15–18 years	55.20	15–18 years	59.00
Females:		*Females:*	
11–14 years	43.80	11–14 years	46.00
15–18 years	45.40	15–18 years	44.00

[1] From Dietary Reference Values for Food Energy and Nutrients for the United Kingdom. Department of Health Report on Health and Social Subjects No. 41. London: HMSO, 1991. Estimated Average Requirement.
[2] United States Recommended Daily Intakes, 1989.

I.3 RECOMMENDATIONS FOR INTAKES OF MINERALS – UK

Age	Calcium		Phosphorus		Magnesium	
	(mmol/day)	(mg/day)	(mmol/day)	(mg/day)	(mmol/day)	(mg/day)
0–3 months	13.1	525	13.1	400	2.2	55
4–6 months	13.1	525	13.1	400	2.5	60
7–9 months	13.1	525	13.1	400	3.2	75
10–12 months	13.1	525	13.1	400	3.3	80
1–3 years	8.8	350	8.8	270	3.5	85
4–6 years	11.3	450	11.3	350	4.8	120
7–10 years	13.8	550	13.8	450	8.0	200
Males:						
11–14 years	25.0	1000	25.0	775	11.5	280
15–18 years	25.0	1000	25.0	775	12.3	300
Females:						
11–14 years	20.0	800	20.0	625	11.5	280
15–18 years	20.0	800	20.0	625	12.3	300

From Dietary Reference Values for Food Energy and Nutrients for the United Kingdom. Department of Health Report on Health and Social Subjects No. 41. London: HMSO, 1991. Reference Nutrient Intake.

RECOMMENDATIONS FOR INTAKES OF MINERALS – USA

Age	Calcium		Phosphorus		Magnesium	
	(mmol/day)	(mg/day)	(mmol/day)	(mg/day)	(mmol/day)	(mg/day)
Infants						
0–6 months	5.25*	210*	3.23*	100*	1.25*	30*
7–12 months	6.75*	270*	8.87*	275*	3.13*	75*
Children						
1–3 years	12.50*	500*	14.84	460	3.33	80
4–8 years	20.00*	800*	16.13	500	5.42	130
Males						
9–13 years	32.50*	1300*	40.32	1250	10.00	240
14–18 years	32.50*	1300*	40.32	1250	17.08	410
Females						
9–13 years	32.50*	1300*	40.32	1250	10.00	240
14–18 years	32.50*	1300*	40.32	1250	15.00	360

*Adequate Intakes (AI).
Dietary Reference Intakes, National Academy of Sciences 1998.

I.4 RECOMMENDATIONS FOR INTAKES OF TRACE ELEMENTS

Age	Iron				Zinc			
	UK[1]		USA[2]		UK[1]		USA[2]	
	(mg/ day)	(μmol/ day)	(mg/ day)	(μmol/ day)	(mg/ day)	(μmol/ day)	(mg/ day)	(μmol/ day)
0–3 months	1.7	30	6.0	106	4.0	60	5.0	75
4–6 months	4.3	80	6.0	106	4.0	60	5.0	75
7–9 months	7.8	140	10.0	177	5.0	75	5.0	75
10–12 months	7.8	140	10.0	177	5.0	75	5.0	75
1–3 years	6.9	120	10.0	177	5.0	75	10.0	150
4–6 years	6.1	110	10.0	177	6.5	100	10.0	150
7–10 years	8.7	160	10.0	177	7.0	110	10.0	150
Males:								
11–14 years	11.3	200	12.0	210	9.0	140	15.0	230
15–18 years	11.3	200	12.0	210	9.5	145	15.0	230
Females:								
11–14 years	14.8	260	15.0	265	9.0	140	12.0	180
15–18 years	14.8	260	15.0	265	7.0	140	12.0	180

Age	Copper			
	UK[1]		USA[2]	
	(mg/day)	(μmol/day)	(mg/day)	(μmol/day)
0–3 months	0.2	5	0.4–0.6	6–9
4–6 months	0.3	5	0.4–0.6	6–9
7–9 months	0.3	5	0.6–0.7	9–11
10–12 months	0.3	5	06–0.7	9–11
1–3 years	0.4	6	0.7–1.0	11–16
4–6 years	0.6	9	1.0–1.5	16–24
7–10 years	0.7	11	1.0–2.0	16–32
Males:				
11–14 years	0.8	13	1.5–2.5	24–40
15–18 years	1.0	16	1.5–2.5	24–40
Females:				
11–14 years	0.8	13	1.5–2.5	24–40
15–18 years	1.0	16	1.5–2.5	24–40

[1]From Dietary Reference Values for Food Energy and Nutrients for the United Kingdom. Department of Health Report on Health and Social Subjects No. 41. London: HMSO, 1991. Estimated Average Requirement.
[2]United States Recommended Daily Intakes 1989.

I.5 RECOMMENDATIONS FOR INTAKES OF ELECTROLYTES – UK

Age	Sodium		Potassium		Chloride	
	(mmol/day)	(mg/day)	(mmol/day)	(mg/day)	(mmol/day)	(mg/day)
0–3 months	9	210	20	800	9	320
4–6 months	12	280	22	850	12	400
7–9 months	14	320	18	700	14	500
10–12 months	15	350	18	700	15	500
1–3 years	22	500	20	800	22	800
4–6 years	30	700	28	1100	30	1000
7–10 years	50	1200	50	2000	50	1800
Males:						
11–14 years	70	1600	80	3100	70	2500
15–18 years	70	1600	90	3500	70	2500
Females:						
11–14 years	70	1600	80	3100	70	2500
15–18 years	70	1600	90	3500	70	2500

From Dietary Reference Values for Food Energy and Nutrients for the United Kingdom. Department of Health Report on Health and Social Subjects No. 41. London: HMSO, 1991. Reference Nutrient Intake.

RECOMMENDATIONS FOR INTAKES OF ELECTROLYTES – USA

Age	Weight[1]	Sodium[1,2]		Chloride[1,2]		Potassium[3]	
	(kg)	(mmol)	(mg)	(mmol)	(mg)	(mmol)	(mg)
0–5 months	4.5	5.22	120	5.14	180	12.82	500
6–11 months	8.9	8.69	200	8.57	300	17.95	700
1 year	11.0	9.78	225	10.00	350	25.64	1000
2–5 years	16.0	13.04	300	14.29	500	35.89	1400
6–9 years	25.0	17.39	400	17.14	600	41.03	1600
10–18 years	50.0	21.74	500	21.43	750	51.28	2000
>18 years[4]	70.0	21.74	500	21.43	750	51.28	2000

[1]No allowance included for large, prolonged losses from the skin through sweat.
[2]There is no evidence that higher intakes confer any health benefit.
[3]Desirable intakes of potassium may considerably exceed these values.
[4]No allowance included for growth. Values for those below 18 years assume a growth rate at the 50th percentile reported by the National Center for Health Statistics and are averaged for males and females. Hamill PV, Drizd TA, Johnson CL et al. Physical Growth: National Centre for Health Statistics percentiles. Am J Clin Nutr 1979;32:607–29.

From Recommended Dietary Allowances, 10th edition. National Academy of Sciences, 1989.

I.6 RECOMMENDATIONS FOR INTAKES OF WATER-SOLUBLE VITAMINS

Age	Vitamin C (mg/day)		Thiamine (B$_1$) (mg/day)		Riboflavin (B$_2$) (mg/day)		Niacin (mg/day)	
	UK[1]	USA[2]	UK[1]	USA[3]	UK[1]	USA[3]	UK[1]	USA[3]
0–6 months	25	30	0.2	0.2	0.4	0.3	3	2.0
7–9 months	25	35	0.2	–	0.4	–	4	–
10–12 months	25	35	0.3	–	0.4	–	5	–
7–12 months	–	–	–	0.3	–	0.4	–	4.0
1–3 years	30	40	0.5	0.5	0.6	0.5	8	6.0
4–6 years	30	45	0.7	–	0.8	–	11	–
4–8 years	–	–	–	0.6	–	0.6	–	8.0
7–10 years	30	45	0.7	–	1.0	–	12	–
Males/females:								
9–13 years	–	–	–	0.9	–	0.9	–	12.0
11–14 years	35	50	0.9/0.7*	–	1.2/1.1*	–	15/12*	–
14–18 years	–	–	–	1.2/1.0*	–	1.3/1.0*	–	16.0/14.0*
15–18 years	40	60	1.1/0.8*	–	1.3/1.1*	–	18/14*	–

Age	Vitamin B$_6$ (mg/day)		Vitamin B$_{12}$ (μg/day)		Folate (μg/day)	
	UK[1]	USA[3]	UK[1]	USA[3]	UK[1]	USA[3]
0–6 months	0.2	0.1	0.3	0.34	50	65
7–9 months	0.3	–	0.4	–	50	–
10–12 months	0.4	–	0.4	–	50	–
7–12 months	–	0.3	–	0.50	–	80
1–3 years	0.7	0.5	0.5	0.90	70	150
4–6 years	0.9	–	0.8	–	100	–
4–8 years	–	0.6	–	1.20	–	200
7–10 years	1.0	–	1.0	–	150	–
Males/females:						
9–13 years	–	1.0	–	1.80	–	300
11–14 years	1.2/1.0*	–	1.2	–	200	–
14–18 years	–	1.3/1.2*	–	2.40	–	400
15–18 years	1.5/1.2*	–	1.5	–	200	–

[1]From Dietary Reference Values for Food Energy and Nutrients for the United Kingdom. Department of Health Report on Health and Social Subjects No. 41. London: HMSO, 1991. Estimated Average Requirement.
[2]United States Recommended Dietary Allowances, 10th edition. National Academy of Sciences, 1989.
[3]Dietary Reference Intakes. National Academy of Sciences, 1998.
*Female Data.

I.7 RECOMMENDATIONS FOR INTAKES OF FAT-SOLUBLE VITAMINS – UK

Age	Vitamin A	Vitamin D	Vitamin E[†]
	(μg retinol equivalents per day)	(μg/day)	(mg α-tocopherol per day)
0–3 months	350	8.5	0.4 mg per gram of
4–6 months	350	8.5	polyunsaturated
7–9 months	350	7.0	fatty acids
10–12 months	350	7.0	
1–3 years	400	7.0	No
4–6 years	400	*	recommendation
7–10 years	500	*	
Males:			
11–14 years	600	*	>4
15–18 years	700	*	>4
Females:			
11–14 years	600	*	>3
15–18 years	600	*	>3

*No recommendations – requirements assumed to be met by synthesis.
[†]No recommendations for Dietary Reference Value – Safe Intake only.
From Dietary Reference Values for Food Energy and Nutrients for the United Kingdom. Department of Health Report on Health and Social Subjects No. 41. London: HMSO, 1991. Reference Nutrient Intake.

I.7 RECOMMENDATIONS FOR INTAKES OF FAT-SOLUBLE VITAMINS – USA

Age	Vitamin A[1]	Vitamin D[2]	Vitamin E[1]
	(μg retinol equivalents per day)	(μg/day) (a, b)	(mg α-tocopherol per day)
0–3 months	375	5*	3
4–6 months	375	5*	3
7–9 months	375	5*	4
10–12 months	375	5*	4
1–3 years	400	5*	6
4–6 years	500	5*	7
7–10 years	700	5*	7
Males:			
11–14 years	1000	5*	10
15–18 years	1000	5*	10
Females:			
11–14 years	800	5*	8
15–18 years	800	5*	8

[1]United States Recommended Daily Intakes, 1989.
[2]United States Dietary Reference Intakes. National Academy of Sciences, 1998.
*Adequate Intakes (AI).

a) As cholecalciferol.
b) In the absence of adequate exposure to sunlight.

I.8 NORMAL FLUID REQUIREMENTS

Age	Weight	Fluid per day
	(kg)	
Preterm	1–2	150–200 ml/kg
0–6 months	2–8	120–150 ml/kg
7–12 months	6–10	100–120 ml/kg
	11–20	1000 ml + 50 ml/kg for each additional kg over 10 kg
	>20	1500 ml + 25 ml/kg for each additional kg over 20 kg (to a max. of 2500 ml/day)

I.9 Nomogram for Determination of Surface Area

I.19. Nomogram for determination of surface area

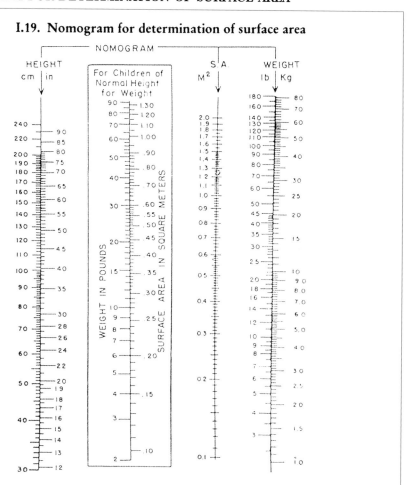

Weight range (kg)	Approximate surface area (m²)
1–5	0.05 × W + 0.05
6–10	0.04 × W + 0.10
11–20	0.03 × W + 0.20
21–70	0.02 × W + 0.40

W = weight (kg).

I.10 ESTIMATION OF BODY SURFACE AREA IN INFANTS AND CHILDREN

Body weight	Surface area	Body weight	Surface area
(kg)	(m²)	(kg)	(m²)
2.0	0.16	11	0.53
2.5	0.19	12	0.56
3.0	0.21	13	0.59
3.5	0.24	14	0.62
4.0	0.26	15	0.65
4.5	0.28	16	0.68
5.0	0.30	17	0.71
5.5	0.32	18	0.74
6.0	0.34	19	0.77
6.5	0.36	20	0.79
7.0	0.38	21	0.82
7.5	0.40	22	0.85
8.0	0.42	23	0.87
8.5	0.44	24	0.90
9.0	0.46	25	0.92
9.5	0.47	30	1.10
10.0	0.49	35	1.20

These estimates are for children with a normal height for age and a normal distribution of fat and lean tissue.

I.11 GIRLS PRETERM 20 WEEKS – EDD

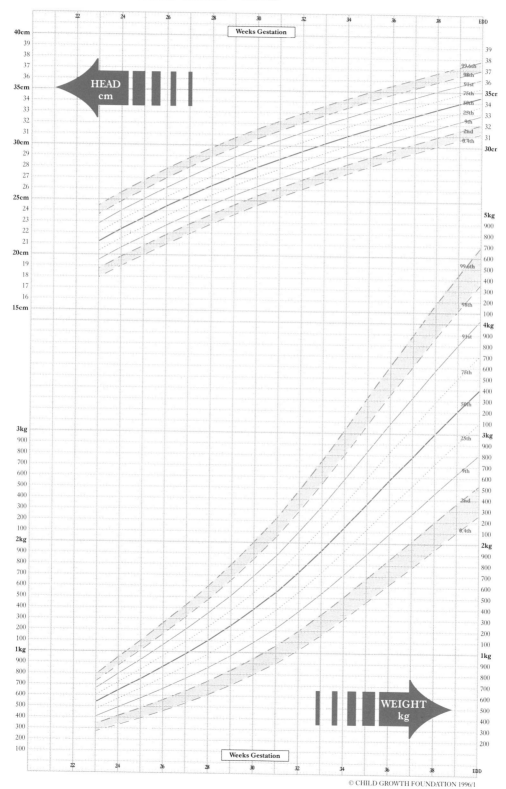

© CHILD GROWTH FOUNDATION 1996/1

I.12 BOYS PRETERM 20 WEEKS – EDD

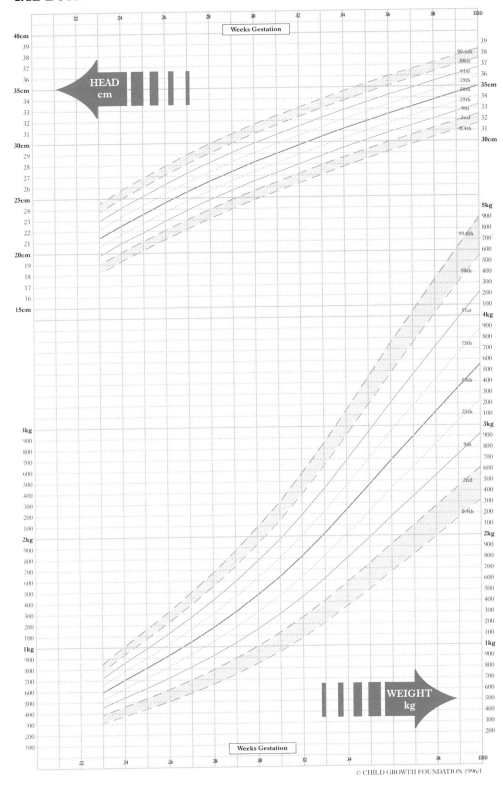

© CHILD GROWTH FOUNDATION 1996/1

I.13 GIRLS PRETERM (30 WKS GESTATION) – 52 WEEKS

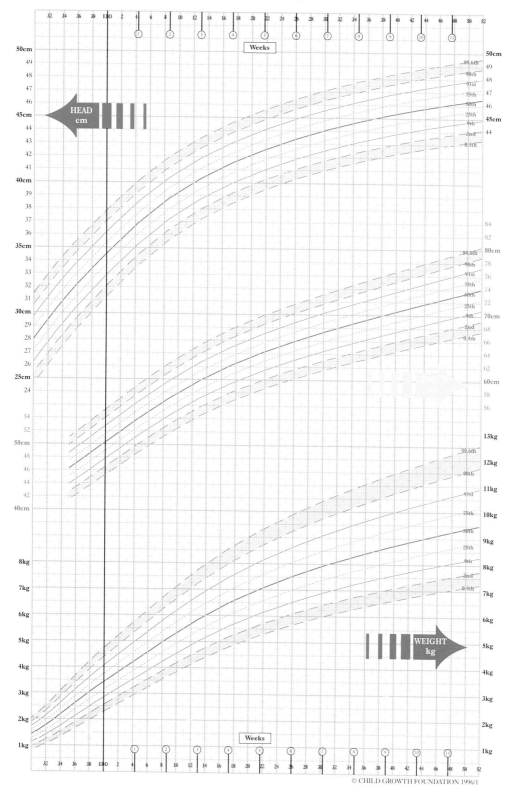

I.14 Boys preterm (30 wks gestation) – 52 weeks

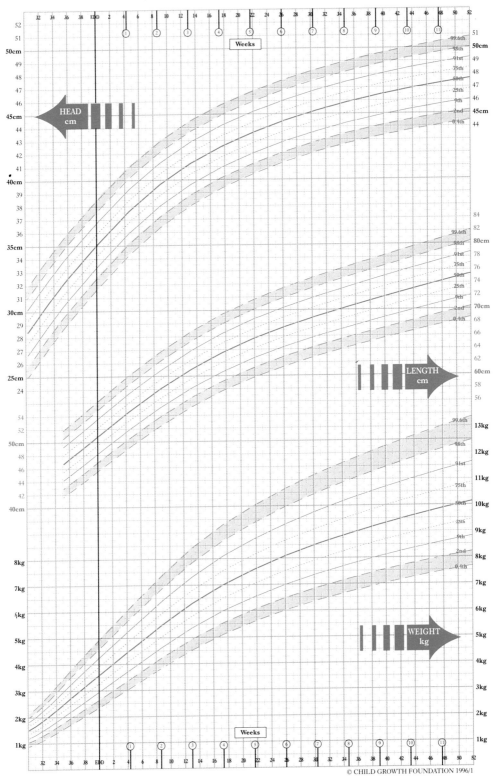

© CHILD GROWTH FOUNDATION 1996/1

I.15 GIRLS 12–24 MONTHS

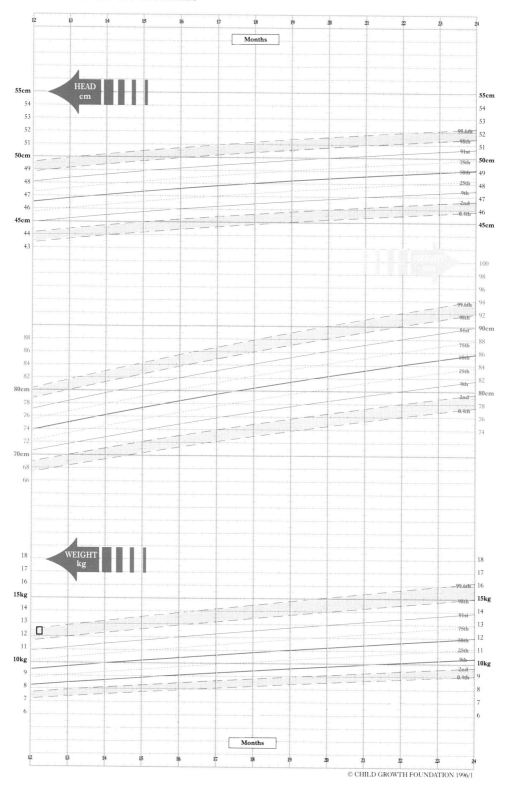

I.16 BOYS 12–24 MONTHS

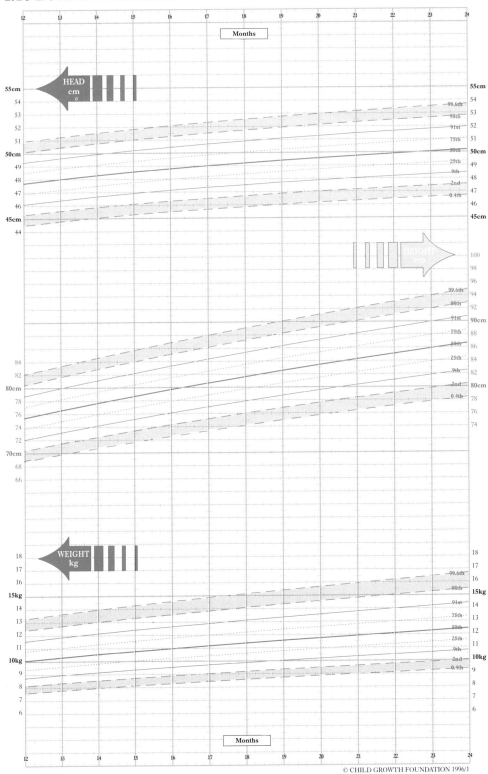

I.17 GIRLS 0–20 YEARS

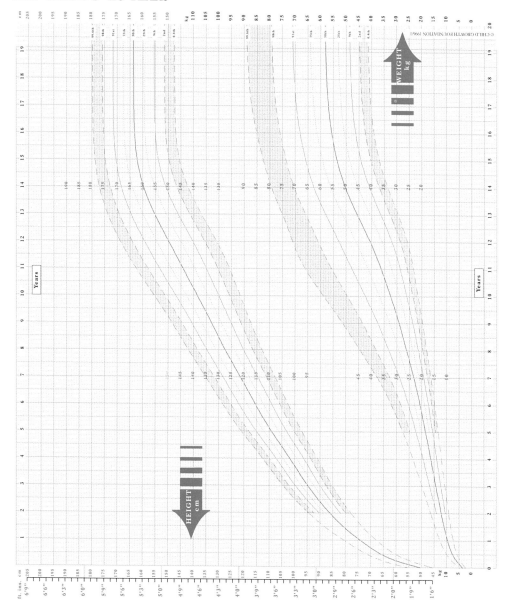

© CHILD GROWTH FOUNDATION 1996/1

I.18 Boys 0–20 years

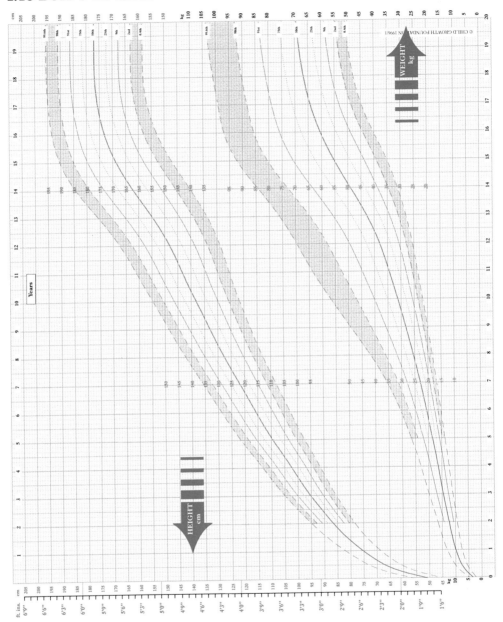

I.19 GIRLS BMI CHART (BIRTH–20 YEARS): UNITED KINGDOM CROSS-SECTIONAL REFERENCE: 2002/1

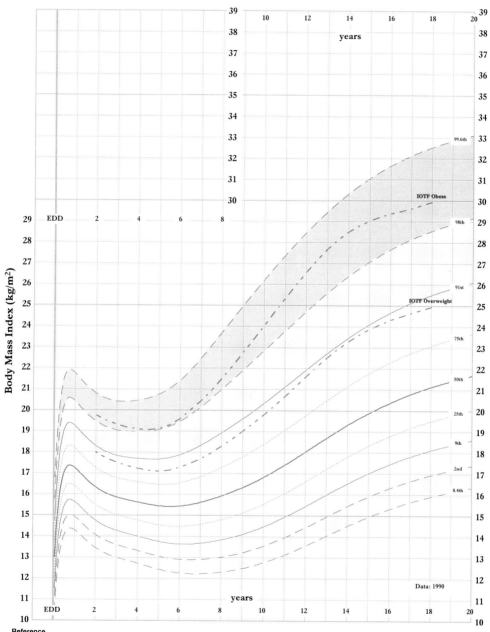

Reference
Body Mass Index reference curves for the UK, 1990 (TJ Cole, JV Freeman, MA Preece) Arch Dis Child 1995; **73**: 25-29
Establishing a standard definition for child overweight and obesity: international survey, (Cole TJ, Bellizi MC, Flegal KM, Dietz WH) BMJ 2000; **320**: 1240-3

I.20 BOYS BMI CHART (BIRTH–20 YEARS): UNITED KINGDOM
CROSS-SECTIONAL REFERENCE: 2002/1

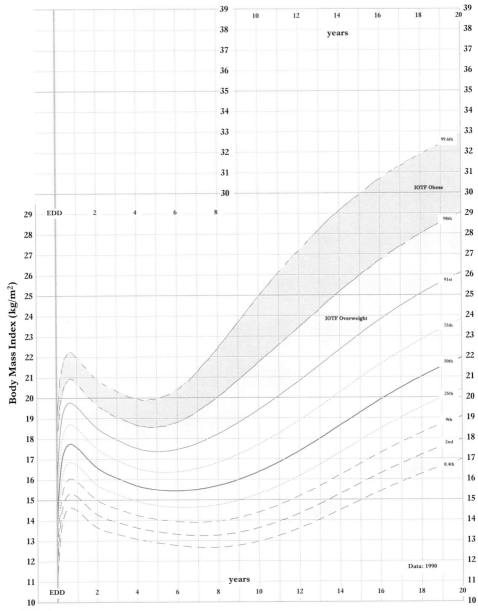

Reference
Body Mass Index reference curves for the UK, 1990 (TJ Cole, JV Freeman, MA Preece) Arch Dis Child 1995; **73**: 25-29
Establishing a standard definition for child overweight and obesity: international survey, (Cole TJ, Bellizi MC, Flegal KM, Dietz WH) BMJ 2000; **320**: 1240-3

© CHILD GROWTH FOUNDATION 1997/1

I.21 WEIGHT-FOR-STATURE PERCENTILES: GIRLS

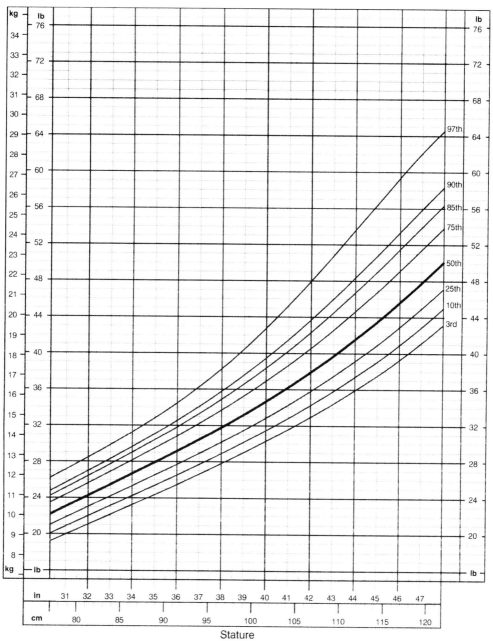

Stature

SOURCE: Developed by the National Center for Health Statistics in collaboration with
the National Center for Chronic Disease Prevention and Health Promotion (2000).

I.22 WEIGHT-FOR-STATURE PERCENTILES: BOYS

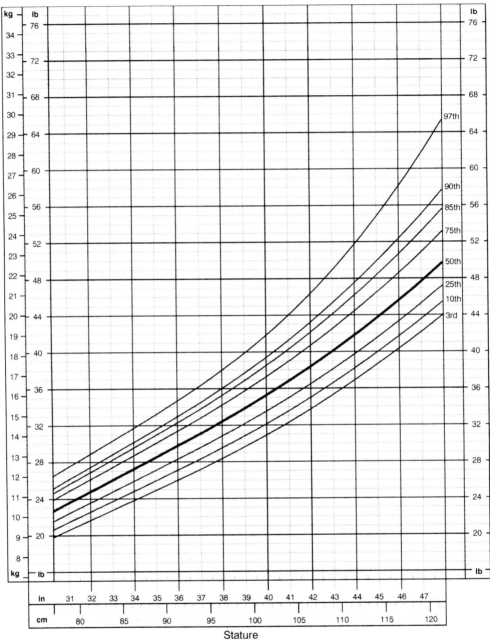

SOURCE: Developed by the National Center for Health Statistics in collaboration with
the National Center for Chronic Disease Prevention and Health Promotion (2000).

I.23 WEIGHT-FOR-LENGTH PERCENTILES: GIRLS, BIRTH TO 36 MONTHS

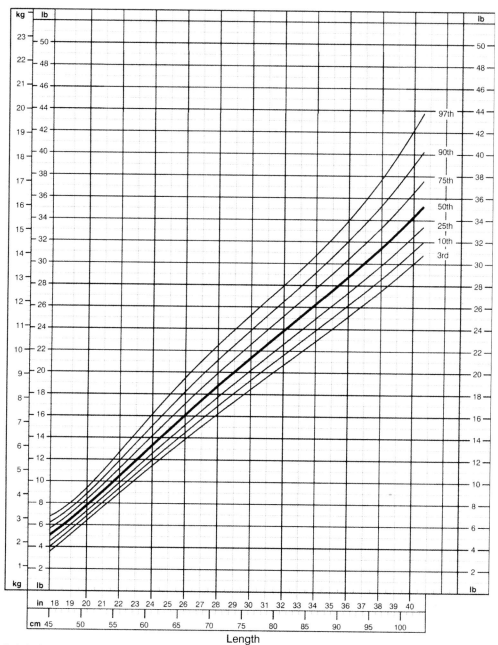

Length

Revised and corrected June 8, 2000.

SOURCE: Developed by the National Center for Health Statistics in collaboration with the National Center for Chronic Disease Prevention and Health Promotion (2000).

I.24 WEIGHT-FOR-LENGTH PERCENTILES: BOYS, BIRTH TO 36 MONTHS

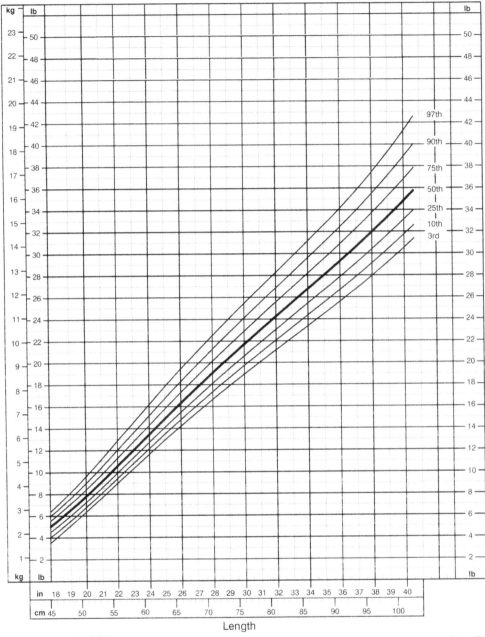

Length

Revised and corrected June 8, 2000.

SOURCE: Developed by the National Center for Health Statistics in collaboration with
the National Center for Chronic Disease Prevention and Health Promotion (2000).

I.25 HEAD CIRCUMFERENCE-FOR-AGE PERCENTILES: GIRLS, BIRTH TO 36 MONTHS

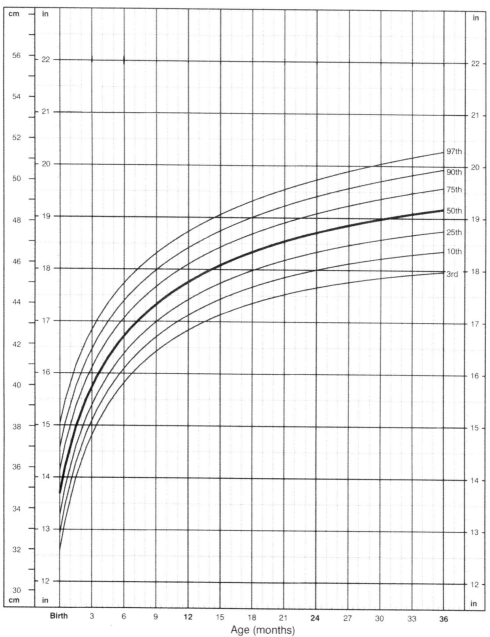

SOURCE: Developed by the National Center for Health Statistics in collaboration with
the National Center for Chronic Disease Prevention and Health Promotion (2000).

I.26 HEAD CIRCUMFERENCE-FOR-AGE PERCENTILES: BOYS, BIRTH TO 36 MONTHS

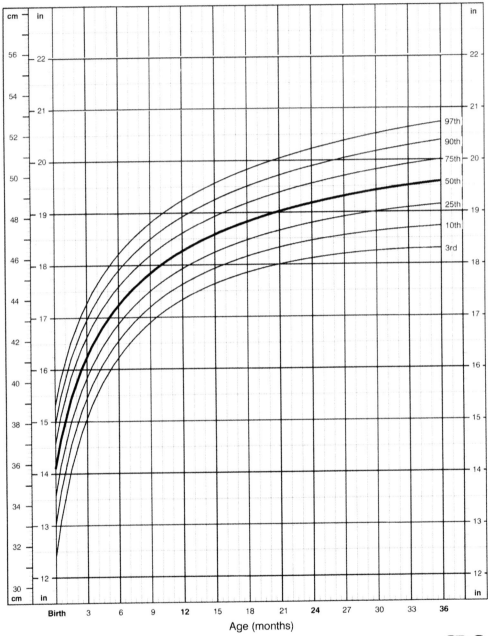

SOURCE: Developed by the National Center for Health Statistics in collaboration with
the National Center for Chronic Disease Prevention and Health Promotion (2000).

I.27 STATURE-FOR-AGE PERCENTILES: GIRLS, 2 TO 20 YEARS

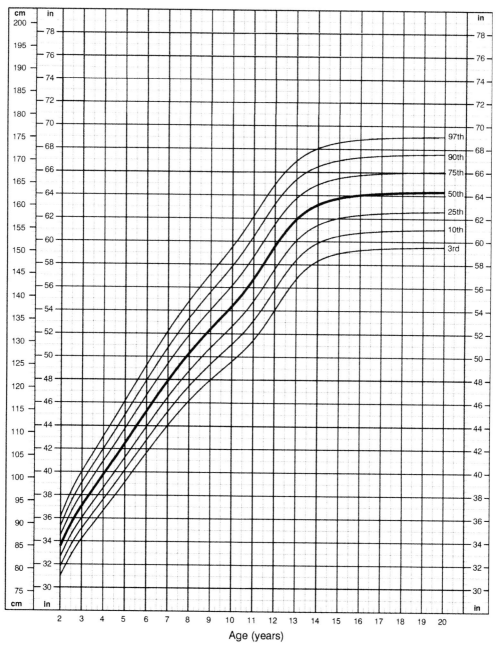

SOURCE: Developed by the National Center for Health Statistics in collaboration with
the National Center for Chronic Disease Prevention and Health Promotion (2000).

I.28 STATURE-FOR-AGE PERCENTILES: BOYS, 2 TO 20 YEARS

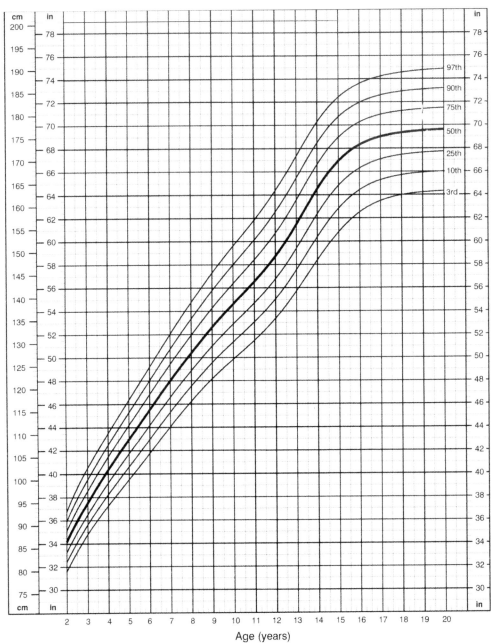

Age (years)

SOURCE: Developed by the National Center for Health Statistics in collaboration with
the National Center for Chronic Disease Prevention and Health Promotion (2000).

I.29 LENGTH-FOR-AGE PERCENTILES: GIRLS, BIRTH TO 36 MONTHS

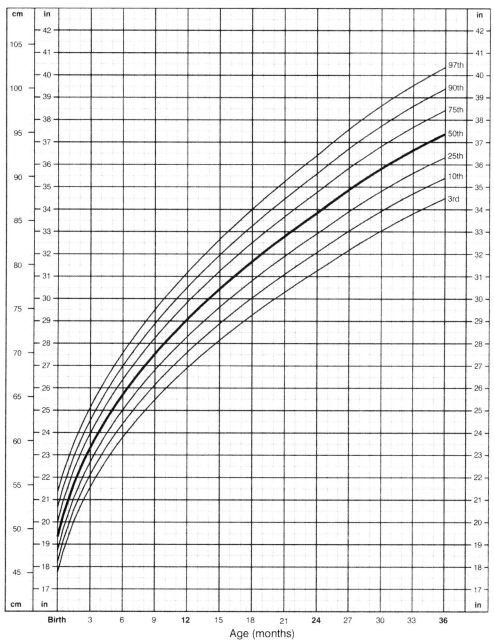

SOURCE: Developed by the National Center for Health Statistics in collaboration with the National Center for Chronic Disease Prevention and Health Promotion (2000).

I.30 LENGTH-FOR-AGE PERCENTILES: BOYS, BIRTH TO 36 MONTHS

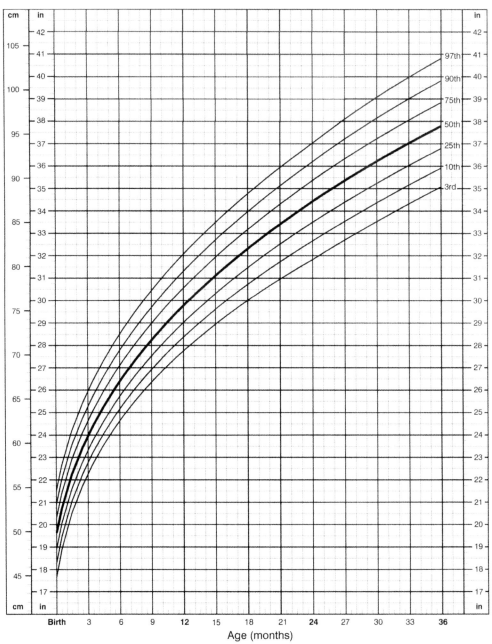

SOURCE: Developed by the National Center for Health Statistics in collaboration with
the National Center for Chronic Disease Prevention and Health Promotion (2000).

I.31 WEIGHT-FOR-AGE PERCENTILES: GIRLS, 2 TO 20 YEARS

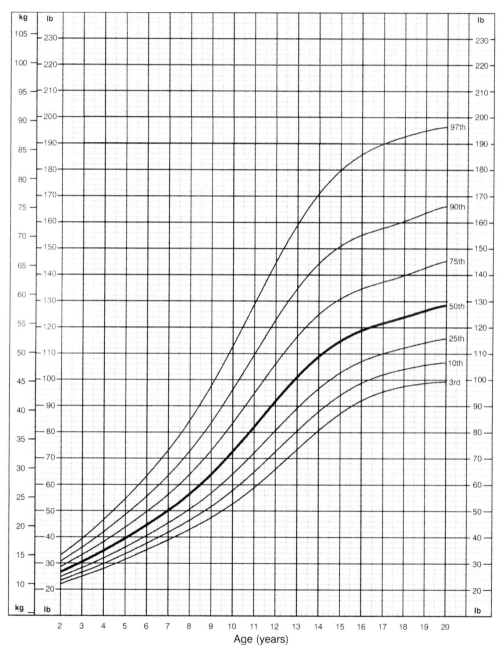

Age (years)

SOURCE: Developed by the National Center for Health Statistics in collaboration with the National Center for Chronic Disease Prevention and Health Promotion (2000).

I.32 WEIGHT-FOR-AGE PERCENTILES: BOYS, 2 TO 20 YEARS

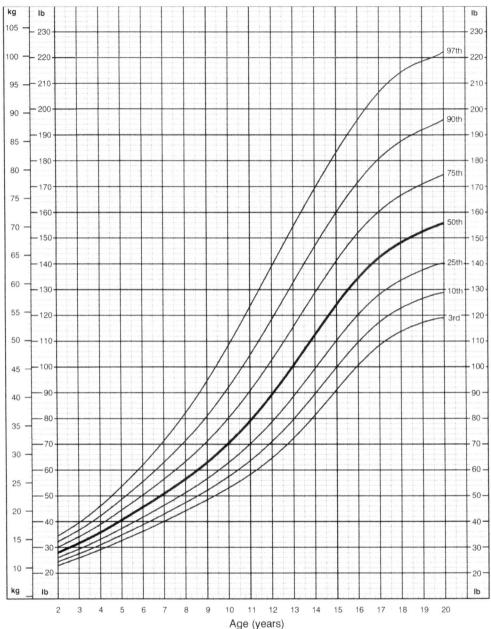

SOURCE: Developed by the National Center for Health Statistics in collaboration with
the National Center for Chronic Disease Prevention and Health Promotion (2000).

I.33 WEIGHT-FOR-AGE PERCENTILES: GIRLS, BIRTH TO 36 MONTHS

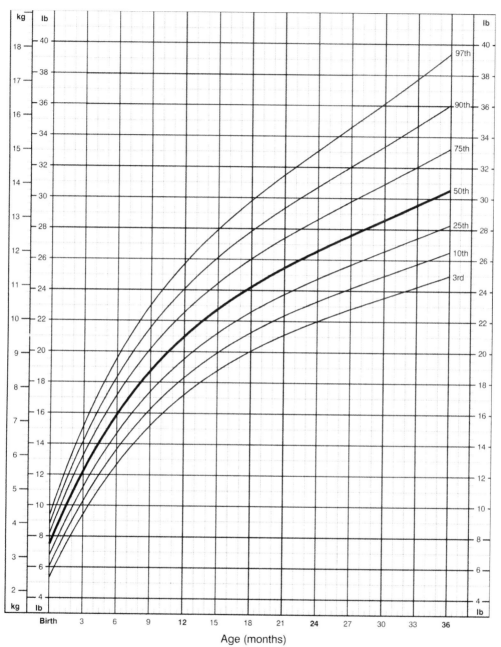

SOURCE: Developed by the National Center for Health Statistics in collaboration with the National Center for Chronic Disease Prevention and Health Promotion (2000).

I.34 WEIGHT-FOR-AGE PERCENTILES: BOYS, BIRTH TO 36 MONTHS

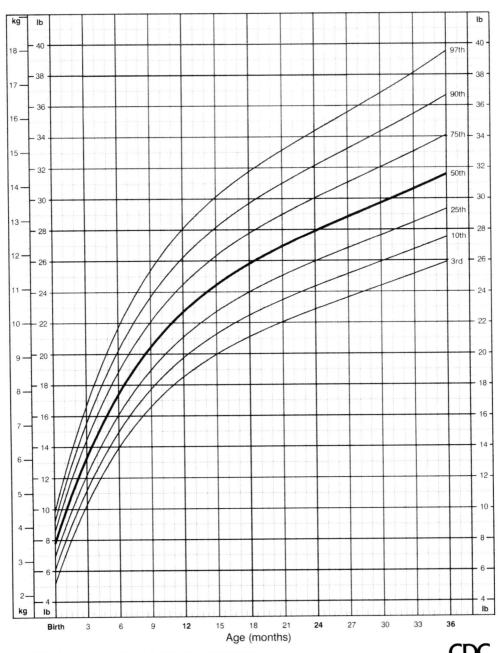

SOURCE: Developed by the National Center for Health Statistics in collaboration with
the National Center for Chronic Disease Prevention and Health Promotion (2000).

I.35 BODY MASS INDEX-FOR-AGE PERCENTILES: GIRLS, 2 TO 20 YEARS

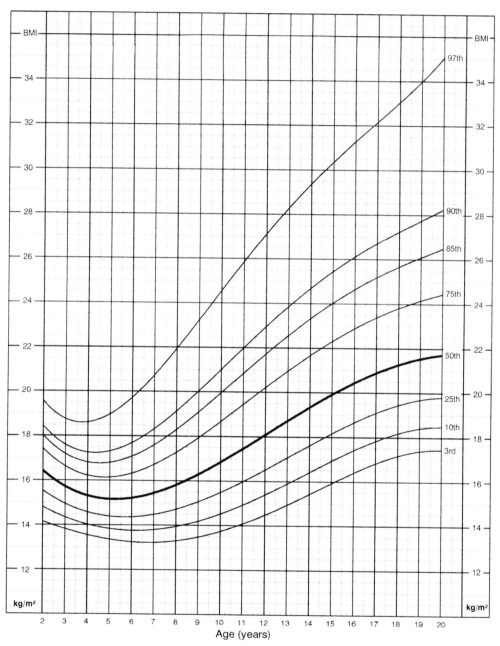

SOURCE: Developed by the National Center for Health Statistics in collaboration with
the National Center for Chronic Disease Prevention and Health Promotion (2000).

I.36 BODY MASS INDEX-FOR-AGE PERCENTILES: BOYS, 2 TO 20 YEARS

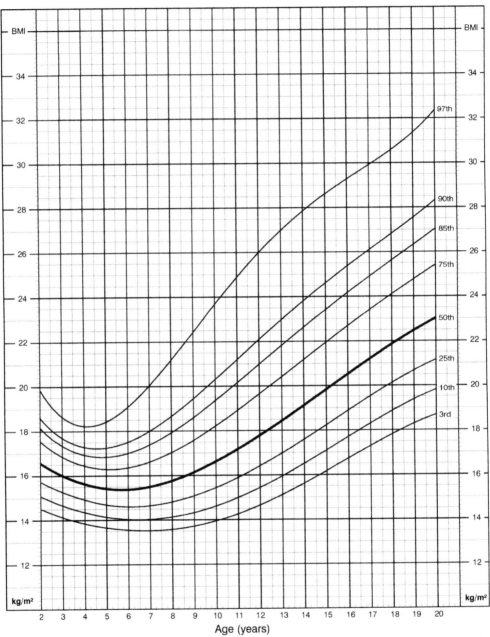

SOURCE: Developed by the National Center for Health Statistics in collaboration with
the National Center for Chronic Disease Prevention and Health Promotion (2000).

appendix II

PREPARATIONS FOR NORMAL AND PREMATURE INFANTS, ORAL AND INTRAVENOUS FLUIDS AND VITAMIN/MINERAL SUPPLEMENTS

II.1 RECOMMENDATIONS FOR COMPOSITION OF INFANT FORMULAS BASED ON COW MILK – CONTENT (PER 100 AVAILABLE KCAL) FOR MACRONUTRIENTS AND VITAMINS

	EEC[1,2]	USA[3]
Energy per 100 ml milk	60–75 kcal (251–314 kJ)	
Protein (g)	1.8–3.0	1.8–4.5
Taurine (μmol)	Minimum 4.2	
L-carnitine (μmol)	Minimum 7.5	
Nucleotides (mg)	Maximum 5	
Lipid (g)	4.4–6.5	3.3–6.0
Linoleic acid (mg)	300–1200	Minimum 300
α-Linoleic acid (mg)	Minimum 5	
Linoleic/α-linoleic ratio	5–15	
LCPUFA – n3 – n6	Maximum 1% total fat Maximum 2% total fat	
Carbohydrate (g)	7–14	
Lactose (g)	Minimum 3.5	
Sucrose (g)	Maximum 20% total carbohydrate	
Vitamin A (μg retinol equivalents)	60–180	75–225
Vitamin D (μg)	1.0–2.5	1.0–2.5
Thiamine (μg) minimum	40	40
Riboflavin (μg) minimum	60	60
Nicotinamide (mg) minimum	0.8	0.8
Pantothenic acid (μg) minimum	300	300
Vitamin B_6 (μg) minimum	35	35
Vitamin B_{12} (μg) minimum	0.1	0.15
Biotin (μg) minimum	1.5	1.4
Folic acid (μg) minimum	4	4
Vitamin C (μg) minimum	8	8
Vitamin K (μg) minimum	4	4
Vitamin E (mg α-tocopherol) minimum	0.5	0.5

[1] EEC Commission Directive 91/321/EEC (OJ No L175, 4.7.91, p.35).
[2] EEC Commission Directive 96/4/EC (OJ No L49, 28.2.96, p.12).
[3] USA Nutrient Requirements for Infant Formula, Final Rule, Federal Register, 1985. Vol. 50:45106–8:21 CFR 107.
  LCPUFA = long-chain polyunsaturated fatty acids

II.2 RECOMMENDATIONS FOR COMPOSITION OF INFANT FORMULAS BASED ON COW MILK – CONTENT (PER 100 AVAILABLE KCAL) FOR MINERALS AND TRACE ELEMENTS

	EEC[1,2]	USA[3]
Sodium (mg)	20–60	20–60
Potassium (mg)	60–145	80–200
Calcium (mg)	Minimum 50*	Minimum 60
Phosphorus (mg)	25–90	Minimum 30
Magnesium (mg)	5–15	Minimum 6
Iron[†] (mg)	0.5–1.5	1.0–2.55
Zinc (mg)	0.5–1.5	Minimum 0.5
Copper (μg)	20–80	Minimum 60
Iodine (μg)	Minimum 5	5–25
Selenium (μg)	Maximum 3	Minimum 3
Manganese (μg)	No recommendation	Minimum 5

[1] EEC Commission Directive 91/321/EEC (OJ No L175, 4.7.91, p. 35).
[2] EEC Commission Directive 96/4/EC (OJ No L49, 28.2.96, p. 12).
[3] USA Nutrient Requirements for Infant Formula, Final Rule, Federal Register, 1985. Vol. 50:45106–8:21 CFR 107.

* Calcium/phosphorus ratio should lie between 1.2 and 2.
[†] Limits apply to formulas with added iron.

II.3 RECOMMENDATIONS FOR THE COMPOSITION (PER 100 AVAILABLE KCAL) OF FOLLOW-UP FORMULAS BASED ON COW MILK THAT DIFFER FROM THOSE FOR STARTER FORMULAS

EEC Recommendations[1,2]	
Energy per 100 ml	60–80 kcal (251–335 kJ)
Protein (g)	2.25–4.5
Lipid (g)	3.3–6.5
Linoleic acid (mg)*	300
Iron (mg)	1–2
Vitamin D (μg)	1–3

[1] EEC Commission Directive 91/321/EEC (OJ No L175, 4.7.91, p. 35).
[2] EEC Commission Directive 96/4/EC (OJ No L49, 28.2.96, p. 12).
* If product is composed of vegetable oils.

Calcium/phosphorus ratio not greater than 2. Other minerals at least the content of cow milk.

II.4 Normal infant formulas

Most normal infant formulas are based on heat-treated cow milk, with the addition of fats, carbohydrates, vitamins and trace elements to provide a composition similar to that of mature human breast milk. Fresh cow or goat milk and dried milk powder based on unmodified whole or skimmed milk are not suitable for infants under the age of 12 months because the protein and renal solute load is undesirably high and because the vitamin and mineral content is not optimum. Such milks can be used if there is no alternative, but the product must be diluted. Appendix II.6 gives suggestions for modification of such milks.

Formulas that have a composition similar to that of human milk are known as modified milks and are considered to be suitable for the feeding of infants from birth onward if the mother is not breastfeeding.

Two main types of modified infant formulas exist: those based on whole milk protein, with a whey:casein ratio of approximately 20:80 (casein dominant), and those based on dialyzed whey protein, usually with a whey:casein ratio of 60:40 (whey dominant), similar to that found in human milk. Provided the protein content of the formula is not higher than the levels recommended, there appears to be little advantage of one type of formula over the other. If an infant is receiving a low-protein diet and the protein intake is close to the minimum, the amino acid pattern found in the whey-based preparations might be more beneficial. This type of formula is usually lower in electrolytes than the non-whey preparations.

The carbohydrate in human milk and the majority of infant formulas is lactose. Some modified formulas contain other carbohydrates, which partially replace lactose; this type of formula may be useful for infants after surgery or where a partial intolerance to lactose is suspected. The fat of human milk is more readily digested and absorbed than that of whole cow milk. For this reason, most modified infant formulas have wholly or partially replaced the butterfat with a mixture of other animal fats or vegetable oils. Formulas that contain animal fat other than butterfat are not suitable for use for infants of Moslem (unless Halal approved), Jewish or Hindu faith.

The standard energy density of feeds is 65–75 kcal (270–315 kJ) per 100 ml. Some manufacturers also produce a dilute (half-strength) formula which should only be used for short periods when grading infants onto full-strength feeds. Formulas with a higher energy concentration than that recommended are also available (see Appendix III.6); however, these should be used with caution as they have a high osmolality and can cause an osmotic diarrhea.

'Follow-up' formulas have been designed for use in infants over the age of 4 months (6 months in the UK). They are usually higher in protein content than modified formulas and contain a higher quantity of minerals, including sodium. Vitamins are added to these milks, and recommendations for their composition are given in Appendix II.3. The use of such formulas is not particularly beneficial for infants who receive a good weaning diet, because unmodified cow's milk is considered by most authorities to be suitable for infants over the age of 12 months. However, for infants who are reluctant with solids, who fail to gain weight or are considered to need additional vitamins, and in areas where fresh pasteurized cow milk is not available, this type of formula will be useful.

Infant milks are available in the form of dried milk powder for reconstitution with water, liquid concentrates and as ready-to-feed products in cartons or pre-measured sterile disposable bottles. The last-mentioned have the advantage of accuracy and hygiene, but are extremely expensive compared with the powder product. Care must be taken to ensure that the person preparing the formula is able to prepare it correctly. Most modified baby milks enclose a scoop or spoon with the package, and the milk is reconstituted using one scoop to either 1 fl oz of water (30 ml) in Europe or 2 fl oz (60 ml) of water in North America. If changing to a different formula, the person in charge of preparation should be aware that the recipe for making up the feed may differ between formulas. Manufacturers market feeds under alternative brand names in different countries. The same brand name may not have the same nutrient composition or the same dilution in different parts of the world. Manufacturer's instructions should always be consulted before preparing a feed. Appendix II.5 groups formulas according to their protein type. Brand names listed as alternatives may not have the same nutrient composition, and information on the packaging should be checked.

The availability of clean water is important in the less developed countries. Every effort must be made to continue breastfeeding if there is any doubt about the quality of the local water. Bottled potable or mineral water is expensive and may be too high in sodium and calcium for use in the preparation of infant feeds, and this should be checked before its use is recommended.

Some countries have made laws to control the nutritional content of milks marketed specifically for infants and young children. Details of legislation for Europe and the USA are given in Appendix II.1. In countries where codification exists, it can be assumed that all milks on sale to the general public will conform to guidelines. However, many less developed countries do not have such legislation and it is common for milks to be sold indicating that they are designed for infants, when they are, in fact, unmodified. The composition of all formulas should be checked against guidelines before being recommended to mothers.

II.5 COMPOSITION OF NORMAL INFANT FORMULAS – PER 100 ML AS FED

Product	Manufacturer	Protein	Fat	
		(g)	(g)	Source
Starter formula – whey:casein 100:0				
Carnation Good Start	Nestlé	1.5	3.5	Palm olein, soy, coconut, safflower oils
Starter formula – whey:casein 70:30				
Nan 1*	Nestlé	1.2	3.4	Palm olein, coconut, canola, corn oils
Starter formula – whey:casein 60:40				
Frisolac H*	Friesland	1.4	3.5	Vegetable oils, milk fat
Enfamil with iron	Mead Johnson	1.5	3.8	Palm, soy, coconut, sunflower oils
Aptamil First*	Milupa	1.4	3.6	Milk fat, corn oil
Premium*	Cow & Gate	1.4	3.5	Vegetable oils, milk fat
Similac PM	Ross	1.5	3.8	Corn, coconut, soy oils
SMA Gold*/SMA	SMA/Wyeth	1.5	3.6	Vegetable oils
Starter formula – whey:casein (approx.) 20:80				
Milumil*	Milupa	1.9	3.1	Milk fat, corn oil
Plus*	Cow & Gate	1.8	3.3	Milk fat, vegetable oils
Similac 20 with iron	Ross	1.6	3.7	Soy, coconut, safflower oils
SMA White*	SMA/Wyeth	1.6	3.6	Vegetable oils
Starter formula – casein predominant				
Lactogen 1	Nestlé	1.5	3.5	Palm olein, coconut, canola, corn oils
Toddler milks/follow-up formulas				
Frisomel*	Friesland	2.2	3.5	Milk fat, vegetable oils
Next Steps	Cow & Gate	2.6	4.2	Palm, soy, coconut, sunflower oils
Forward*	Milupa	2.3	3.1	Milk fat, corn oil
Carnation Follow-Up Formula	Nestlé	1.8	2.8	Palm olein, soy, coconut, safflower oils
Nan 2*	Nestlé	2.2	2.9	Palm olein, coconut, canola, corn oils
Step Up*	Cow & Gate	2.8	3.5	Milk fat, vegetable oils
Toddlers Best**	Ross	2.6	4.7	Soy oil
Progress*	SMA/Wyeth	2.2	3.0	Vegetable oils
Lactogen 2	Nestlé	2.4	2.7	Palm olein, coconut, canola, corn oils
Neslac	Nestlé	2.7	2.6	Milk fat, corn, canola high oleic, sunflower oils

II.5 – CONTINUED

Product	Carbohydrate		Energy		Iron		Similar products[†]
	(g)	Type	(kcal)	(kJ)	(µmol)	(mg)	
Starter formula – whey:casein 100:0							
Carnation Good Start	7.6	Lactose/ maltodextrin	68	284	17.85	1.00	
Starter formula – whey:casein 70:30							
Nan 1*	7.5	Lactose	67	280	14.28	0.80	
Starter formula – whey:casein 60:40							
Frisolac H*	7.4	Lactose	67	280	11.07	0.62	
Enfamil with iron	7.0	Lactose	68	284	22.85	1.28	Enfamil (low iron) Enfamil LIPIL
Aptamil First*	8.3	Lactose	68	284	12.50	0.70	Aptamil 1, Pre Aptamil
Premium*	7.5	Lactose	67	280	8.92	0.50	Nutrilon Premium, Bebelac 1
Similac PM	6.9	Lactose	68	284	2.67	0.15	
SMA Gold*	7.2	Lactose	67	280	14.28	0.80	S-26 SMA[‡]
Starter formula – whey:casein (approx.) 20:80							
Milumil*	8.1	Lactose, maltodextrin, starch, sucrose	67	283	12.50	0.70	Milumil 2 KF (sucrose free), Milumil
Nan 2*	8.0	Lactose	67	280	20.35	1.10	Beba 2, Nidal 2
Plus*	8.0	Lactose, maltodextrin	70	293	23.75	1.33	Nutrilon Plus, Bebelac 2
Similac 20 with iron	7.2	Lactose	68	284	21.42	1.20	
SMA White*	7.0	Lactose	67	280	14.28	0.80	SMA[‡]
Starter formula – casein predominant							
Lactogen 1	7.4	Lactose	67		14.28	0.80	Beba 1, Guigoz 1, Nidal 1
Toddler milks/follow-up formulas							
Frisomel*	8.6	Lactose, sucrose	72	301	19.64	1.10	
Next Steps	10.0	Lactose, corn syrup	67	280	21.60	1.21	Enfagrow, Kindercal (106 kcal/100 ml)
Forward*	10.7	Lactose, sucrose, starch	80	333	16.07	0.90	Milupino, Kindermilch
Carnation Follow-Up Formula	8.9	Corn syrup, lactose, maltodextrin	68	284	23.03	1.21	Neslac
Step Up*	8.6	Lactose, maltodextrin	72	301	23.21	1.30	Follow-On
Toddlers Best**	11.9	Sucrose, fructose	68	284	32.14	1.80	Also soy-based Toddlers Best
Progress*	7.8	Lactose	67	281	22.67	1.27	Promil
Lactogen 2	8.2	Lactose, maltodextrin	67	281	19.64	1.10	Guigoz 2
Neslac	8.2	Lactose, sucrose, maltodextrin, honey	67	281	21.42	1.20	

Always check with manufacturers for product changes/most up to date product composition.
*Not available in the USA.
**Available in the USA but slightly different formulation.
[†]Products described as 'similar' may be the same product marketed under a different product name in another country. Alternatively they may contain different ingredients, such as starch or sucrose. It is important to check the ingredients and nutrient content listed on the package.
[‡]The composition of SMA differs in different parts of the world. The product may be whey dominant or casein dominant.

II.6 MILKS NOT ADAPTED AS INFANT FORMULAS

Manufacturers of infant formulas have generally designed the milk so as to meet the requirements of the small infant. Where possible, a normal or specialized milk should be used. However, in situations where such formulas are not available through economic or geographic reasons, other milks can be used to provide adequate nutrition.

Cow milk

This must be pasteurized or boiled before it is fed to an infant. Undiluted cow milk is not recommended for infants of less than 12 months of age because of its high protein and sodium content. A diluted formula can be used if a suitable alternative is not available.

Preparation of diluted formula: To each 70 ml of boiled cow milk add 30 ml of boiled water. In addition, carbohydrate (glucose, glucose polymer, maltodextrin or sucrose) should be added at a level of 5 g per 100 ml of diluted feed.

This adapted formula falls within the EEC and USA guidelines for the major nutrients (see Appendix II.1), but is deficient in iron, retinol, cholecalciferol, ascorbic acid and nicotinic acid, and these should be supplemented if cow milk is to be fed for a period longer than a few days.

Canned evaporated whole milk

The composition of evaporated milk is subject to the regulations in force in the country where it is marketed. The figures given in Appendix II.7 are for milks available in the UK. In North America, evaporated milk contains more water and the content of all nutrients is about 1% lower than the figures in the table. Other regulations may affect the nutrient content of evaporated milk: in some countries, iron and/or cholecalciferol may be added. Evaporated milk is not recommended for feeding to infants of less than 12 months of age, but where whole milk is not available or where the quality of the milk is in doubt, a diluted formula can be prepared.

Preparation of diluted formula: To each 25 ml of evaporated milk add 75 ml of boiled water. In addition, carbohydrate (glucose, glucose polymer, maltodextrin or sucrose) should be added at a level of 5 g per 100 ml of diluted feed.

This adapted formula falls within the EEC and USA guidelines with the same exceptions as for whole cow milk (see Appendix II.2). Care should be taken to ascertain whether iron and/or cholecalciferol have already been added to the product. The total intake of cholecalciferol should not exceed 2 μg/100 kcal.

Canned, condensed, skimmed or sweetened cow milk

This type of product is generally not suitable for adaptation into a feed for infants.

Goat milk

This should always be boiled or pasteurized before it is fed to an infant. Undiluted goat milk is not recommended for feeding to infants of less than 12 months of age, but where there is no suitable alternative, a diluted formula can be devised.

Preparation of diluted formula: To each 70 ml of boiled goat milk add 30 ml of boiled water. In addition, carbohydrate (glucose, glucose polymer, maltodextrin or sucrose) should be added at a level of 4 g per 100 ml of diluted feed.

The nutrient content of this adapted formula will fall within the EEC and USA guidelines for the major nutrients (see Appendix II.1). However, the vitamin and mineral content of milk from domestic goats, particularly when they are reared in less than ideal surroundings, is not well known. It would seem advisable to give a complete vitamin supplement under these circumstances. The folic acid content of goat milk is known to be particularly low, and a vitamin supplement should always include folate.

Sheep milk

This should always be boiled or pasteurized before it is fed. Undiluted sheep milk is not recommended for feeding to infants of less than 12 months of age, but where there is no suitable alternative, a diluted formula can be devised.

Preparation of diluted formula: To each 50 ml of boiled sheep milk add 50 ml of boiled water. In addition, carbohydrate (glucose, glucose polymer, maltodextrin or sucrose) should be added at a level of 5 g per 100 ml of diluted feed.

The nutrient content of this diluted formula exceeds EEC guidelines for protein but falls within the USA guidelines. Fat and carbohydrate contents both fall within guidelines. The vitamin and mineral content of milk from domestic sheep, particularly when they are reared in less than ideal surroundings, is not well known. It would seem advisable to give a complete vitamin supplement under these circumstances.

II.7 COMPOSITION OF NON-ADAPTED MILKS (PER 100 ML)

Milk	Protein	Fat	Carbohydrate	Energy		Sodium	
	(g)	(g)	(g)	(kcal)	(kJ)	(mmol)	(mg)
Cow milk	3.3	3.8	4.7	65	272	2.17	49.91
Diluted cow milk formula	2.3	2.6	8.3	66	275	1.52	34.96
Canned evaporated milk	8.6	9.0	11.3	158	660	7.80	179.40
Diluted evaporated milk formula	2.1	2.2	7.8	60	250	1.95	44.85
Goat milk	3.3	4.5	4.6	71	296	1.80	41.40
Diluted goat milk formula	2.3	3.1	7.2	66	275	1.26	28.98
Sheep milk	5.4	6.0	5.1	95	397	1.91	43.93
Diluted sheep milk formula	2.7	3.0	7.5	68	284	0.96	22.08

See Appendix II.6 for full details regarding use of these products.

II.8 RENAL SOLUTE LOAD OF MILKS

$$\text{PRSL* (mOsm/l)} = \frac{\text{Protein (g/l)}}{0.175} + \text{Na (mmol/l)} + \text{K (mmol/l)} + \text{Cl (mmol/l)} + \text{P (mmol/l)}$$

	PRSL* (mOsm/l)
Mature human milk	90
Whey-dominant formula	95
Casein-dominant formula	110
Preterm formula	150
High-energy formula (Appendix III)	240
Cow milk	225

PRSL* = potential renal solute load

II.9 ORAL REHYDRATION SOLUTIONS

Oral rehydration solutions (ORS) or oral electrolyte solutions (OES) are used for oral rehydration therapy (ORT) in diarrhea. The prime aim of administering the ORS is to prevent or minimize dehydration; secondary aims are to correct acid–base and electrolyte disturbances.

The most important ingredients are sodium and glucose, ideally in equimolar quantities in order to promote maximum water absorption from the gut. The recommended sodium content for well-nourished children in western countries is 45–50 mmol/l; for malnourished children, WHO recommends a sodium content of 90 mmol/l. Since many forms of acute diarrheal disease cause a temporary impairment of carbohydrate absorption, it is preferable that the quantity of carbohydrate does not exceed 25 g/l. The inclusion of potassium, chloride and base is not necessary for the optimal absorption of water, although they perform useful functions. Renal losses of potassium are likely to be increased in situations where sodium is being conserved, leading to hypokalemia. Increased lactate and ketone production can cause the development of acidosis and the inclusion of a base such as citrate at a level of about 30 mmol/l helps to buffer the changes in blood pH. The overall osmolarity of the ORS should be 270–310 mOsm/l.

The inclusion of larger organic molecules such as amino acids and oligopeptides, which partially replace glucose, has not shown any clear advantages over conventional ORS formulas. The inclusion of a starch compound as a source of glucose appears to have some advantages in older children and in those with a secretory-type diarrhea. The inclusion of the infant or child's normal diet during acute diarrhea is discussed on page 131.

ORS are generally available in single-dose packages or sachets (they are also available as a ready-to-feed solution), which are reconstituted with 100 ml or 200 ml of water. Where no manufactured product is available, a 'home-prepared' recipe can be used (see Appendix II.10), although a potassium source should also be included where possible.

It is important that the water used to prepare the ORS is microbiologically safe and is boiled before use. The ORS should be prepared immediately prior to feeding as it is subject to bacterial contamination if stored at ambient temperatures for more than 1–2 h.

II.10 COMPOSITION OF ORAL REHYDRATION SOLUTIONS

Product	Manufacturer	Sodium		Potassium	
		(mmol/l)	(mg/l)	(mmol/l)	(mg/l)
Alhydrate*	Nestlé	60	1380	20	780
Dioralyte*	Rhone-Poulenc Rorer	60	1380	20	780
Dioralyte Relief*	Rhone-Poulenc Rorer	60	1380	20	780
Infalyte	Mead Johnson	50	1150	25	975
Pedialyte	Ross	45	1035	20	780
Rehydrat*	Searle	50	1150	20	780
Rehydralyte	Ross	75	1725	20	780
WHO rehydration salts		90	2070	20	780
EquaLYTE	Ross	78	1794	22	858
Resol	Wyeth-Ayerst	50	1150	20	780
Ricelyte	Mead Johnson	50	1150	25	975

Product	Chloride		Base	Carbohydrate	
	(mmol/l)	(mg/l)	(mmol/l)	(g/l)	Type
Alhydrate*	60	2100	Citrate 18	80	Maltodextrin/ sucrose
Dioralyte*	60	2100	Citrate 20	16	Glucose
Dioralyte Relief*	50	1750	Citrate 10	30	Rice starch[†]
Infalyte	45	1575	Citrate 30	30	Rice syrup/ glucose
Pedialyte	50/35	1750/1225	Citrate 30	25	Glucose
Rehydrat*	50	1750	Bicarb 20 Citrate 9	50	Sucrose Glucose Fructose
Rehydralyte	60/65	2100/2275	Citrate 30	25	Glucose
WHO rehydration salts	80	2800	Citrate 30	20	Glucose
EquaLYTE	68	2380	Citrate 30	25	Glucose
Resol	50	1750	Citrate 34	20	Glucose
Ricelyte	45	1575	Citrate 34	20	Rice syrup solids

*Not available in the USA.
[†]Contains aspartame.

Composition of a homemade oral rehydration solution

Salt 5.0 g, glucose or sucrose 25 g, water to make up to 1000 ml.

This solution provides 85 mmol Na^+ and Cl^- and 92 mmol glucose per liter.

The solution contains no potassium or base and should only be used where there is no alternative. Fruit such as banana can provide additional potassium (100 g provides 9 mmol potassium and 20 g carbohydrate).

Water must be from a clean source and must be boiled before making up the solution.

II.11 REALIMENTATION FORMULAS

These formulas have been designed to act as an intermediate stage between clear oral fluids and full milk feeds or normal solid diet during diarrhea or protein–energy malnutrition. They are usually lower in lactose and higher in electrolytes than normal infant formulas. Although these products can be useful in the above-mentioned conditions, they are expensive and are unlikely to be available to infants and children who would derive the most benefit from them.

HN25   Milupa

Casein based, low in lactose and fat. Carbohydrates derived from banana, apple, corn and rice. Gluten free. Complete feed, no supplements recommended. Meets Food and Agriculture Organisation (FAO) criteria. Manufacturer recommends a maximum of 7–10 days' use as sole source of nutrients.

HN25 type	Protein	Fat	Carbohydrate		Energy		Sodium		Potassium	
	(g)	(g)	Total (g)	Lactose (g)	(kcal)	(kJ)	(mmol)	(mg)	(mmol)	(mg)
100 g granules	18.5	8.4	64.9	0.6	409	1712	12.0	276.0	20.0	780.0
100 ml feed	2.6	1.2	9.1	0.1	58	243	1.7	39.1	2.8	109.2

II.12 Thickening agents for milk feeds

Agents that form a gel when mixed with liquid and therefore increase the viscosity of the liquid are used for infants and children with dysphagia or regurgitation. Two types of thickening agents are available commercially: those based on pre-gelatinized starch and gums derived from seeds and beans.

Both types of products can be added to cold liquids. Starch gels are more stable and can be added to formulas some time before they are consumed: gums usually need to be added at the time of consumption.

Thickening agents based on starch gels contribute absorbable energy and need to be included as part of the energy and carbohydrate of the formula.

Products marked with an asterisk(*) are not available in the USA.

Instant Carobel*   Cow & Gate**

Powder derived from carob seed. Free from gluten and lactose.

Dosage: 2–3 level scoops (1.16–1.74 g) to each 100 ml feed.

Nestargel*   Nestlé**

Powder derived from carob seed. Low in protein, gluten free.

Dosage: 1 level scoop (1 g) to each 100 ml feed.

Thixo D*   Sutherland**

Powder derived from modified maize starch. Gluten free.

Dosage: 1 heaped scoop (15 ml) per 170 ml feed.

Thick and Easy*   Fresenius Kabi**

Powder derived from modified maize starch. Free from gluten and lactose.

Dosage: 1 tablespoon (approx. 4.5 g) to each 100 ml feed.

Vitaquick*   Vitaflo**

Powder derived from modified maize starch.

Dosage: 2–4 level scoops (10–20 ml) to each 100 ml feed.

Baby rice cereal   **Various**

Commercially available weaning cereal, gluten free. May contain soya oil.

Dosage: 1–3 teaspoons to each 100 ml feed.

Composition (per 100 g) of thickening agents for feeds

Product	Energy		Protein	Fat	Carbohydrate	Type
	(kcal)	(kJ)	(g)	(g)	(g)	
Instant Carobel*	251	1065	2.4	0.45	59	Carob gum
Nestargel*	38	159	6	0.8	Nil	Carob gum
Thixo D*	392	1641	0.5	0.2	97	Maize starch
Thick and Easy*	372	1562	Nil	Nil	92.6	Maize starch
Vitaquick*	400	1674	Trace	Trace	95	Maize starch
Rice cereal	380	1560	20	10	180	Rice cereal

*Not available in the USA.

II.13 Formulas designed as antireflux feeds

These feeds are designed to reduce regurgitation in infants with mild reflux. They are nutritionally complete and have a similar nutrient profile to standard infant formulas. There is some evidence that whey-dominant formulas empty from the stomach more rapidly than casein-dominant milks and, theoretically, might be advantageous. When reconstituted with water, these feeds have a thicker consistency than standard milks. This is due to the replacement of part of the sugar content of the feed with a pre-gelatinized starch or, in one feed, to the addition of a hemi-cellulose gum that forms a gel.

Products marked with an asterisk (*) are not available in the USA.

Frisovom 1*   **Friesland Nutrition**
Nutritionally complete, casein-dominant formula thickened with carob bean gum, designed for infants with reflux.

Enfamil AR   **Mead Johnson**
Nutritionally complete, casein-dominant formula thickened with rice starch.

Nan AR*   **Nestlé**
Nutritionally complete, casein-dominant formula thickened with cornstarch.

Nutrilon AR*   **Nutricia**
Nutritionally complete, casein-dominant formula thickened with cornstarch.

SMA Staydown*   **SMA**
Nutritionally complete casein-dominant formula thickened with corn starch

Composition (per 100 ml normal dilution) of formulas designed as antireflux feeds

Product	Energy		Protein	Fat	Carbohydrate	Thickener
	(kcal)	(kJ)	(g)	(g)	(g)	
Frisovom 1*	64	268	1.40	3.4	7.60	Carob bean gum
Enfamil AR	69	289	1.70	3.5	7.50	Rice starch
Nan AR*	67	281	1.74	3.1	7.93	Cornstarch
Nutrilon AR*	66	276	1.72	2.9	8.18	Cornstarch
SMA Staydown*	67	280	1.60	3.6	7.00	Cornstarch

Product	Na		K		Calcium		Iron	
	(mmol)	(mg)	(mmol)	(mg)	(mmol)	(mg)	(μmol)	(mg)
Frisovom 1*	0.87	20.01	1.59	62.01	0.03	48.0	10.71	0.60
Enfamil AR	1.04	23.92	2.20	85.80	1.38	55.0	14.28	0.80
Nan AR*	1.04	23.92	2.00	78.00	1.55	62.0	14.28	0.80
Nutrilon AR*	1.16	26.68	2.06	80.34	1.78	71.1	10.00	0.56
SMA Staydown*	0.95	22.00	2.05	80.00	1.40	56.0	14.28	0.80

*Not available in the USA.

II.14 VITAMIN AND MINERAL SUPPLEMENTS

Oral preparations available in the UK

Product	Manufacturer	Contents	
Abidec drops	Warner Lambert	0.6 ml contains:	
		Vitamin A	1200 μg
		Thiamin HCL	1 mg
		Riboflavin	0.4 mg
		Nicotinamide	5 mg
		Pyridoxine HCL	0.5 mg
		Ascorbic acid	50 mg
		Ergocalciferol	10 μg
Ketovite tablets	Yamanouchi Pharma	One tablet contains:	
		Ascorbic acid	16.6 mg
		Riboflavin	1 mg
		Thiamin HCL	1 mg
		Pyridoxine HCL	0.33 mg
		Nicotinamide	3.3 mg
		Calcium pantothenate	1.16 mg
		α-tocopherol acetate	5 mg
		Inositol	50 mg
		Biotin	0.17 mg
		Folic acid	0.25 mg
		Acetomenaphtone	0.5 mg
Ketovite liquid	Yamanouchi Pharma	(Sup liquid: sugar free)	per 5 ml liquid:
		Vitamin A	750 μg
		Vitamin D	10 μg
		Choline chloride	150 mg
		Cyanocobalamin	12.5 μg
Phlexy Vits (per 7 g)*	SHS	Vitamin A	800 μg
		Vitamin D_3	10 μg
		Vitamin E	9 IU/6.6 mg
		Vitamin C	50 mg
		Vitamin K_1	70 μg
		Thiamine	1.2 mg
		Riboflavin	1.4 mg
		Niacin	20 mg
		Vitamin B_6	1.6 mg
		Folacin	700 μg
		Vitamin B_{12}	5 μg
		Biotin	150 mg
		Pantothenic acid	5 mg
		Calcium	100 mg
		Phosphorus	775 mg
		Magnesium	300 mg
		Iron	15 mg
		Zinc	11 mg
		Manganese	1.5 μg
		Copper	1.5 mg
		Iodine	150 μg
		Molybdenum	70 μg
		Chromium	30 μg
		Selenium	75 μg

*Also available in the USA.

Pediatric Seravit Powder (Scientific Hospital Supplies)

	Flavored per 100 g	Unflavored per 100 g	Unflavored per 14 g*	Flavored per 17 g†	Unflavored per 17 g†
Energy (kcal/kJ)	268/1122	300/1256	42/176	46/193	51/214
Protein (g)	Nil	Nil	Nil	Nil	Nil
Carbohydrate (g)	67	75	11	11	13
Fat (g)	Nil	Nil	Nil	Nil	Nil
Vitamins					
Vitamin A (mg)	4.2	4.2	0.59	0.71	0.71
Vitamin E (mg)	29	29	4.06	4.93	4.93
Vitamin C (mg)	400	400	56	68	68
Thiamine (mg)	3.2	3.2	0.45	0.54	0.54
Riboflavin (mg)	4.4	4.4	0.62	0.75	0.75
Pyridoxine (mg)	3.4	3.4	0.48	0.58	0.58
Nicotinamide (mg)	35	35	4.9	5.95	5.95
Pantothenic acid (mg)	17	17	2.38	2.89	2.89
Inositol (mg)	700	700	98	119	119
Choline (mg)	350	350	49	59.5	59.5
Vitamin D_3 (μg)	55.5	55.5	7.77	9.44	9.44
Vitamin B_{12} (μg)	8.6	8.6	1.20	1.46	1.46
Folic acid (μg)	303	303	42.42	51.51	51.51
Biotin (μg)	214	214	29.96	36.38	36.38
Vitamin K_1 (μg)	166	166	23.24	28.22	28.22
Minerals					
Sodium (mmol/mg)	0.86/19.78	0.86/19.78	0.12/2.76	0.15/3.45	0.15/3.45
Potassium (mmol/mg)	0.78/30.42	Trace	Trace	0.13/5.07	Trace
Chloride (mmol/mg)	0.56/19.6	1.12/39.2	0.16/5.6	0.10/3.5	0.19/6.65
Calcium (mmol/mg)	64.25/2570	64.25/2570	8.99/359.8	10.92/436.9	10.92/436.9
Phosphorus (mmol/mg)	55.29/1714	55.29/1714	7.74/239.96	9.39/291.38	9.39/291.38
Magnesium (mmol/mg)	14.87/357	14.87/357	2.08/49.98	2.52/60.69	2.52/60.69
Trace elements					
Iron (mmol/mg)	1.23/69	1.23/69	0.17/9.66	0.21/11.73	0.21/11.73
Copper (mmol/mg)	0.07/4.6	0.07/4.6	0.01/0.64	0.01/0.78	0.012/0.78
Zinc (mmol/mg)	0.71/46	0.71/46	0.09/6.44	0.12/7.82	0.12/7.82
Iodine (μg)	332	332	46.48	56.44	56.44
Manganese (mg)	4.6	4.6	0.64	0.78	0.78
Molybdenum (μg)	351	351	49.14	59.67	59.67
Chromium (μg)	137	137	19.18	23.29	23.29
Selenium (μg)	137	137	19.18	23.29	23.29

*Recommended dose for infants aged 0–6 months; flavored product is not recommended for this age group.
†Recommended dose for infants aged 6–12 months.

Seravit Powder (Scientific Hospital Supplies)

	Per 100 g	Per 25 g (adult dose)
Energy (kcal/kJ)	320/1340	80/335
Protein (g)	Nil	Nil
Carbohydrate (g)	80	20
Fat (g)	Nil	Nil
Vitamins		
Vitamin A (μg)	6500	1625
Vitamin D_3 (μg)	38	9.5
Vitamin E (mg)	166	41.5
Vitamin C (mg)	566	141.5
Vitamin K_1 (μg)	3920	980
Thiamine (mg)	11.6	2.9
Riboflavin (mg)	11.6	2.9
Niacin (mg)	83.2	20.8
Vitamin B_6 (mg)	15	3.75
Folic acid (μg)	1660	415
Vitamin B_{12} (μg)	36	9
Biotin (μg)	1160	290
Pantothenic acid (mg)	40	10
Choline (mg)	1832	458
Inositol (mg)	184	46
Minerals		
Sodium (mmol/mg)	Trace	Trace
Potassium (mmol/mg)	Trace	Trace
Chloride (mmol/mg)	Trace	Trace
Calcium (mmol/mg)	Trace	Trace
Phosphorus (mmol/mg)	51.61/1600	12.90/400
Magnesium (mmol/mg)	52.08/1250	13.02/312.5
Trace elements		
Iron (mmol/mg)	1.49/83.2	0.37/20.8
Copper (mmol/mg)	0.13/8.2	0.03/2.05
Zinc (mmol/mg)	1.28/83.2	0.32/20.8
Manganese (mmol/mg)	0.23/12.4	0.06/3.1
Iodine (μg)	666	166.5
Molybdenum (μg)	666	166.5
Chromium (μg)	90	22.5

Modified Seravit Powder (Scientific Hospital Supplies)

	Per 100 g	Per scoop (5.5 g)
Energy (kcal/kJ)	252/1055	14/58
Protein (g)	Nil	Nil
Carbohydrate (g)	63	3.46
Fat (g)	Nil	Nil
Vitamins		
Vitamin A (μg)	3200	180
Vitamin D_3 (μg)	19	1.04
Vitamin E (mg)	83	4.56
Vitamin C (mg)	283	15.6
Vitamin K_1 (μg)	1960	108
Thiamine (mg)	5.8	0.3
Riboflavin (mg)	5.8	0.3
Niacin (mg)	41.6	2.3
Vitamin B_6 (mg)	7.5	0.41
Folic acid (μg)	833	45.8
Vitamin B_{12} (μg)	18	0.99
Biotin (μg)	583	32.1
Pantothenic acid (mg)	20	1.1
Choline (mg)	916	50.4
Inositol (mg)	92	5.1
Minerals		
Sodium (mmol/mg)	109/2507	6/138
Potassium (mmol/mg)	103/4017	5.7/222.3
Chloride (mmol/mg)	133/4655	7.3/255.5
Calcium (mmol/mg)	100/4000	5.5/220
Phosphorus (mmol/mg)	129.03/4000	7.09/220
Magnesium (mmol/mg)	26.04/625	1.43/34.4
Trace elements		
Iron (mmol/mg)	0.74/41.6	0.04/2.29
Copper (mmol/mg)	0.06/4.1	0.003/0.22
Zinc (mmol/mg)	0.64/41.6	0.04/2.29
Manganese (mmol/mg)	0.11/6.2	0.006/0.34
Iodine (μg)	333	18.3
Molybdenum (μg)	333	18.3
Chromium (μg)	45	2.47

Pediatric Renal Seravit Powder (Scientific Hospital Supplies)

	Per 100 g	Per 8 g	Per 12 g
Energy (kcal/kJ)	344/1440	28/115	41/173
Protein (g)	Nil	Nil	Nil
Carbohydrate (g)	86	6.9	10.3
Fat (g)	Nil	Nil	Nil
Vitamins			
Vitamin A (μg)	7400	592	888
Vitamin D_3 (μg)	97	7.76	11.6
Vitamin E (mg)	50	4	6
Vitamin C (mg)	700	56	84
Vitamin K_1 (μg)	290	23.2	34.8
Thiamine (mg)	5.5	0.44	0.66
Riboflavin (mg)	7.6	0.61	0.91
Niacin (mg)	61	4.88	7.32
Vitamin B_6 (mg)	6	0.48	0.72
Folic acid (μg)	530	42.4	63.6
Vitamin B_{12} (μg)	15	1.2	1.8
Biotin (μg)	375	30	45
Pantothenic acid (mg)	30	2.4	3.6
Choline (mg)	612	49	73.4
Inositol (mg)	1224	97.9	146.9
Minerals			
Sodium (mmol/mg)	<1.74/40.02	<0.14/3.22	<0.21/4.83
Potassium (mmol/mg)	Nil added	Nil added	Nil added
Chloride (mmol/mg)	<1.12/39.2	<0.09/3.15	<0.13/4.55
Calcium (mmol/mg)	Nil added	Nil added	Nil added
Phosphorus (mmol/mg)	Nil added	Nil added	Nil added
Magnesium (mmol/mg)	26.04/625	2.08/50	3.13/75
Trace elements			
Iron (mmol/mg)	2.14/120	0.17/9.6	0.26/14.4
Copper (mmol/mg)	0.13/8	0.01/0.64	0.02/0.96
Zinc (mmol/mg)	1.23/80	0.09/6.4	0.15/9.6
Manganese (mmol/mg)	0.15/8	0.01/0.64	0.02/0.96
Iodine (μg)	580	46.4	69.6
Molybdenum (μg)	615	49.2	73.8
Selenium (μg)	240	19.2	28.8
Chromium (μg)	240	19.2	28.8

Preparations available in the USA

Product	Contents	
Vi-Daylin & Poly-Vi-Sol[a]*	Vitamin A	450 μg
Dose: 0–3 years = 1 ml	Vitamin D	10 μg
	Vitamin E	3.42 mg
	Ascorbic acid	35 mg
	Thiamine	0.5 mg
	Riboflavin	0.6 mg
	Niacin	8 mg
	Vitamin B$_6$	0.4 mg
	Vitamin B$_{12}$	1.5 (20[a]) μg
Vi-Daylin ADC & Trivisol	Vitamin A	450 μg
Dose: 0–3 years = 1 ml	Vitamin D	10 μg
	Ascorbic acid	35 mg
Centrum[b] & Theragran[c]	Vitamin A	1500 μg
	Vitamin D	10 μg
	Vitamin E	20 mg
	Vitamin K	(25[b]) μg
	Ascorbic acid	(60[b]) (90[c]) mg
	Thiamine	(1.5[b]) (3[c]) mg
	Riboflavin	(1.7[b]) (3.4[c]) mg
	Niacin	20 mg
	Vitamin B$_6$	(2[b]) (3[c]) mg
	Vitamin B$_{12}$	(6[b]) (9[c]) μg
	Folic acid	400 μg
	Pantothenic acid	10 mg
	Biotin	30 μg
	Iron	(0.32/18[b]) (0.48/27[c]) mmol/mg
	Magnesium	1.81/100 mmol/mg
	Calcium	(4.05/162[b]) mmol/mg
	Zinc	0.23/15 mmol/mg
	Copper	0.03/2 mmol/mg
	Phosphorus	(3.51/109[b]) (1/31[c]) mmol/mg
	Potassium	(1.02/40[b]) (0.19/7.5[c]) mmol/mg
	Iodine	1.18/150 $\mu mol/\mu g$
	Manganese	(0.04/2.5[b]) (0.09/5[c]) mmol/mg
	Chloride	(1.03/36.3[b]) (0.21/7.5[c]) mmol/mg
	Chromium	(0.48/25[b]) (0.28/15[c]) $\mu mol/\mu g$
	Molybdenum	(0.26/25[b]) (0.15/15[c]) $\mu mol/\mu g$
	Selenium	(0.25/20[b]) (0.12/10[c]) $\mu mol/\mu g$
	Nickel	(0.08/5[b]) $\mu mol/\mu g$
	Tin	(0.08/10[b]) $\mu mol/\mu g$
	Silicon	(0.07/2[b]) mmol/mg
	Vanadium	(0.19/10[b]) $\mu mol/\mu g$
	Boron	(0.01/150[b]) mmol/μg

[a] Poli-Vi-Sol
[b] Centrum
[c] Theragran
*Also available with iron

IRON PREPARATIONS

Preparations available in the UK

Oral preparations	Manufacturer	Contents
Fersamal syrup Dilutent: syrup Life of diluted mixture: 14 days	Goldshield	5 ml contains: 140 mg Ferrous fumarate (0.80 mmol/45 mg iron)
Plesmet syrup	Link	10 ml contains: 282 mg Ferrous glycine sulfate (0.89 mmol/50 mg iron)
Ferrous sulfate mixture To be taken well diluted with water	Paediatric BP	5 ml contains: 60 mg Ferrous sulfate (0.21 mmol/12 mg iron)
Sytron Elixir Dilutent: water for preparations Life of diluted elixir: 14 days	Link	10 ml contains: 380 mg Sodium iron edetate (equivalent to 0.98 mmol/55 mg iron)
Injectable preparations		
Jectofer	Astra	Iron sorbitol injection 5% (equivalent to 0.89 mmol/50 mg iron) per ml

POTASSIUM PREPARATIONS

Preparations available in the UK

Oral preparations	Manufacturer	Contents	
Slow-K (slow release)	Alliance	Each tablet contains: Potassium chloride (provides 8 mmol/312 mg K⁺)	600 mg
Sando-K tablets (effervescent)	HK Pharma	Each tablet contains: Potassium bicarbonate Potassium chloride (12 mmol/468 mg K⁺ and 8 mmol/280 mg Cl⁻)	400 mg 600 mg
Kay-Cee-L syrup (sugar free) Do not dilute	Geistlich	Potassium chloride (equivalent to 1 mmol/39 mg K⁺) per ml	75 mg
Potassium citrate mixture for infants Dose: 4–8 ml, well diluted with water	BPC 1959	Potassium citrate Citric acid monohydrate Benzoic acid solution Amaranth solution Syrup Chloroform water	731.2 mg 146.4 mg 0.083 ml 0.033 ml 1.33 ml to 4 ml
Injectable preparations			
Strong potassium chloride solution	BP 1973	A sterile 15% solution of potassium chloride in water for injection pH 5–7; 10 ml contains approx. 20 mmol (780 mg) of potassium and of chloride and must be diluted before use with not less than 50 times its volume of sodium chloride 0.9% injection or other suitable dilutent	
Potassium chloride, sodium chloride and glucose intravenous infusion	BP	A sterile solution of potassium chloride 0.17–0.19% and sodium chloride 0.17–0.19%. Anhydrous glucose 3.8–4.2% in water for injection	

Preparations available in the USA

Oral preparations	Manufacturer	Contents
Potassium chloride elixir	USP	Rum-K 10 mmol K⁺ and Cl⁻ per 5 ml (sugar free) Cena-K 13.3 mmol K⁺ and Cl⁻ per 5 ml (sugar free)
Injectable preparations		
Potassium chloride injection	USP	A sterile solution in water for injections pH 4–8. To be diluted before use
Potassium phosphate injection	USP	4.4 mmol of K⁺ 3 mmol of HPO₄²⁻ (provided by potassium phosphate dibasic 236 mg and potassium phosphate monobasic 224 mg/ml)

CALCIUM PREPARATIONS

Preparations available in the UK

Oral preparations	Manufacturer	Contents	
Sandocal 400 1 tablet = 400 mg (10 mmol)	Novartis	Each tablet contains: Calcium lactate gluconate Calcium carbonate Citric acid	930 mg 700 mg 1.189 g
Calcium-Sandoz Dilutent: syrup Life of diluted elixir: 14 days	Alliance	5 ml contains: Calcium glubionate Calcium lactobionate (108 mg calcium or 2.7 mmol Ca^{2+}/5 ml)	1.09 g 0.727 g
Injectable preparations			
Calcium chloride injection	BP	(13.4% w/v CaCl$_2$) 2H$_2$O 1.34 g in 10 ml 9.12 mmol Ca^{2+} in 10 ml 18.23 mmol Cl$^-$ in 10 ml	
Calcium gluconate	BP	Calcium gluconate 10% (5 and 10 ml ampoules) 2.25 mmol (90 mg) Ca^{2+} in 10 ml	

Preparations available in the USA

Oral preparations	Manufacturer	Contents
Calcium gluconate tables	USP	Tablets containing anhydrous calcium gluconate
Injectable preparations		
Calcium gluconate injections	USP	A sterile solution of anhydrous calcium gluconate in water for injections; it may contain small amounts of calcium saccharate or other suitable calcium salts as stabilizers; sodium hydroxide may be added to adjust the pH to 6–8.2
Calcium gluceptate injections	USP	A sterile solution of calcium gluceptate in water for injections; it contains the equivalent of 17–19 mg (0.42–0.47 mmol) Ca^{2+} in each milliliter, pH 5.6–7

MAGNESIUM SALTS

Preparations available in the UK

Injectable preparations	Manufacturer	Contents
Magnesium sulfate 20%	BP	10 ml contains: 8.14 mmol/195.36 mg Mg^{2+}
Magnesium sulfate 50%	BP	10 ml contains: 20.4 mmol/489.6 mg Mg^{2+}

Preparations available in the USA

Oral preparations	Manufacturer	Contents
Magnesium gluconate tablets (USP)	GYN (Amfre-Grant)	Each gram represents approximately 2.2 mmol (52.8 mg) of magnesium
Injectable preparations		
Magnesium sulfate	USP	A sterile solution of magnesium sulfate in water for injections; pH of 5% solution 5.5–7

MINERAL SUPPLEMENTS**

Aminogran Mineral Mixture (UCB)

Mineral	Unit	Per 100 g	Per 8 g (recommended dose)
Potassium	mmol/mg	210/8190	17/663
Calcium	mmol/mg	202.5/8100	16.25/650
Phosphorus	mmol/mg	193.54/6000	15.48/480
Sodium	mmol/mg	170/3910	14/322
Magnesium	mmol/mg	40/960	3.2/76.8
Iron	mmol/mg	1.12/63	0.08/5.0
Zinc	mmol/mg	0.73/48	0.06/4.0
Copper	mmol/mg	0.20/13	0.01/1.0
Manganese	μmol/mg	72.7/4	7.27/0.4
Iodine	μg	Trace	
Aluminium	μg	Trace	
Cobalt	μg	Trace	
Molybdenum	μg	Trace	

Metabolic Mineral Mixture (SHS)

Mineral	Unit	Per 100 g	Per 8 g[*]
Sodium	mmol/mg	172/3956	13.8/317.4
Potassium	mmol/mg	212/8268	16.97/661.83
Calcium[†]	mmol/mg	205/8200	16.4/656
Magnesium	mmol/mg	40.41/970	3.20/77
Chloride	mmol/mg	51/1785	4.08/142.8
Phosphorus	mmol/mg	192.25/5960	15.38/477
Iron	mmol/mg	1.12/63	0.09/5.04
Copper	mmol/mg	0.20/13	0.01/1.04
Zinc	mmol/mg	0.73/48	0.05/3.84
Manganese	μmol/mg	0.10/5.7	8.36/0.46
Iodine	μmol/μg	5.98/760	0.47/60.8
Molybdenum	μmol/μg	1.56/150	0.12/12.0

*Recommended daily dose for infants weighing >5.5 kg; infants weighing <5.5 kg should receive 1.5 g/kg/day.
**Not available in the USA.
†Calcium-free product also available.

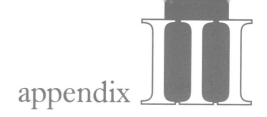

appendix III

ENTERAL FEEDING AND FEEDS WITH INCREASED PROTEIN/ENERGY DENSITY

III.1 PRODUCTS USED FOR ENTERAL FEEDING

Complete feeds containing the required quantities of minerals and micronutrients may be recommended as an oral or a tube feed; it is important to determine whether a feed of this type is palatable before recommending it to be taken orally. The products described as supplementary feeds are usually palatable as they are intended to be taken orally.

Where a feed is intended to form a major part of the child's diet it is important not only that it is nutritionally complete but also that it does not provide excess quantities of nutrients that may potentially be harmful. Feeds designed for adults are too high in protein and fat-soluble vitamins for the young or malnourished child. Over the age of 6 years, or above a weight of 20 kg, a standard adult feed (1 kcal/ml or 4.2 kJ/ml) is usually suitable, provided there is no renal or hepatic impairment. High-energy adult feeds (1.5 kcal/ml or 6.3 kJ/ml) usually provide excess protein. For infants under the age of 6 years or below a weight of 20 kg, or where renal and liver function is not optimum, a pediatric feed should be used. Where feeds are taken orally as a supplement to the diet and do not provide more than 50% of the fluid requirement, standard adult sip feeds (1 kcal/ml or 4.2 kJ/ml) can be used from the age of 2 years or a weight of 10 kg.

Products may be in the form of a powder, that is reconstituted with water or milk. These have the advantages of economy and ease of transport and storage; however, if they are to be reconstituted by untrained personnel, there is a danger both of contamination due to poor hygiene practices and of inaccuracies occurring. Ready-to-feed products are normally marketed in sterile containers and require no reconstitution. Although these feeds are expensive and are difficult to transport and store, they have the advantage of accuracy and ease of use. Where sip feeds are not available, liquid supplements can be prepared using domestic ingredients (see Appendix III.10). These provide protein and energy but do not contain a full range of minerals, vitamins and trace elements, so a supplement may be required.

III.2 COMPLETE FEEDS FOR CHILDREN WHO WEIGH <20 KG

Products marked with an asterisk (*) are not available in the USA.

Frebini Original*   Fresenius Kabi

A 1 kcal/ml (4.2 kJ/ml) nutritionally complete feed based on whole milk. The fat source is derived from medium-chain triglycerides (MCTs) and soy oil, and the carbohydrate source is maltodextrin. Recommended for children aged 1–6 years or 8–20 kg in weight. Free from gluten, fiber, carrageenan and lactose. Recommended for tube feeding.

Kindercal/Enfagrow*   Mead Johnson

A 1 kcal/ml (4.2 kJ/ml) nutritionally complete feed based on whey protein. The fat source is a combination of vegetable oil and MCT. The carbohydrate source is a combination of maltodextrin and sucrose. Contains soy fiber. Free from lactose and gluten. Vanilla flavor. Can be used as an oral drink.

Nutren Junior   Nestlé

A 1 kcal/ml (4.2 kJ/ml) nutritionally complete feed based on milk proteins. The fat source is a combination of vegetable oil and MCT (25%). The carbohydrate source is free from gluten and lactose. Can be used as an oral drink. Also available with fiber. Available in vanilla and unflavored. Unflavored can be mixed with flavor packets.

Nutrini*   Nutricia

A 1 kcal/ml (4.2 kJ/ml) nutritionally complete feed based on whole milk. The fat source is derived from vegetable oil and the carbohydrate source is maltodextrin. Recommended for children aged 1–6 years or 8–20 kg in weight. Free from gluten and lactose. Recommended for tube feeding.

Also available – Nutrini Extra and Nutrini Multifibre:
Nutrini Extra is an energy-dense feed providing 1.5 kcal/ml (6.3 kJ/ml).
Nutrini Multifibre contains a mixture of six types of fibers (soy polysaccharide, arabic gum, resistant starch, inulin, cellulose, oligofructose), which provides 0.8 g fiber/100 ml.

Paediasure   Abbott

A 1 kcal/ml (4.2 kJ/ml) nutritionally complete feed based on whey protein. The fat source is a combination of vegetable oil and MCT and the carbohydrate sources maltodextrin and sucrose. Recommended for children aged 1–6 years or 10–20 kg in weight. Free from gluten and lactose. Flavors available are chocolate, vanilla, banana and strawberry. Recommended as an oral drink.

Also available – Paediasure Fibre, Paediasure Plus, and Paediasure Plus Fibre.
Paediasure Fibre contains non-starch polysaccharide and provides 0.50 g fiber/100 ml. Paediasure Plus is an energy dense feed providing 1.5 kcal/ml (6.3 kJ/ml). Paediasure Plus Fibre is an energy-dense feed providing 1.5 kcal/ml (6.3kJ/ml) and 0.75g fiber. Vanilla flavor. Recommended for tube feeding.

---

*These products are availbale in strawberry, vanilla, and banana flavors as a sip feed and in vanilla flavor as a tube feed.

Composition of enteral feeds (per 100 ml of feed)

Product	Protein	Fat	Carbohydrate	Energy		Fiber
	(g)	(g)	(g)	(kcal)	(kJ)	(g)
Frebini Original*	2.5	4.4	12.5	100	419	–
Kindercal	3.0	4.4	13.5	106	444	0.63
Nutren Junior	3.0	4.2	12.7	100	419	–
Nutren Junior with fiber	3.0	4.2	12.7	100	419	0.60
Nutrini*	2.8	4.4	12.3	100	420	–
Nutrini Extra*	4.1	6.7	18.5	150	630	–
Nutrini Multifibre*	2.8	4.4	12.3	100	420	0.8
Paediasure	2.8	5.0	11.2	101	422	–
Paediasure fibre	2.8	5.0	11.2	101	422	0.50
Pediasure USA	3.0	5.0	11.2	101	422	0.50

Product	Na		K		Iron		Calcium	
	(mmol)	(mg)	(mmol)	(mg)	(μmol)	(mg)	(mmol)	(mg)
Frebini Original*	2.2	50.0	2.6	100.0	16.07	0.9	1.50	60
Kindercal	1.6	36.8	3.3	128.7	19.64	1.1	2.12	85
Nutren Junior	2.0	46.0	3.3	132.0	25.0	1.4	2.50	100
Nutren Junior with fiber	2.0	46.0	3.3	132.0	25.0	1.4	2.50	100
Nutrini*	2.6	60.0	2.8	110.0	17.85	1.0	1.50	60
Nutrini Extra*	3.9	90.0	4.2	165.0	26.78	1.5	2.25	90
Nutrini Multifibre*	2.6	60.0	2.8	110.0	17.85	1.0	1.50	60
Paediasure	2.6	60.0	2.8	110.0	17.85	1.0	1.40	56
Paediasure fibre	2.6	60.0	2.8	110.0	17.85	1.0	1.40	56
Pediasure USA	1.6	36.8	3.3	128.7	25.0	1.4	2.40	96

*Not available in the USA

III.3 FORMULAS DESIGNED FOR PREMATURE AND LOW-BIRTH-WEIGHT INFANTS

Products designed to meet the needs of preterm or low-birth-weight infants from birth up until the time of discharge from hospital are generally in a ready-to-feed format and contain approximately 80 kcal (335 kJ) per 100 ml feed. Formulas have a higher nutrient density than standard milks. Some are supplemented with iron; others require a full supplement to be given. Formulas for the preterm infant post-discharge may be in a ready-to-feed or powder format; they are generally reduced in nutrient density compared with formulas for hospitalized infants, though are still more nutrient dense than standard milks. Post-discharge formulas marketed in the USA and Europe need to comply with current regulations governing the composition of standard formulas (see Appendix II.2).

Preterm formulas are designed based upon both the Tsang consensus recommendations and the European Society for Paediatric Gastroenterology and Nutrition Committee on Nutrition (ESPGAN-CON) recommendations as listed in the table below.

Nutrient	Tsang /100 kcal Infant <1000 g	Tsang /100 kcal Infant ≥ 1000 g	ESPGAN /100 kcal	Comments
Protein g	3.0–3.16	2.5–3.0	2.25–3.10	Amino acid content of the protein should not be less than breast milk
Fat: Total g			4.4–6.0	Not more than 40% medium-chain triglycerides should contain monounsaturated fatty acids
Linoleic g Linolenic g C18:2/C18:3	0.44–1.70 0.11–0.44 ≥ 5	0.44–1.70 0.11–0.44 ≥ 5	0.5–1.2 >0.055 5–15	
Long chain polyunsaturated fatty acids			Desirable additives	n–6 LCP 1–2% of total fatty acids n–3 LCP 0.5–1% of total fatty acids
Total Carbohydrate			7–14	Not more than 11 g/100 ml; acceptable carbohydrates are lactose, glucose, starch hydrolysates, and sucrose
Lactose g	3.16–9.5	3.16–9.8	3.2–12.0	Not more than 8 g/100 ml
Oligomers g	0–7.0	0–7.0		
Vitamin A μg	583–1250	583–1250	90–150	May be advisable to supplement 200–1000 μg/day
Vitamin D μg	125–333 Aim 400 IU/d	125–333 Aim 400 IU/d	not exceeding 3 μg	Cholecalciferol or ergocalciferol preferred; supplement to a total of 20–40 μg
Vitamin E μg	5–10	5–10	4–15	α-tocopherol:polyunsaturated fat ratio should be at least 0.9 mg/g

Nutrient	Tsang /100 kcal Infant <1000 g	Tsang /100 kcal Infant ≥ 1000 g	ESPGAN	Comments
Vitamin K μg	6.66–8.33	6.66–8.33	4–15	
Vitamin B1 μg	150–200	150–200	20–250	
Vitamin B2 μg	200–300	200–300	60–600	
Niacin mg	3–4	3–4	0.8–5.0	
Pantothenic Acid mg	1.0–1.5	1.0–1.5	>0.3	
Vitamin B6 μg	125–175	125–175	35–250	15 mg per gram of protein
Biotin μg	3–5	3–5	>1.5	
Folic Acid μg	21–42	21–42	>60	
Vitamin B12 μg	0.25	0.25	>0.15	
Vitamin C mg	15–20	15–20	7–40	
L-Carnitine mg	~2.4	~2.4	>1.2	
Sodium mg	38–58	38–58	23–53	Infants <34 weeks gestation may require additional supplementation
Potassium mg	65–100	65–100	90–152	
Chloride mg	59–89	59–89	57–89	
Calcium mg	100–192	100–192	70–140	Calcium:phosphorus ratio 1.4–2.0
Phosphorous mg	50–117	50–117	90	
Magnesium mg	6.6–12.5	6.6–12.5	<12	
Iron mg	1.67	1.67	1.5	Infants should achieve an iron intake of 2.0–2.5 mg/kg daily from age 8 weeks (max. 15 mg/day); iron supplements may be required
Zinc μg	833	833	550–1100	
Copper μg	100–125	100–125	90–120	
Manganese μg	6.3	6.3	1.5–7.5	
Iodine μg	25–50	25–50	10–45	
Taurine mg	3.75–7.50	3.75–7.50		
Inositol mg	27.0–67.5	27.0–67.5		
Choline mg	12.0–23.4	12.0–23.4		

ESPGAN Committee on Nutrition of the Preterm Infant. Nutrition and feeding of preterm infants. Acta Paediatr Scand Suppl 1987;336:1–14.

ESPGAN Committee on Nutrition. Comment on the content and composition of lipids in infant formulas. Acta Paediatr Scand 1991;80:887–96.

Tsang RC, Lucas A, Uauy R, Zlotkin S, eds. Consensus recommendations. Nutritional needs of the preterm infant. Scientific basis and practical guidelines. Baltimore: Williams and Wilkins, 1993.

III.4 COMPOSITION OF FORMULAS DESIGNED FOR PREMATURE AND LOW-BIRTH-WEIGHT INFANTS (PER 100 ML OF FEED)

Product	Manufacturer	Countries available	Protein*	Fat	
			(g)	(g)	Type
For hospital use					
Prematil	Milupa	Europe	2.40	4.40	Vegetable oils
Pre-Aptamil with Milupan	Milupa	UK	2.40	4.40	Vegetable oils
Similac Special Care 20	Ross	USA	1.83	3.67	MCT, soy, coconut
Similac Special Care 24	Ross	USA	2.20	4.41	MCT, soy, coconut
Frisopré	Friesland Nutrition	Asia, Europe, Far East and Middle East	1.90	4.00	Vegetable oils, fish oils
Enfamil Premature 20	Mead Johnson	USA	2.00	3.50	MCT, soy, coconut
Enfamil Premature 24	Mead Johnson	USA	2.40	4.10	MCT, soy, coconut
Neosure	Abbott	USA	1.90	4.00	Coconut, soy, MCT
Nutriprem	Cow & Gate	UK	2.20	4.40	Vegetable oils, fish oils
PreNan	Nestlé	UK, Middle East, Europe Asia, Latin America	2.32	4.16	MCT, high oleic sunflower, palm olein, canola, sunflower, fish, egg lecithin
SMA low birth weight	SMA	UK	2.00	4.40	Vegetable oils, MCT
Post-discharge formulas					
Similac Neosure	Ross	USA	1.70	3.70	Soy, coconut, MCT
Nutriprem 2	Cow & Gate	UK	1.80	4.10	Vegetable oils
Premcare	Farleys	UK	1.85	3.96	Vegetable oils, fish oils
Enfacare	Mead Johnson	USA	1.90	3.80	Sunflower oil, MCT, coconut oil

*All have whey: casein ratio 60:40
MCT = medium-chain triglycerides

III.4 CONTINUED

Product	Carbohydrate		Energy		Iron	
	(g)	Type	(kcal)	(kJ)	(µmol)	(mg)
For hospital use						
Prematil	7.9	Lactose, maltodextrin	80	335	16.07	0.90
Pre-Aptamil with Milupan	7.9	Lactose, maltodextrin	80	335	16.07	0.90
Similac Special Care 20	7.2	Lactose, glucose polymers	68	284	21.42	1.20
Similac Special Care 24	8.6	Lactose, glucose polymers	81	339	21.42	1.20
Frisopré	7.9	Maltodextrin, lactose	75	314	8.92	0.50
Enfamil Premature 20	7.5	Corn syrup, lactose	68	284	26.78	1.50
Enfamil Premature 24	9.0	Corn syrup, lactose	81	339	26.78	1.50
Neosure	7.6	Corn syrup, lactose	74	310	23.21	1.30
Nutriprem	8.0	Maltodextrin, lactose	80	335	16.07	0.90
PreNan	8.6	Lactose, maltodextrin	80	335	21.42	1.20
SMA low birth weight	8.6	Lactose, maltodextrin	82	343	14.28	0.80
Post-discharge formulas						
Similac Neosure	6.9	Glucose polymers, lactose	80	335	5.35	0.30
Nutriprem 2	7.5	Lactose	74	310	19.64	1.10
Premcare	6.2	Lactose, maltodextrin	72	301	11.60	0.65
Enfacare	8.2	Lactose, maltodextrin	74	310	23.21	1.30

*All have whey:casein ratio 60:40
MCT = medium-chain triglycerides

III.5 BREAST-MILK FORTIFIERS

For the low-birth-weight or sick infant, breast milk is the most beneficial feed, although as the sole source of nutrition it may not provide sufficient protein, energy or other nutrients to sustain rapid or catch-up growth. Where the infant is unable to suckle directly from the breast and the mother is expressing milk, a fortifier may be added to increase the nutrient density. Fortified breast milk does not offer the same degree of protection against necrotizing enterocolitis as unfortified milk. The use of fortifiers for infants at risk of the condition may be contraindicated.

Breast-milk fortifiers are available in powder form and are usually packaged to facilitate the addition of small quantities (3–4 g) to 100 ml of expressed breast milk. They provide additional protein and energy, but vary in the degree of micronutrient supplementation included. Iron is generally not included in these products.

Fortifiers should be added to the breast milk as close as possible to the time of feeding. Breast milk that has been fortified does not retain its anti-infective properties and the growth of harmful bacteria may occur if the fortifier is added before milk is stored. Enzymes present in raw breast milk break down the carbohydrate and fat in the supplement, and feed osmolality increases with storage if the fortifier is added early.

Products marked with an asterisk (*) are not available in the USA.

Eoprotin*   Milupa
Mixture of whey protein, caseinate and amino acids. The carbohydrate source is glucose syrup. Separate supplementation with iron and vitamins is required.

Enfamil Human Milk Fortifier   Mead Johnson
Based on whey protein. The carbohydrate source is glucose polymers and lactose. Supplemented with vitamins and minerals.

FM85*   Nestlé
Based on extensively hydrolysed whey protein. The carbohydrate source is maltodextrin. Supplemented with vitamins and minerals.

Nutriprem*   Cow & Gate
Mixture of whey protein hydrolysate and casein hydrolysate. The carbohydrate source is maltodextrin. Separate supplementation with iron and vitamins is required.

SMA Breast Milk Fortifier*   SMA
Based on whey protein. The fat source is derived from soybean oil and the carbohydrate source is maltodextrin. Supplemented with vitamins and some minerals. Further supplementation will be required.

Similac Human Milk Fortifier   Ross
Based on whey protein concentrate and non-fat dried milk. The fat source is MCT oil and the carbohydrate source is corn syrup. Extra supplementation with iron and vitamins will be required.

Check with manufacturers for preparation instructions.

Composition of breast-milk fortifiers

Product	Energy		Protein	Carbohydrate	Fat
	(kcal)	(kJ)	(g)	(g)	(g)
Mature human milk per 100 ml	69	288	1.3	7.2	4.1
3 g Eoprotin* +100 ml milk	80	334	1.9	9.3	4.1
4 g Enfamil +100 ml milk	84	349	2.0	10.0	4.1
5 g FM85 +100 ml milk	85	355	2.3	10.6	4.1
3 g Nutriprem* +100 ml milk	79	330	2.0	9.2	4.1
4 g SMA Fortifier* + 100 ml milk	85	357	2.3	9.8	4.3

Product	Sodium		Calcium		Osmolality when added to breast milk
	(mmol)	(mg)	(mmol)	(mg)	mOsm/l
Mature human milk per 100 ml	0.65	14.95	0.85	34	
3 g Eoprotin* +100 ml milk	0.65	14.95	1.78	71	330–340
4 g Enfamil +100 ml milk	0.97	22.31	3.20	128	351
5 g FM85 +100 ml milk	0.91	20.95	2.70	109	370
3 g Nutriprem* +100 ml milk	0.92	21.16	2.35	94	361
4 g SMA Fortifier* + 100 ml milk	1.41	32.43	3.10	125	344

*Not available in the USA.

III.6 HIGH NUTRIENT DENSITY FEEDS FOR INFANTS

Infants who have increased nutrient requirements or who are restricted in their fluid intake are unlikely to thrive on a standard infant formula containing 65–70 kcal (272–293 kJ) per 100 ml. Since requirements of all nutrients are increased, it is important to use a feed with a high nutrient density rather than merely adding an energy supplement such as carbohydrate and/or fat. In order for catch-up growth to occur, approximately 9% of the total energy should derive from protein, i.e. for every 100 kcal (419 kJ) there should be a minimum of 2.2 g of protein. Requirements for minerals, particularly sodium, are also increased, and feeds should provide a minimum of 0.8–1.0 mmol of sodium per 100 kcal (419 kJ).

Ready-to-feed, high nutrient density products have been designed to meet the requirements of the growing infant. They are recommended for infants from birth and can be used until normal weight and height are achieved or until the infant is ready to go onto a pediatric feed (age 1 year or weight 8–10 kg – see Appendix III.1). Ready-to-feed concentrated infant formulas are available in the USA as 24 kcal/oz formulas.

If ready-to-feed products are not available, a concentrated infant formula recipe can be used (Appendix III.7), though care should be taken to ensure that the milk powder is not concentrated further than is recommended in the recipe.

Infatrini   Nutricia

A 1 kcal/ml (4.2 kJ/ml) nutritionally complete feed based on skimmed milk powder and whey powder. Protein:energy ratio is 10.4%. The renal solute load is 280 mOsm/l. The fat source is derived from vegetable oils and the carbohydrate source is maltodextrin. Recommended for infants from birth to 12 months or up to 8 kg in body weight. Not suitable for infants who are intolerant to lactose and/or cow milk protein. Free from gluten. Recommended for tube or oral feeding.

SMA High Energy   SMA

A 0.91 kcal/ml (3.8 kJ/ml) nutritionally complete feed based on skimmed milk and whey. Protein:energy ratio is 8.8%. The renal solute load is 126 mOsm/l. The fat source is derived from vegetable oils and the carbohydrate source is lactose. Recommended for infants from birth to 18 months. Contains added nucleotides. Free from gluten. Suitable for tube or oral feeding.

Composition of high nutrient density feeds (per 100 ml product)

Product	Protein (g)	Fat (g)	Carbohydrate (g)	Energy (kcal)	(kJ)
Infatrini	2.6	5.4	10.4	100	419
SMA High Energy	2.0	4.9	9.8	91	382

Product	Na (mmol)	(mg)	K (mmol)	(mg)	Fe (μmol)	(mg)	Ca (mmol)	(mg)
Infatrini	1.00	23.0	2.60	101.4	13.39	0.75	2.00	80
SMA High Energy	0.95	22.0	2.25	88.0	19.64	1.10	1.42	57

III.7 HIGH NUTRIENT DENSITY FEEDS PREPARED FROM STANDARD FORMULAS

Recipe for 1000 ml	Protein	Fat	Carbohydrate	Energy		Sodium	
	(g)	(g)	(g)	(kcal)	(kJ)	(mmol)	(mg)
150 g powder, whey-based infant formula	17.2	44.0	81.0	770	3224	8.5	195.5
10 g glucose polymer/sugar	–	–	10.0	40	167	–	–
Water to make up to 1000 ml	–	–	–	–	–	–	–
Total per 100 ml	**1.7**	**4.4**	**9.1**	**81**	**339**	**0.85**	**19.55**

Renal solute load = 147 mOsm/l
Protein energy 8.4%

Recipe for 1000 ml	Protein	Fat	Carbohydrate	Energy		Sodium	
	(g)	(g)	(g)	(kcal)	(kJ)	(mmol)	(mg)
170 g powder, whey-based infant formula	19.5	50.0	92.0	870	3643	9.6	220.8
20 g glucose polymer/sugar*	–	–	20.0	80	335	–	–
Water to make up to 1000 ml	–	–	–	–	–	–	–
Total per 100 ml	**1.95**	**5.0**	**11.2**	**95**	**398**	**0.96**	**22.08**

*If additional carbohydrate is not tolerated, 20 ml of 50:50 oil:water emulsion or 10 ml of oil can be used instead.

Renal solute load = 166 mOsm/l
Protein energy 8.2%

III.8 HIGH-ENERGY AND HIGH-PROTEIN MILK DRINKS PREPARED FROM HOME INGREDIENTS

1.	20 g milk powder 180 ml full cream/whole milk **Provides 13 g protein and 190–215 kcal (795–900 kJ)***	Purée/blend together
2.	100 ml canned evaporated milk 100 ml full cream/whole milk 5 g sugar or glucose polymer **Provides 12 g protein and 245 kcal (1026 kJ)**	Stir together
3.	30 g ice cream 10 g milk powder 160 ml full cream/whole milk **Provides 10 g protein and 200 kcal (837 kJ)**	Stir together
4.	100 g natural yogurt 10 g sugar or glucose polymer 100 ml full cream/whole milk **Provides 9 g protein and 160 kcal (670 kJ)**	Stir together Or 100 g sweetened yogurt and omit sugar
5.	30 g thick (heavy/double) cream 170 ml full cream/whole milk **Provides 6 g protein and 245 kcal (1026 kJ)**	Stir together
6.	100 g soft canned fruit (e.g. peaches) 20 g milk powder 80 ml full cream/whole milk **Provides 10 g protein and 190–220 kcal (795–921 kJ)***	Purée/blend together

*Higher energy value using dried whole milk powder; lower value assumes skimmed milk powder.
All of the above recipes may be flavored with milkshake syrup or milkshake powder to taste.

III.9 HIGH-ENERGY AND HIGH-PROTEIN SOUPS

1.	30 g soft cooked meat 100–120 ml meat or vegetable soup **Provides approx. 8–10 g protein and 150–170 kcal (628–712 kJ)**	Purée/blend together
2.	20 g dried milk powder 100–120 ml vegetable soup **Provides approx. 8–10 g protein and 150–170 kcal (628–712 kJ)**	Purée/blend together
3.	80 g canned baked beans* 100–120 ml tomato soup **Provides approx. 6–7 g protein and 120–160 kcal (502–670 kJ)**	Purée/blend together
4.	40 g thick (heavy/double) cream 100–120 ml vegetable-type soup **Provides approx. 2–4 g protein and 240–260 kcal (1005–1089 kJ)**	Purée/blend together – do not boil after adding the cream

*Instead of baked beans, 80 g of the following cooked pulses/beans can be used: chickpeas, lentils, kidney beans or soybeans.

III.10 HIGH-ENERGY FRUIT DRINKS

These drinks all provide approximately 120 kcal (502 kJ) per 200 ml serving. A negligible amount of protein is provided by drinks 1–3.

1.	190 ml natural unsweetened fruit juice 10 g sugar or glucose polymer	Stir together
2.	100 g soft canned fruit (e.g. peaches) 10 g sugar or glucose polymer 90 ml water	Purée/blend together
3.	20 ml fruit-flavored squash or cordial drink* 25 g sugar or glucose polymer 160 ml water	Stir together
4.	40 g ice cream 150 ml cola or fizzy drink/soda **Provides 1.5 g protein**	Stir together just before drinking

*Alternatively a reconstituted powder fruit flavored drink could be used.

These drinks are not nutritionally complete and will need a micronutrient and iron supplement. The following can be used as a basis: formula milk, follow-up formula, whey/casein-based infant formula.

III.11 MAINTENANCE FEED (1 l) FOR CHILDREN WITH SEVERE PROTEIN–ENERGY MALNUTRITION

Dried skimmed milk (g)	Sugar (g)	Oil (g)
15	100	40

Mix with water to make up to 1 litre (1000 ml)
Provides 80 kcal (335 kJ) and 0.5 g protein per 100 ml

This feed contains insufficient protein and micronutrients to achieve growth. It should only be used for a few days until the child is able to tolerate a normal infant formula or a feed that is nutritionally complete.

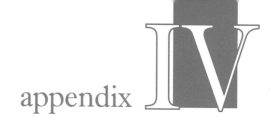

appendix IV

DIETS USED IN THE TREATMENT OF GASTROINTESTINAL AND ALLERGIC CONDITIONS AND DISORDERS OF FAT METABOLISM

IV.1 FORMULAS WITH A REDUCED LACTOSE CONTENT

Formulas with a reduced lactose content are based on cow milk and may be whey dominant or casein dominant. The fat source is either vegetable oils or a mixture of butterfat and vegetable oils, similar to standard infant formulas.

In most formulas, the lactose has been replaced with maltodextrin or glucose polymers, with a residual lactose content of <10 mg/100 ml. Galactomin 19 contains fructose as the carbohydrate source and is free of glucose.

They are complete formulas and supply adequate quantities of all nutrients when consumed in appropriate quantities. They are designed for use in alactasia due to gastroenteritis, gut surgery or certain drugs. Because of the small amount of residual lactose, they are generally not recommended for the treatment of galactosemia, where a soy-based formula is preferred.

Products marked with an asterisk (*) are not available in the USA.

AL110*   Nestlé

Casein-based, very-low-lactose formula. Whey-adapted (whey:casein ratio 60:40). Gluten free. Complete formula, no supplements recommended. Powder which requires reconstitution.

Enfamil Lactofree   Mead Johnson

Casein-dominant formula which is also lactose and sucrose free. Complete formula, no supplements recommended. Powder which requires reconstitution.

Galactomin 17*   SHS

Casein-based formula with minimal amounts of lactose and galactose. Complete formula, no supplements recommended. Powder which requires reconstitution.

Galactomin 19*   SHS

Casein-based formula with minimal amounts of lactose, galactose and glucose. The carbohydrate source is fructose. Complete formula, no supplements recommended. Powder which requires reconstitution.

Similac Lactose Free   Ross

The carbohydrate sources are corn syrup and sucrose. The fat sources are coconut and soy oils. Complete formula. Powder which requires reconstitution.

SMA LF*   SMA

Whey-dominant, clinically lactose free feed. Complete formula, no supplements recommended. Powder which requires reconstitution.

Check with manufacturers for preparation instructions.

IV.2 COMPOSITION OF LACTOSE-FREE AND LOW-LACTOSE MILKS (PER 100 ML NORMAL DILUTION)

Milk	Protein	Fat	CHO	Energy		Sodium		Potassium		Osmolality
	(g)	(g)	(g)	(kcal)	(kJ)	(mmol)	(mg)	(mmol)	(mg)	(mOsm/kg)
AL110*	1.7	3.3	7.5	67	281	1.00	23.00	2.00	78.00	170
Enfamil Lactofree	1.5	3.6	7.2	68	285	0.87	20.01	1.89	73.71	200
Galactomin 17*	1.9	3.4	7.2	67	281	1.20	27.60	2.50	97.50	210
Galactomin 19*	1.9	4.0	6.4	69	289	0.90	20.70	1.70	66.30	407
Similac Lactose Free	1.4	3.6	7.2	68	285	0.87	20.01	1.85	72.15	230
SMA LF*	1.5	3.6	7.2	67	281	0.70	16.00	1.79	70.00	198

*Not available in USA.
CHO = carbohydrate.

Check with manufacturers for full details of product.

IV.3 FORMULAS BASED ON SOY

Soy formulas adapted for use in infants have as their protein source soy isolate supplemented with L-methionine, L-carnitine and taurine. The fat content is mainly derived from vegetable oils. The carbohydrate is derived from starch, starch hydrolysates, maltodextrin and glucose polymer. Soy-based infant feeds are free of milk protein, lactose and gluten. They are fortified with a full range of micronutrients and minerals. Because of the presence of phytate, minerals and trace elements are less well absorbed from soy compared with milk-based formulas; the level of fortification in soy formulas is correspondingly higher to overcome this. Soy formulas contain natural phyto-estrogens, which have caused concerns because of their potential hormone-like actions. However, soy phyto-estrogens have been shown to have a low affinity for human estrogen receptors and a low potency. Because of the high risk of developing an allergy to soy proteins, they should only be used if clinically indicated. Infant soy formulas are not recommended for preterm infants weighing <1800 g.

Unmodified soy milks sold for general use are unsuitable for infants under the age of 1 year. They are likely to contain unmodified soy protein and may not include adequate minerals, particularly calcium.

Products marked with an asterisk (*) are not available in the USA.

Alsoy*   **Nestlé**
Nutritionally complete, soy-based formula. Powder which needs to be reconstituted. Also available in concentrated and ready-to-feed form in some markets.

Infasoy*   **Cow & Gate**
Nutritionally complete, soy-based formula. Powder which needs to be reconstituted.

Isomil   **Ross/Abbott**
Nutritionally complete, soy-based formula. Powder which needs to be reconstituted.

Isomil DF   **Ross/Abbott**
Nutritionally complete, soy-based formula. Concentrated liquid. Contains soy fiber.

Prosobee/Enfamil Prosobee   **Mead Johnson**
Nutritionally complete, soy-based formula. Powder which needs to be reconstituted.

Soya Formula*   **Farley's**
Nutritionally complete, soy-based formula. Powder which needs to be reconstituted.

Wysoy*   **SMA**
Nutritionally complete, soy-based formula. Powder which needs to be reconstituted.

Check with manufacturers for preparation instructions.

IV.4 COMPOSITION OF SOY MILKS (PER 100 ML NORMAL DILUTION)

Milk	Protein	Fat	CHO	Energy		Sodium		Potassium		Osmolality
	(g)	(g)	(g)	(kcal)	(kJ)	(mmol)	(mg)	(mmol)	(mg)	(mOsm/kg)
Alsoy	1.9	3.3	7.5	67	281	0.97	22.00	2.00	78.00	200
Infasoy*	1.8	3.6	6.7	66	276	0.78	17.94	1.66	64.74	200
Isomil	1.8	3.7	6.9	68	285	1.30	29.90	1.95	76.05	240
Isomil DF	1.7	3.7	6.8	68	285	1.30	29.90	1.87	72.93	240
Prosobee	2.0	3.6	6.6	68	285	1.06	24.38	2.07	80.73	180
Soya Formula*	1.1	3.8	7.0	70	293	1.08	24.84	1.92	74.88	122
Wysoy/Nursoy	1.8	3.6	6.9	67	280	0.83	19.00	1.85	72.00	189

*Not available in USA.
CHO = carbohydrate.

Check with manufacturers for full details of product.

IV.5 FORMULAS CONTAINING HYDROLYZED PROTEIN

Infant formulas based on protein hydrolysate fall broadly into two types: extensively hydrolyzed and partially hydrolyzed (hypoallergenic) formulas.

Formulas may be based on a number of protein sources – cow milk (whey or casein), soy or collagen derived from meat. The protein is subjected to hydrolysis by proteolytic enzymes, heat treatment and ultrafiltration, in order to reduce the whole protein to short-chain peptides. This reduces the number of epitopes present in the protein, but does not eliminate them entirely. Of the extensively hydrolyzed formulas, the ones based on casein tend to be the least allergenic. Whey-based formulas are likely to have a larger proportion of peptides greater than 6.0 kD, a size that is thought to be allergenic. Extensively hydrolyzed formulas are free of lactose; partially hydrolyzed fomulas do contain lactose. The extensively hydrolyzed preparations contain medium-chain triglycerides (MCTs), while the fat composition of the partial hydrolysates resembles that of normal milk.

Extensively hydrolyzed formulas are suitable for treatment of proven or suspected milk protein allergy. Partial hydrolysates should not be used as a form of treatment. They are designed for use in infants thought to be at risk of developing food allergy, although their effectiveness in prevention is still a subject of controversy.

All formulas meet guidelines for nutritional composition and, unless otherwise indicated, are suitable as complete feeds for infants.

Products marked with an asterisk (*) are not available in the USA.

Hydrolyzed-protein formulas for use in infants and young children

Extensive hydrolysates

Alfaré*   **Nestlé**
Nutritionally complete formula based on milk (whey) protein. The fat component is derived from MCTs and vegetable oils. Contains 50% MCT and 50% long-chain triglyceride (LCT). The carbohydrate source is maltodextrin. Powder which requires reconstitution.

Alimentum   **Ross**
Nutritionally complete formula based on casein. The fat component is 50% MCT and 50% vegetable oils. The carbohydrate sources are sucrose and modified tapioca starch.

Pepdite 0–2*   **SHS**
Nutritionally complete formula based on non-milk (soy and meat) protein. The fat component is mainly coconut fat, peanut oil and animal fat. Contains 2.6% MCT and 97.4% LCT. The carbohydrate source is dried glucose syrup. Powder which requires reconstitution.

MCT Pepdite 0–2*   **SHS**

Nutritionally complete formula based on non-milk (soy and meat) protein. Contains 83% MCT and 17% LCT. The carbohydrate source is dried glucose syrup. Powder which requires reconstitution.

It is recommended that MCT Pepdite 0–2 be supplemented with walnut oil in the range of 1–5 ml per 100 g powdered product to achieve the recommended minimum intake for linolenic acid.

Pepdite 1+   **SHS**

Nutritionally complete semi-elemental formula with 44% free amino acids and 56% peptides. Contains 35% MCT and 65% LCT. Carbohydrate source is corn syrup. Powder which requires reconstitution.

Pepdite 2+*   **SHS**

Nutritionally complete formula based on non-milk (soy and meat) protein. Contains 35% MCT and 65% LCT. The carbohydrate source is dried glucose syrup. For use in children over 2 years of age. Powder which requires reconstitution.

MCT Pepdite 2+*   **SHS**

Nutritionally complete formula based on non-milk (soy and meat) protein. Contains 83% MCT and 17% LCT. The carbohydrate source is dried glucose syrup. For use in children over 2 years of age. Powder which requires reconstitution.

It is recommended that MCT Pepdite 2+ be supplemented with walnut oil in the range of 1–5 ml per 100 g powdered product to achieve the recommended minimum intake for linolenic acid.

Nutramigen   **Mead Johnson**

Milk protein (casein) based nutritionally complete formula. The fat source is palm olein, coconut oil, soy oil and sunflower oil. Contains 2.9% MCT and 97.1% LCT. The carbohydrate source is glucose syrup. Available as ready-to-feed product or as powder requiring reconstitution.

Pepti-Junior*   **Cow & Gate**

Milk protein (whey) based nutritionally complete formula. The fat source is MCT oil and corn oil. Contains 50% MCT and 50% LCT. The carbohydrate source is glucose syrup. Powder which requires reconstitution.

Pregestimil   **Mead Johnson**

Milk protein (casein) based nutritionally complete formula. The fat source is MCT oil, corn oil, soy oil and safflower oil. Contains 55% MCT and 45% LCT. The carbohydrate source is glucose syrup. Available as ready-to-feed product or as powder requiring reconstitution.

Prejomin*   **Milupa**

Nutritionally complete formula based on non-milk (soy and porcine collagen) protein. The fat source is vegetable fat. Contains 6% MCT and 94% LCT. The carbohydrate source is maltodextrin. Powder which requires reconstitution.

Partial hydrolysates

Aptamil 1 HA*   **Milupa**

Nutritionally complete formula based on whole milk. The fat source is vegetable oils and egg. The carbohydrate source is lactose and maltodextrin. Available as ready-to-feed product and as powder which requires reconstitution.

Carnation Good Start   **Nestlé**

Nutritionally complete formula based on whey protein. The fat source is coconut and vegetable oils. The carbohydrate source is lactose and maltodextrin. Powder which requires reconstitution. Also available in concentrated and ready-to-feed form in some markets.

Nan HA*   **Nestlé**

Nutritionally complete formula based on whey hydrolysate. The fat source is coconut and vegetable oils. The carbohydrate source is lactose and maltodextrin. Available as ready-to-feed product and as powder which requires reconstitution.

Hydrolysates for use in older children

Peptamen Junior   **Nestlé**

Isotonic, nutritionally complete formula based on whey hydrolysate. The fat source is derived from vegetable oils and MCTs. The carbohydrate source is maltodextrin and cornstarch. Used for oral or tube feeding.

Check with manufacturers for preparation instructions.

IV.6 COMPOSITION OF HYDROLYZED MILKS

Composition of extensively hydrolyzed protein formulas (per 100 ml normal dilution)

| Milk | Protein | Fat | Fatty acid distribution % total fatty acids | | CHO | Energy | |
	(g)	(g)	Total MCFA	Total LCFA	(g)	(kcal)	(kJ)
Alfaré*	2.20	3.2	50.0	50.0	7.0	65	272
Alimentum	1.90	3.8	50.0	50.0	6.9	67	281
Pepdite 0-2*	2.07	3.4	2.6	97.4	7.8	71	297
MCT Pepdite 0-2*	2.07	2.7	83.0	17.0	8.8	68	286
Pepdite 1+	3.10	5.0	35.0	65.0	10.6	100	420
Pepdite 2+*	2.76	3.5	35.0	65.0	11.4	89	373
MCT Pepdite 2+*	2.76	3.6	83.0	17.0	11.8	91	381
Nutramigen	1.90	3.4	2.9	97.1	7.4	68	285
Peptamen Junior	3.00	3.8	60.0	40.0	13.8	100	445
Pepti Junior*	1.78	3.6	50.0	50.0	6.6	66	276
Pregestimil	1.90	3.8	55.0	45.0	6.9	68	285
Prejomin*	2.00	3.6	6.0	94.0	8.6	75	314

| Milk | Sodium | | Potassium | | Osmolality |
	(mmol)	(mg)	(mmol)	(mg)	(mOsm/kg)
Alfaré*	1.70	39.10	2.08	81.12	220
Alimentum	1.30	29.90	2.05	79.95	370
Pepdite 0-2*	1.50	34.50	1.47	57.33	224
MCT Pepdite 0-2*	1.50	34.50	1.40	54.60	277
Pepdite 1+	1.80	41.40	3.40	132.60	430
Pepdite 2+*	1.82	41.86	2.64	102.96	319
MCT Pepdite 2+*	1.82	41.86	2.64	102.96	335
Nutramigen	1.39	31.97	1.89	73.71	290
Peptamen Junior	2.00	46.00	3.38	132.00	260
Pepti Junior*	0.90	20.70	1.70	66.30	210
Pregestimil	1.39	31.97	1.89	73.71	330
Prejomin*	0.17	3.91	2.35	91.65	220–230

*Not available in USA.
CHO = carbohydrate

Composition of partially hydrolyzed protein formulas (per 100 ml normal dilution)

Milk	Protein	Fat	CHO	Energy	
	(g)	**(g)**	**(g)**	**(kcal)**	**(kJ)**
Aptamil 1 HA*	1.60	3.60	7.20	67	281
Good Start	1.50	3.50	7.60	68	284
Nan HA*	1.51	3.41	7.56	67	281

Milk	Sodium		Potassium		Osmolality
	(mmol)	**(mg)**	**(mmol)**	**(mg)**	**(mOsm/kg)**
Aptamil 1 HA*	1.30	29.9	2.10	81.90	305
Good Start	0.70	16.1	1.68	65.52	265
Nan HA*	0.70	16.1	1.69	65.91	275

*Not available in USA.
CHO = carbohydrate.

IV.7 FORMULAS CONTAINING MEDIUM-CHAIN TRIGLYCERIDES

Medium-chain triglycerides (MCTs) are oils containing fatty acids with a chain length of C_8–C_{12}. The energy value of MCTs is 8.3 kcal/g (34.8 kJ/g) [cf. 9 kcal/g (37.7 kJ/g) for other triglycerides]. Fatty acids with these chain lengths normally constitute approximately 1% of naturally occurring fats. Commercially, MCT is derived from coconut oil. Because of their particle size, MCTs are more easily hydrolyzed than other triglycerides and, once absorbed, enter directly into the bloodstream via the hepatic portal vein, thus providing a rapidly utilizable source of energy even in conditions where there is impairment of fat digestion and absorption.

MCTs exert a higher osmotic pressure than other triglycerides; hence, care must be taken not to introduce MCTs too rapidly into the diet, as abdominal cramps, nausea and diarrhea may result.

Two types of formula are available that contain whole milk protein and that have had a proportion of the long-chain triglycerides (LCTs) replaced by MCTs. Caprilon and Portagen are designed for infants with malabsorption and are approximately 75–80% MCTs and 20–25% LCTs. Monogen has a lower LCT content and is mainly intended for use in infants with inborn errors of fat metabolism or infants with a severe intolerance to LCT (e.g. in chylothorax).

Both types of feeds are suitable for use from birth and are fortified with appropriate minerals, vitamins and trace elements. All products are free of both gluten and lactose.

Products marked with an asterisk (*) are not available in the USA.

Caprilon* SHS
Whey-dominant, nutritionally complete formula. The fat source is 75% MCT with 23% soy oil. The carbohydrate source is glucose syrup.

Monogen* SHS
Nutritionally complete, low-fat, whole-protein powdered supplement. The fat source is coconut oil and walnut oil. Contains 93% MCT. The carbohydrate source is glucose syrup.

Portagen Mead Johnson
Nutritionally complete, casein-based formula. The fat source is 86% MCT and 24% corn oil. The carbohydrate source is corn syrup and sucrose.

IV.8 COMPOSITION (PER 100 ML NORMAL DILUTION) OF FORMULAS CONTAINING MEDIUM-CHAIN TRIGLYCERIDES

	Protein	Fat	LCTs	MCTs	CHO	Energy	
	(g)	(g)	(g)	(g)	(g)	(kcal)	(kJ)
Caprilon*	1.50	3.6	0.90 (25%)	2.70 (75%)	7.0	66	276
Monogen*	2.00	2.0	0.14 (7%)	1.86 (93%)	12.0	74	310
Portagen	2.40	3.2	0.45 (14%)	2.75 (86%)	7.8	68	285

	Sodium		Potassium		Osmolarity
	(mmol/l)	(mg/l)	(mmol/l)	(mg/l)	(mOsm/kg)
Caprilon*	0.8	18	1.70	66	233
Monogen*	1.5	35	1.50	59	280
Portagen	1.6	37	2.12	83	230

*Not available in USA.
LCTs = long-chain triglycerides; MCTs = medium-chain triglycerides; CHO = carbohydrate.

IV.9 USES OF MEDIUM-CHAIN TRIGLYCERIDES

Medium-chain triglyceride (MCT) preparations are available as oils and water-miscible emulsions (Appendix IV.16) and with the MCTs incorporated into milk formulas (Appendices IV.7 and IV.8). For older children, foods containing a small amount of MCT should be given initially, and the portion size or MCT quantity built up over a period of days. Tolerance to the high osmolality develops with time.

For older children and adults, MCT oil can be used for cooking in a similar way to other edible oils. It can be used for frying to add variety and energy to the diet, although the technique of cooking with MCTs is slightly different to that when using other oils. It has a low smoke point compared with other oils used for cooking, and care must be taken that it does not burn. The optimal cooking temperature for MCTs is 160°C, compared with 210°C for corn oil.

Foods need to be cooked for a few minutes longer than normal because of the lower temperature used. If MCTs are heated above 20°C, they develop a bitter taste and an unpleasant odor and hence should be discarded.

As a consequence of the lower cooking temperature, the color of items such as fried potato is paler than that of foods cooked in other oils. Users should be warned not to cook for too long in the hope of achieving a more intense color, as foods will become dry and hard in texture. Fat-containing foods such as bacon or meat can be fried using MCTs, but because these foods will leak long-chain triglycerides into the MCTs, the oil should be discarded after use. It can be re-used once or twice if it has been used for fat-free items such as potato or bread. MCTs can also be used to make cakes, cookies and pastry by following recipes that use oils, such as corn oil, in place of solid fats.

IV.10 MINIMAL-FAT REGIMENS

If a minimal-fat (LCT) complete feed such as Monogen is not available, a modular regimen can be used (see Appendix IV.12). A whey-based module is preferable, but, if unavailable, one based on skimmed milk can be used. However, such products contain extremely high levels of sodium and may be unsuitable for young infants. Care should be taken to ensure that excess sodium, potassium, calcium and phosphorus are not included and a full nutritional breakdown of the protein module should be examined before a micronutrient supplement is prescribed. If the amount of long-chain fat in the feed is less than 1.0 g/100 ml, it is unlikely that sufficient essential fatty acids will be provided and a supplement of walnut oil should be considered.

Walnut oil provides the most plentiful supply of linoleic and α-linolenic acids in an appropriate ratio for human requirements. It is recommended that 1% of total energy should be provided as linoleic acid and 0.2% as α-linolenic acid. Walnut oil contains 61 g of linoleic acid and 12 g of α-linolenic acid per 100 g of fat. In a feed that contains inadequate quantities of essential fatty acids, 0.2 ml of walnut oil should be added for each 100 kcal. For example, for a feed with an energy density of 76 kcal/100 ml (see Appendix IV.12), 0.16 ml of oil should be added to each 100 ml of feed. If each bottle or feed container has a volume of 200 ml, 0.32 ml of oil should be added to each. The receptacle should be shaken several times during the feed to ensure dispersal.

Since 50% of dietary energy in a normal infant formula is derived from fat, minimal-fat feeds are low in energy unless very high concentrations of carbohydrate are added or MCT is used.

IV.11 MINIMAL-FAT FEED FOR INFANTS

Component	Quantity	Protein (g)	Fat (g)	CHO (g)	Energy (kcal)	Energy (kJ)
Maxipro*/Casec or Propac	3 g/3.2 g	2.4	0.2	Trace	12	50
Glucose polymer	12 g	–	–	12.0	48	201
Walnut oil	0.12 ml	–	0.1	–	1	4
Sodium chloride solution	–	–	–	–	–	–
Potassium chloride solution	–	–	–	–	–	–
Paediatric Seravit*/ Phlexy vits	1 g	–	–	–	–	–
Water	To make up to 100 ml	–	–	–	–	–
Total	**100 ml**	**2.4**	**0.3**	**12.0**	**61**	**255**

Component	Sodium (mmol)	Sodium (mg)	Potassium (mmol)	Potassium (mg)	Calcium (mmol)	Calcium (mg)
Maxipro*/Casec or Propac	0.17	3.9	Trace	Trace	0.38	15
Glucose polymer	–	–	–	–	–	–
Walnut oil	–	–	–	–	–	–
Sodium chloride solution	2.00	46.0	–	–	–	–
Potassium chloride solution	–	–	2.0	78.0	–	–
Paediatric Seravit*/ Phlexy vits	–	–	–	–	0.65	26
Water	–	–	–	–	–	–
Total	**2.17**	**49.9**	**2.0**	**78.0**	**1.03**	**41**

*Not available in USA.
CHO = carbohydrate

IV.12 MINIMAL-FAT FEED WITH ADDED MEDIUM-CHAIN TRIGLYCERIDES

Component	Quantity	Protein	Fat	CHO	Energy	
		(g)	(g)	(g)	(kcal)	(kJ)
Maxipro*/Casec or propac	3 g/3.2 g	2.4	0.20	Trace	12	50
Glucose polymer	10 g	–	–	10.0	40	167
Walnut oil	0.16 ml	–	0.16	–	1	4
MCT oil or Liquigen	3ml or 6 ml	–	3.00	–	24	100
Sodium chloride solution	–	–	–	–	–	–
Potassium chloride solution	–	–	–	–	–	–
Paediatric Seravit*/Phlexy vits	1 g	–	–	–	–	–
Water	To make up to 100 ml	–	–	–	–	–
Total	**100 ml**	**2.4**	**3.36**	**10.0**	**77**	**321**

Component	Sodium		Potassium		Calcium	
	(mmol)	(mg)	(mmol)	(mg)	(mmol)	(mg)
Maxipro*/Casec or propac	0.17	3.9	Trace	Trace	0.38	15
Glucose polymer	–	–	–	–	–	–
Walnut oil	–	–	–	–	–	–
MCT oil or Liquigen	–	–	–	–	–	–
Sodium chloride solution	2.0	46.0	–	–	–	–
Potassium chloride solution	–	–	2.0	78	–	–
Paediatric Seravit*/Phlexy vits	–	–	–	–	0.65	26
Water	–	–	–	–	–	–
Total	**2.17**	**49.9**	**2.0**	**78**	**1.03**	**41**

*Not available in USA.
CHO = carbohydrate; MCT = medium-chain triglyceride

IV.13 Low-fat milk drinks with medium-chain triglycerides for older children

Moderate protein

	Protein	Fat	Energy		Sodium	
	(g)	(g)	(kcal)	(kJ)	(mmol)	(mg)
30 ml cow milk or 15 ml evaporated milk or 4 g dried whole milk powder	1.0	1.1 (LCT)	20	84	0.6	13.8
6 g skimmed milk powder	2.1	Trace	20	84	1.5	34.5
8 ml Liquigen** (p. 417) or 4 ml MCT oil	–	4.0 (MCT)	33*	138*	Trace	Trace
8 g glucose polymer or sugar or milkshake flavoring	–	–	32	134	Trace	Trace
Water to make up to 100 ml	–	–	–	–	–	–
Total	**3.1**	**5.1**	**105**	**440**	**2.1**	**48.3**

*MCT energy value = 8.3 kcal/g (35 kJ/g)
**Not available in USA
LCT = long-chain triglyceride; MCT = medium-chain triglyceride

High protein

	Protein	Fat	Energy		Sodium	
	(g)	(g)	(kcal)	(kJ)	(mmol)	(mg)
30 ml cow milk or 15 ml evaporated milk or 4 g dried whole milk powder	1.0	1.1 (LCT)	20	84	0.6	13.8
15 g skimmed milk powder	5.2	Trace	49	205	3.9	89.7
8 ml Liquigen** (p. 417) or 4 ml MCT oil	–	4.0 (MCT)	33*	138*	Trace	Trace
4 g glucose polymer or sugar or milkshake flavoring	–	–	16	67	Trace	Trace
Water to make up to 100 ml	–	–	–	–	–	–
Total	**6.2**	**5.1**	**118**	**494**	**4.5**	**103.5**

*MCT energy value = 8.3 kcal/g (35 kJ/g)
**Not available in USA.
LCT = long-chain triglyceride; MCT = medium-chain triglyceride

Low sodium
To reduce the sodium content of either of these recipes, substitute a modular protein with a low electrolyte content, such as Maxipro HBV, Promod, Casec or Propac (p. 418).

IV.14 MODULAR FEEDING PREPARATIONS

Despite the large numbers of specialized formulas that are available, there are many occasions when no preparation appears to be exactly suitable or when the preparation is not available.

In these cases it is possible to formulate a recipe using modules that supply one or more of the major nutrients: a feed can be 'tailored' to match an individual's requirements and idiosyncrasies. However, the formulation and preparation of modular feeds require a great deal of time and expertise, so it is wise to try a number of the large range of complete feeds available in the first instance.

Most of the complete specialized formulas available on the market adhere to the World Health Organisation (WHO) recommendations for a complete baby milk for all nutrients. An adequate volume of the full-strength recipe of any of these products will contain sufficient vitamins, minerals and trace elements. There is no such safeguard when individual modules are used. Some formulations will contain no added micronutrients; others, designed primarily for use in adults, will contain a balance of vitamins and minerals that is unsuitable for the young child. Care must be taken to ensure that minimum recommendations for all nutrients (Appendix I) are met.

Protein

Protein modules may consist of whole unmodified protein such as milk or meat protein, or they may be reduced in allergenicity by hydrolysis; alternatively, a mixture of essential and non-essential amino acids may provide the nitrogen source.

For infants and children who require a modular feed because of malabsorption it is unlikely that feeds based on unmodified whole or skimmed milk will be tolerated. The feed based on whole meat, comminuted chicken (not available in USA) does appear to be well tolerated and has the advantage of a low osmolality.

It is important when devising a modular feed that excess protein is not given. With protein intakes over 6.0 g per kilogram of actual body weight, it is essential to check blood urea nitrogen values once or twice weekly to avoid uremia.

Carbohydrate

Carbohydrate modules can consist of monosaccharides such as glucose or fructose, which require no hydrolysis by digestive enzymes. Glucose absorption is by a sodium-dependent carrier process and is optimized if there is a small quantity (10.0 mmol/l) of sodium chloride in the solution. Fructose absorption is not sodium dependent, but care should be taken when using fructose as the sole carbohydrate source as it can provoke a lactic acidosis. The disadvantage of using monosaccharides is that they have a higher osmolality than disaccharides or oligosaccharides (see Table below). If monosaccharides are used, an equal mixture of glucose and fructose is better tolerated than just one carbohydrate.

A disaccharide such as sucrose, lactose or dextrose has a lower osmolality than glucose or fructose, but, in malabsorptive states where luminal disaccharidases are likely to be impaired, they are unlikely to be well tolerated.

Most carbohydrate modules are oligosaccharides based on hydrolyzed starch or corn syrup. The osmolality of the products depends upon the length of the glucose polymers, which in turn depends upon the source of the starting material, but in general they have a considerably lower osmolality than mono- or disaccharides (see Table below). Although they do not require digestion by intraluminal enzymes, they do require hydrolysis before they can be transported across the gut mucosal cell. In severe malabsorption, particularly where glucose is a problem, glucose polymers may not be tolerated.

Where it is not possible to achieve a carbohydrate concentration of 5 g/100 ml enteral feed in very small infants (<5 kg) or 3 g/100 ml enteral feed in older infants and children, it is important that intravenous glucose is continued in order to prevent hypoglycemia.

Osmotic effects of carbohydrates

Number of glucose units	20–2500	10–20	5–10
Carbohydrate	Starch	Dextrin	Maltodextrin
	Polysaccharides	Polysaccharides	Polysaccharides
			Oligosaccharides
		Glucose polymers	Glucose polymers
Grams of carbohydrate per 100 ml which has osmolality of 250 mosmol (iso-osmolar)	Insoluble	24 g	24 g
Number of glucose units	1–10	3–5	1–2
Carbohydrate	Liquid glucose	Corn syrup	Sugar, mono- and disaccharides
	Oligosaccharides	Oligosaccharides	
	Glucose polymers	Glucose polymers	
Grams of carbohydrate per 100 ml which has osmolality of 250 mosmol (iso-osmolar)	10 g	7.5 g	5 g

Lipid

Products such as canola or corn oil, or other locally available oils, can be used as a source of fat to add to a modular regimen. The disadvantage of using oils is that they are not water miscible and will separate to form a layer on top of the feed. The feeding container needs to be shaken vigorously several times during the course of a feed in order to disperse this oil layer. In addition, oil will adhere to the internal surface of the feeding container and will result in a lower nutrient density of feed.

Commercially available lipid modules have been emulsified so that they are water miscible. Lipid emulsions usually consist of either long-chain fats derived from vegetable oils or medium-chain fats mainly derived from coconut oil. They comprise a 50% oil/water emulsion, so that each 100 ml of product contains 50 g of lipid.

Some preparations, particularly if high in medium-chain triglycerides, contain no linoleic acid and will not meet requirements for essential fatty acids. If there is no intravenous source of essential fatty acids then an additional quantity of walnut oil will provide such in a small quantity of lipid.

Products marked with an asterisk (*) are not available in the USA.

Protein modules

Derived from whole milk protein

Casec Powder   **Mead Johnson**

Calcium caseinate with no added vitamins or minerals. High calcium and low sodium content.

Casilan 90*   **Heinz**

Calcium caseinate with no added vitamins or minerals. High calcium and minimal sodium content.

Maxipro   **SHS**

Whey protein supplemented with amino acids. No added vitamins or minerals. Low calcium and sodium content.

Promod   **Abbott**

Whey protein with soy lecithin. No added vitamins or minerals.

Protifar*   **Nutricia**

Casein-based skimmed milk concentrate. Very low lactose and low fat content. No added vitamins or minerals.

ProViMin   **Ross**

Casein based with added vitamins and minerals.

Skimmed milk powder

Not designed as a module for infants. No added vitamins or minerals – high in calcium, phosphate, sodium and potassium.

Vitapro*   **Vitaflo**

Based on whey protein. Free from gluten and sucrose. No added vitamins and minerals.

Hydrolyzed protein

Pepdite Module (code 767)   **SHS**

Based on non-milk protein (soy and pork) and supplemented with amino acids. No added vitamins or minerals apart from sodium and potassium.

Meat-based products

Comminuted chicken*   **Cow & Gate**

Liquidized ground chicken meat in water. Contains some fat but no carbohydrate. No added vitamins or minerals.

Amino acids

Complete Amino Acid Mixture (code 124)   **SHS**

Powdered mixture of essential and non-essential amino acids. No added vitamins or minerals.

Lipid modules

Calogen*

SHS

Water miscible source of fat in the form of LCT emulsion from peanut oil. Can be taken undiluted, or diluted with either milk or water. Available as unflavored or strawberry flavor.

Corn oil/sunflower oil/safflower oil/canola oil

Mainly long-chain unsaturated fatty acids that contain linoleic and oleic acids. If included in quantities greater than 5 g daily, should provide adequate essential fatty acids. These are oils that are not emulsified.

Liquigen*

SHS

Water miscible source of fat in the form of MCT emulsion. Should be taken diluted. Easily flavored, e.g. with milkshake syrups.

MCT Oil

Mead Johnson

Mainly medium-chain saturated fatty acids. Does not contain essential fatty acids and is not emulsified.

Microlipid

Sherwood Medical

50% oil/water emulsion of safflower oil. Water miscible. Contains linoleic acid and should provide adequate quantities of essential fatty acids if 5 g/day are included.

Modules containing more than one nutrient

Protein & fat

Pro-Cal*

Vitaflo

Based on skimmed milk powder. The fat source is derived from vegetable oils and carbohydrates are derived from lactose.

Product 3232A

Mead Johnson

Monosaccharide- and disaccharide-free powder which is a casein-based hydrolysate. The fat source is derived from MCTs and LCTs. The carbohydrate source is modified tapioca starch. This is a complete feed apart from carbohydrate.

Ross Carbohydrate Free (RCF) Concentrated Liquid

Abbott

Soy protein isolate which contains long-chain vegetable fats and a trace of carbohydrate. Free from lactose. A complete feed apart from carbohydrate. Manufacturers advise the addition of an iron supplement.

Protein & carbohydrate

Protifar Powder*

Nutricia

Casein-based milk powder. The carbohydrate source is lactose. No added vitamins or minerals.

Fat & carbohydrate

Product 80056 Powder   **Mead Johnson**

Protein-free powder. Contains glucose polymers and modified tapioca starch. The fat source is corn oil. Vitamins and minerals are added. Manufacturers advise adequate protein, sodium, potassium and chloride must also be supplied.

Duocal   **SHS**

Protein-free powder. The carbohydrate source is hydrolyzed starch. The fat source is derived from vegetable oils. 35% of the total lipid content is in the form of MCTs. No added vitamins, minerals or trace elements.

Also available – Duocal liquid and Duobar.

Quickcal*   **Vitaflo**

Based on hydrogenated vegetable oil and lactose. No added vitamins or minerals.

Pro-Phree   **Abbott**

Protein-free powder. The carbohydrate source is hydrolyzed starch. The fat source is derived from vegetable oils. Vitamins and minerals are added.

IV.15 COMPOSITION OF PROTEIN MODULES (PER 100 g POWDER)

Product	Protein	Fat	CHO	Energy	
	(g)	(g)	(g)	(kcal)	(kJ)
Casec	88.0	2.0	–	370	1549
Casilan*	90.0	2.0	Trace	383	1604
Complete Amino Acid Mixture code 124	82.0	–	–	328	1373
Maxipro	80.0	6.0	<5.0	394	1650
Pepdite Module (code 767)	86.0	–	–	346	1449
Promod	75.0	6.9	7.5	392	1658
Protifar*	88.5	1.0	0.5	370	1549
ProViMin	73.0	1.4	2.0	313	1310
Skimmed milk powder	37.0	1.3	53.0	355	1486
Vitapro*	75.0	6.0	9.0	388	1624
Meat based					
Comminuted chicken*	7.0–8.0	2.5–3.5	–	51–64	214–268

Product	Sodium		Calcium		Supplementation
	(mmol)	(mg)	(mmol)	(mg)	
Casec	5.16	118.7	40.00	1600	Full supplementation required except calcium
Casilan*	0.30	6.9	30.00	1200	As for Casec
Complete Amino Acid Mixture code 124	–	–	–	–	Full supplementation required
Maxipro	5.60	129.0	12.50	500	Full supplementation required
Pepdite Module (code 767)	–	–	–	–	As for Casec
Promod	7.83	180.0	10.55	422	Full supplementation required
Protifar*	1.30	30.0	33.75	1350	As for Casec
ProViMin	5.20	120.0	60.00	2400	No
Skimmed milk powder	23.90	552.0	29.75	1190	Full vitamin supplementation and iron required
Vitapro*	10.00	230.0	10.00	400	As for Casec
Meat based					
Comminuted chicken*	0.40	9.2	0.23	9	Full supplementation required

*Not available in the USA.
CHO = carbohydrate

IV.16 COMPOSITION OF TWO-NUTRIENT MODULES (PER 100 g POWDER OR PER 100 ml LIQUID CONCENTRATE)

Product	Protein	Fat			CHO	Energy	
		Total	LCTs	MCTs			
	(g)	(g)	(g)	(g)	(g)	(kcal)	(kJ)
80056	–	22.5	22.5	-	72.0	490	2052
3232A	22.0	33.0	15.0	18.0	33.0	500	2093
Duocal	–	22.3	14.8	7.5	72.7	492	2060
Quickcal*	4.6	77.0	77.0	–	17.0	780	3266
Pro-Cal*	13.5	56.2	56.2	–	26.8	667	2793
Protifar*	88.5	1.0	–	–	0.5	377	1578
Ross Carbohydrate Free (RCF)	4.0	7.2	7.2	–	0.1	81	339

Product	Sodium		Calcium		Supplementation
	(mmol)	(mg)	(mmol)	(mg)	
80056	3.1	73	13.50	540	Requires sodium
3232A	15.6	359	17.98	719	Not required
Duocal	1.2	28	0.75	30	Requires full supplementation
Quickcal*	4.3	99	<0.006	<0.25	Requires full supplementation
Pro-Cal*	10.7	246	9.00	360	Requires full supplementation
Protifar*	1.3	30	33.75	1350	Requires full supplementation except calcium
Ross Carbohydrate Free (RCF)	2.6	60	3.50	140	Requires iron

*Not available in the USA.
CHO = carbohydrate.
LCT = long-chain triglyceride.
MCT = medium-chain triglyceride.

IV.17 COMPOSITION OF NON-PROTEIN MODULES

Product (manufacturer)	Form	Fat (g)	Carbohydrate (g)	Energy (kcal)	(kJ)	Sodium (mmol)	(mg)
Carbohydrate per 100 g powder							
Caloreen* (Nestlé)	Hydrolyzed cornstarch	–	96	400	1675	<1.8	<41.4
Glucose	Glucose	–	100	400	1675	<1.0	<23.0
Fructose	Fructose	–	100	400	1675	<1.0	<23.0
Maxijul* (SHS)	Maltodextrin	–	95	380	1591	<0.86	<19.78
Moducal (Mead Johnson)	Hydrolyzed cornstarch	–	100	376	1574	3.0	69.0
Polycal* (Nutricia)	Glucose polymer	–	96	380	1501	<0.3	6.9
Polycose (Abbott)	Glucose polymers	–	94	376	1598	4.78	109.94
Vitajoule* (Vitaflo)	Maltodextrin	–	96	380	1591	<1.9	<43.7
Fat per 100 ml liquid							
Alembicol D* (Alembic)	MCT	100	–	908	3802	Trace	Trace
Calogen* (SHS)	LCT arachis oil emulsion	50	–	450	1884	0.9	20.7
Liquigen* (SHS)	MCT emulsion	52	–	407	1704	1.7	39.1
Microlipid (Sherwood Medical)	Safflower oil emulsion	50	–	450	1884	Trace	Trace
Vegetable oils	e.g. safflower, corn, walnut oils	100	–	900	3768	–	–

*Not available in USA.
LCT = long-chain triglyceride.
MCT = medium-chain triglyceride.

IV.18 FULL-STRENGTH MODULAR FEED USING MEAT PROTEIN

Feed	Quantity	Protein (g)	Fat (g)	CHO (g)	Energy (kcal)	Energy (kJ)
Comminuted chicken*	30 g	2.3	0.1	–	18	75
Calogen*	6 ml	–	3.0	–	27	113
Moducal	7 g	–	–	7.0	28	117
Metabolic Mineral Mixture*	1 g (max. 8 g daily)	–	–	–	–	–
Water	To make up to 100 ml	–	–	–	–	–
Total	**100 ml**	**2.3**	**3.1**	**7.0**	**73**	**305**

Feed	Sodium (mmol)	Sodium (mg)	Potassium (mmol)	Potassium (mg)	Calcium (mmol)	Calcium (mg)	Iron (mmol)	Iron (mg)
Comminuted chicken*	Trace	Trace	Trace	Trace	–	–	–	–
Calogen*	–	–	–	–	–	–	–	–
Moducal	–	–	–	–	–	–	–	–
Metabolic Mineral Mixture*	1.7	39.1	2.1	81.9	2.05	82	0.01	0.69
Water	–	–	–	–	–	–	–	–
Total	**1.7**	**39.1**	**2.1**	**81.9**	**2.05**	**82**	**0.01**	**0.69**

* Not available in USA.
CHO = carbohydrate

Plus: 3 Ketovite tablets and 5 ml Ketovite Liquid* daily (to provide vitamins).

IV.19 HIGH-ENERGY MODULAR FEED

Many infants will not thrive unless they receive an energy intake approaching 140 kcal (586 kJ) per kilogram actual body weight. Feeds that supply more than 1.0 kcal/ml (4.2 kJ/ml) are not well tolerated, so a generous fluid intake of 150–200 ml/kg may be required.

Feed	Quantity	Protein (g)	Fat (g)	CHO (g)
Comminuted chicken*	40 g	3.0	0.13	–
Calogen*	8 ml	–	4.00	–
Moducal	10 g	–	–	10.0
Metabolic Mineral Mixture*	1 g	–	–	–
Water	To make up to 100 ml	–	–	–
Total	**100 ml**	**3.0**	**4.13**	**10.0**

Feed	Energy (kcal)	(kJ)	Sodium (mmol)	(mg)	Potassium (mmol)	(mg)
Comminuted chicken*	24	100	Trace	Trace	Trace	Trace
Calogen*	36	151	–	–	–	–
Moducal	40	167	–	–	–	–
Metabolic Mineral Mixture*	–	–	1.7	39.1	2.1	81.9
Water	–	–	–	–	–	–
Total	**100**	**418**	**1.7**	**39.1**	**2.1**	**81.9**

*Not available in USA.
CHO = carbohydrate

Plus: 3 Ketovite tablets & 5 ml Ketovite Liquid* daily (to provide vitamins).

IV.20 ELEMENTAL OR CHEMICALLY DEFINED FORMULAS

This type of formula is designed to bypass the normal digestive processes, as it is said to be 'predigested'. The use of elemental feeds should be considered as a safer alternative to intravenous nutrition wherever bowel sounds are present but gut function is likely to be poor. Because there is no intact protein, these formulae are hypoallergenic and can also be used if there is intolerance to milk and other protein or as the basis for an elimination diet for food allergy (see Chapter 17 and Appendix IV.39).

The protein consists of short-chain peptides or free amino acids that require little or no hydrolysis by intestinal peptidases. Preparations containing peptides are considered to have advantages over amino acid preparations because they have a lower osmolality and are thought to be more rapidly absorbed, although clinical trials have failed to demonstrate any convincing benefits of one type of feed over the other.

Carbohydrate is generally in the form of hydrolyzed cornstarch or short-chain glucose polymers. Such products are almost all free of lactose and other disaccharides.

Elemental formulas are usually low in fat, though there should be a small amount of linoleic acid present to prevent the development of a deficiency of essential fatty acids. Where extra triglyceride is present, a proportion of it is in the form of medium-chain triglycerides (MCTs).

There are several products available in powder or ready-to-feed form. Alternatively, a modular preparation can be designed using a protein source that consists of peptides or amino acids (see Appendix IV.14).

There have been few reports on the long-term use of elemental or chemically defined diets in children in situations where no 'natural' foods are taken. If such a regimen is to be used for more than 3–4 weeks, careful monitoring of growth and other nutritional parameters should be undertaken on a regular basis.

Although such products have been found to be useful in situations such as short gut, inflammatory bowel disease and pre- and post surgery to the gut, they have several disadvantages. Consideration should be given to the use of a non-elemental formula that has been adapted to overcome a specific digestive problem, such as low-lactose or low-fat formulas, before an elemental feed is started.

The major disadvantage of elemental products is the high osmolality caused by the large number of small particles in the formula. Introduction of elemental feeds should be very slow, and the initial feed must be a small volume of a dilute formula. Even quarter-strength feeds may have the same osmolality as a full-strength normal milk feed.

In sick and young children, the suggested starting formula is one-eighth strength for at least 12 h, increasing to quarter strength only if there are no symptoms such as vomiting, abdominal discomfort or diarrhea. Half-strength feeds should be continued for at least 24 h, and progression from half- to full-strength feeds should be carried out particularly slowly because the feed will be hyperosmolar at this concentration. A three-quarter strength feed will be necessary for at least 24 h, and an intermediate dilution between three-quarter and full strength may be required.

A further disadvantage of elemental formulas is the unpalatable taste of most products. This is unlikely to cause major problems in infants feeding from a bottle, but older children will need considerable persuasion to take this type of feed from a cup. Toddlers may accept the feed more readily from a feeding bottle or beaker, and older children through a straw. If the feed is chilled prior to offering it to the child, the taste is less obvious. Flavorings are available for some products, or milkshake flavoring can be added. Both types of flavorings will increase the osmolality and the allergenicity of the feed.

Selected elemental formulas

Elecare   Abbott/Ross
Suitable for use in children aged 1–3 years. Nutritionally complete in 1000 ml. Thirty-three percent of fat calories as medium-chain triglycerides (MCTs).

Elemental 028   SHS*
Designed for use in adults. Use with caution in children aged 1–5 years. Unsuitable for infants under 1 year. Free of lactose, sucrose, gluten, milk and all intact protein. The protein component contains essential and non-essential amino acids. The fat source is mainly long-chain triglycerides (LCTs). The carbohydrate source is sugar and dried glucose syrup.

Also available: Pediatric Elemental 028, Elemental 028 Extra (powder) and Elemental 028 Extra Liquid (0.85 kcal/ml; 3.56 kJ/ml). Flavored and unflavored versions.

Neocate/Neocate Infant Formula   SHS*
Suitable for use from birth. Powder with a protein component containimg essential and non-essential amino acids. The carbohydrate source is dried glucose syrup. Contains 5% MCT and 95% LCT.

Neocate Advance/Neocate Junior/Neocate 1 +   SHS*
Suitable for use from 1–10 years. Powder with a protein component containing essential and non-essential amino acids. The carbohydrate source is dried glucose syrup. Contains 35% MCT and 65% LCT.

Vivonex Pediatric   Novartis
Suitable for use from 1–10 years. Powder with a protein component containing essential and non-essential amino acids. Carbohydrate source is maltodextrin and modified starch. Contains MCT oil and soybean oil.

*SHS products vary in name and composition in different countries. Check with manufacturer for current specifications.
Check with manufacturers for preparation instructions.

IV.21 COMPOSITION OF ELEMENTAL OR CHEMICALLY DEFINED FORMULAS (PER 100 ML NORMAL DILUTION)

Product	Energy		Protein equivalent	Carbohydrate	Fat
	(kcal)	(kJ)	(g)	(g)	(g)
Elecare	98	410	3.00	10.7	4.8
Elemental 028 (unflavored)*	76	318	2.00	14.1	1.3
Elemental 028 Extra (unflavored)*	85	356	2.50	11.0	3.5
Neocate	71	298	1.95	8.1	3.5
Neocate Advance	100	419	2.50	14.6	3.5
Neocate One +	100	419	2.50	14.6	3.5
Pediatric E028	100	419	2.50	14.6	3.5
Vivonex Pediatric	80	335	2.40	13.0	2.4

Product	Sodium		Potassium		Osmolality
	(mmol)	(mg)	(mmol)	(mg)	(mOsm/kg)
Elecare	1.95	44.85	3.80	148.2	596
Elemental 028 (unflavored)*	2.20	50.60	2.40	93.6	496
Elemental 028 Extra (unflavored)*	2.70	62.10	2.40	93.6	502
Neocate	0.78	18.00	1.63	63.0	360
Neocate Advance	2.60	59.80	3.00	117.0	636
Neocate One +	0.87	20.00	2.40	93.6	610
Pediatric E028	0.86	20.00	2.30	93.0	820
Vivonex Pediatric	1.70	39.10	3.10	120.9	360

*Not available in the USA.
SHS products vary in name and composition in different countries. Check with manufacturer for current specifications.

IV.22 FULL-STRENGTH MODULAR FEED USING HYDROLYSATE

Product	Quantity	Protein	Fat	Carbohydrate	Energy	
		(g)	(g)	(g)	(kcal)	(kJ)
Pepdite Module 767*	2.5 g	2.1	–	–	9	38
Glucose polymer	8 g	–	–	8.0	32	134
Lipid emulsion, e.g. Calogen	8 ml	–	4.0	–	36	151
Paediatric Seravit	1 g	–	–	–	–	–
Water	To make up to 100 ml	–	–	–	–	–
Total	**100 ml**	**2.1**	**4.0**	**8.0**	**77**	**323**

Product	Sodium		Potassium		Calcium	
	(mmol)	(mg/100 ml)	(mmol)	(mg/100 ml)	(mmol)	(mg)
Pepdite Module 767*	0.9	19	0.5	20	0.75	3
Glucose polymer	–	–	–	–	–	–
Lipid emulsion, e.g. Calogen	–	–	–	–	–	–
Paediatric Seravit	–	–	–	–	2.05	82
Water	–	–	–	–	–	–
Total	**0.9**	**19**	**0.5**	**20**	**2.80**	**85**

*Generally used in UK and Europe.

IV.23 LACTOSE CONTENT OF FOODS

Foods with a high lactose content (>1 g/100 g)	Foods with a low lactose content (<1 g/100 g)	Foods free of lactose
Milks of all species	Hard cheese	Most coffee whiteners/creamers
Milk-based desserts	Double/heavy cream	Soy milks
Single/light cream	Butter	Margarines prepared from vegetable products
Yogurt	Margarines	Ghee
Ice cream	Some processed meat and fish dishes (e.g. burgers, sausages, fish fingers/sticks, chicken nuggets)	Oils
Some processed infant savory dishes		Cooking fats
Creamed soups	Toffee	Saccharin
Some artificial sweeteners	Filled chocolate products	Cyclamate
Milk chocolate	Some fizzy drinks/sodas and 'pop'	Glucose
Processed milk/cheese-based fruit, vegetable and pasta dishes	Some adult breakfast cereals	Fructose
	Some breads	Sucrose
White sauce (sweet and savory)	Cookies/biscuits/crackers and baked goods	Jam/jelly
Most infant breakfast cereals and rusks	Cakes and pastry	Jelly/jello
	Pancakes	Clear fruit-type sweets and gums
	Muffins	Gelatin
	Some flavored potato-crisps and savory snacks	Most fruit drinks
		Vegetables
		Potatoes
		Peas
		Beans
		Lentils
		Nuts
		Fruit
		Rice
		Wheat
		Barley
		Oats
		Maize
		Sago
		Semolina
		Tapioca
		Cornflour
		Cornstarch
		Cornmeal
		Some breads
		Most breakfast cereals
		Pasta

IV.24 FOODS THAT MAY CONTAIN MILK

Protein foods: sausages, burgers, frozen and canned meat and fish in sauce, meat and fish coated with batter or breadcrumbs.

Cereal products: infant cereals and rusks, biscuits and cookies/crackers, milk bread, buns, cakes, pancakes, muffins, pastries, canned spaghetti with cheese.

Dairy products: margarines, canned, dehydrated and frozen desserts and ice creams, canned and dehydrated baby desserts, powdered coffee whiteners and cream substitutes, malted milks.

Fruit and vegetables: canned and dehydrated vegetables in sauce.

Confectionery: milk chocolate, filled chocolates and chocolate bars, toffees and soft sweets or candies, lemon curd, chocolate-type spreads.

Miscellaneous: canned and dehydrated soups, mustard, pickles in sauce, flavored potato-crisps/chips and similar snack items, salad dressings.

IV.25 TERMS FOR MILK PRODUCTS USED IN FOOD LABELING

Buttermilk	Casein	Lactose	Milk solids	Whey
Butterfat, butter solids, milk fat, animal fat, artificial cream, artificial butter flavor.	Caseinates hydrolyzed casein.		Non-fat milk solids	Hydrolyzed whey, vegetarian whey

IV.26 GLUCOSE AND GALACTOSE CONTENT OF FOODS

Foods with a high glucose or galactose content (>1 g/100 g)	Foods with a low glucose or galactose content (<1 g/100 g)	Foods free of glucose and galactose
Milk-based foods	Hard cheese	Oils
Lactose-based artificial sweeteners	Double/heavy cream	Cooking fats
Sucrose and foods containing sucrose	Butter	Ghee (clarified butter)
Starch and foods containing starch	Margarine	Meat
Root vegetables	Liver	Poultry
Starchy vegetables	Shellfish	Fish
Peas	Green leafy vegetables	Eggs
Beans	Asparagus	Saccharin
Lentils	Bamboo shoots	Cyclamate
Nuts	Brussels sprouts	Fructose (levulose) powder
Most fruits and fruit drinks	Celery	Aspartame
Rice	Herbs	Salt
Wheat	Marrow	Pepper
Oats	Mushrooms	Vinegar
Maize	Squash	Spices
Barley	Cantaloupe melon	Essences
Soy	Lemon	Food colorings
Sago		Gelatin
Semolina		Sugar-free gelatin desserts
Tapioca		Sugar-free drinks
Breakfast cereal		
Bread		
Baked goods		
Pasta		

IV.27 FRUCTOSE CONTENT OF FOODS

Foods with a high fructose content (>1 g/100 g)	Foods with a low fructose content (<1 g/100 g)	Foods free of fructose
Some infant formulas	Potato (old)	Milk
Some soy milks	Nuts	Cream
Flavored yogurts	Olives	Cheese
Milk-based desserts	Avocado pear	Butter
Ice cream	Green leafy vegetables	Plain (unflavored) yogurt
Sucrose and foods containing sucrose, i.e. preserves and confectionery/candy	Asparagus	Margarine
	Bamboo shoots	Ghee
Root vegetables	Broccoli	Fats
Sweetcorn	Brussels sprouts	Oils
Tomato	Cauliflower	Meat
Peas	Celery	Poultry
Beans	Mushrooms	Fish
Lentils	Squash	Eggs
Most fruits and fruit drinks	Herbs	Glucose
Corn (maize)	Cranberries	Glucose polymer
Soy	Lemon	Dextrin
Soy flour	Loganberries	Saccharin
Some infant and adult breakfast cereals	Rhubarb	Cyclamate
		Rice
Biscuits/cookies/crackers and baked goods		Wheat
Rusks		Oats
		Barley
		Cornflour/cornstarch
		Pasta
		Most breads and flours
		Salt
		Pepper
		Vinegar
		Spices
		Gelatin

IV.28 SUCROSE AND STARCH CONTENT OF FOODS

Foods containing added sucrose	Foods containing starch	Foods containing natural sucrose	Foods free or low in sucrose and starch
Processed milk-based desserts and puddings	Soy beans	Some brands of pure honey	Milk
Ice cream	Soy flour	Root vegetables*	Cream
Processed meat	Peas	(e.g. carrot, turnip)	Cheese
products*	Beans	Tomato	Butter
(e.g. sausages,	Lentils	Onion	Ghee
burgers)	Nuts	Banana*	Margarines
Processed fish	Potato	Fruits	Fats
products*	Plain potato-crisps	Unsweetened fruit	Oils
(e.g. fish fingers)	Savory snacks	juice	Meat
Some artificial	Rice		Poultry
sweeteners	Wheat		Offal
Sweets/candies	Oats		Fish
Jam/jelly	Barley		Eggs
Jelly/jello	Maize		Glucose
Preserves	Tapioca		Lactose
Some honey	Sago		Fructose
Canned vegetables	Semolina		Saccharin
and bean dishes*	Pasta		Cyclamate
Some flavored	Bread		Aspartame
potato-crisps* and	Pastry		Green leafy
savory snacks*	Cornflour/cornstarch		vegetables
Baked goods*			Asparagus
(e.g. biscuits,			Celery
cookies, cakes)			Cauliflower
Canned pasta* and			Green beans
milk puddings*			Marrow
Some adult and			Mushrooms
infant breakfast			Lemon
cereals*			Blackberries
Fruit drinks			Cherries
Sauces and ketchups			Cranberries
Fizzy drinks, 'pop'			Currants
			Gooseberries
			Grapes
			Raspberries
			Strawberries
			Salt
			Pepper
			Herbs
			Spices
			Vinegar
			Gelatin
			Spirits
			(e.g. gin, whisky)

* These foods also contain starch.

IV.29 FOODS FREE OF LACTOSE AND SUCROSE

Glucose (dextrose), fructose (levulose) powders
Margarines prepared entirely from vegetable products
Ghee
Cooking fats
Cooking oils
Gelatin
Meat
Poultry
Fish
Offal
Eggs
Salt
Pepper
Herbs
Spices (not monosodium glutamate)
Potato*
Grapes
Cherries
Rhubarb[†]
Green leafy vegetables
Green beans
Celery[†]
Mushrooms
Cauliflower
Broccoli[†]
Rice*
Wheat*
Oats*
Barley*
Cornflour/cornstarch*
Sago*
Semolina*
Tapioca*
Some adult and infant type breakfast cereals (check ingredients)*
Most varieties of bread (check ingredients)*

*Contain starch
[†]Contain traces of sucrose

IV.30 HIGH-FAT AND LOW-FAT FOODS

Foods with a high fat content (>6 g per average adult-size portion)	Foods with a moderate fat content (2–6 g per average adult-size portion)	Foods with a low fat content (<2 g per average adult-size portion)	Minimal-fat foods (<0.5 g per average adult-size portion)
Doughnuts	Biscuits/cookies	Breakfast cereals	White flour
Whole milk	Pastry	Brown and wholemeal flours	Cornflour/cornstarch
Cream	Cakes		Cornmeal
Beef	Semi-skimmed milk	Bread	Grits
Pork	1% or 2% milk	Low-fat yogurt	White rice
Lamb	Ice cream	Prawns/shrimp	Rice cakes
Sausages	Chicken	Tuna (canned in water or brine)	Pasta
Hamburgers	Turkey		Rice noodles
Meat pies	Oily fish	Dried soya mince	Skimmed milk
Egg	Packet soups	Cottage cheese	White fish (e.g. cod, plaice)
Cheese	Low-fat spreads/margarine	Quark	Egg white
Nuts	Salad dressings		All fresh, frozen and canned fruits and vegetables
Butter	Avocado pear		Boiled sweets/ hard candy
Margarine	Olives		Jelly sweets
Cooking fats and oils	Toffee		Marshmallow
Fried foods	Malted milk powders		Clear fruit sweets and candies
Chocolate	Malted milk drinks		Fizzy drinks/sodas
			Fruit juice drinks
			Fruit squash
			Jelly/jello
			Jam/jelly
			Honey
			Sugar
			Herbs
			Spices
			Condiments
			Ketchup
			Vinegar

IV.31 FAT CONTENT OF FOODS

Food	Fat content (g per 100 g food)
Beef steak (lean)	6.0
Chicken (light meat)	5.0
Gammon (lean)	5.5
Ham	5.0
Turkey (white meat)	2.0

Food	Fat content (g per 25 g food)
Cornflakes	0.2
Puffed wheat	0.3
Rice Krispies	0.2
Weetabix	0.7
Bread – white	0.4
Bread – wholemeal	0.7

Cereals with a chocolate coating have a higher fat content.

IV.32 CHOLESTEROL CONTENT OF SELECTED FOODS

High cholesterol (>100 mg per average adult-size portion)	Cholesterol/ 100 g food	Moderate cholesterol (20–100 mg per average adult-size portion)	Cholesterol/ 100 g food
	(mg)		(mg)
Cream, double/heavy	130	Cream, single/light	55
Egg, whole	385	Ice cream, dairy	31
Kidney	400	Milk, whole	14
Liver	370	Butter and ghee	230
Lamb and mutton, raw	110	Cheese, cheddar	100
Beefburgers, raw	96	Cheese, stilton	105
Cod roe (fried)	500–700	Beef, raw	59
Shrimps, raw	200	Pork, raw	69
		Chicken, raw	57
		Frankfurters	46
		Sausage beef, raw	40
		Salami	79
		Cod, raw	46
		Plaice, raw	42
		Tuna, canned	50
		Sardines, canned	76
		Crab, canned	72
		Prawns, boiled	81

Low cholesterol (up to 20 mg per average adult-size portion)	Cholesterol/ 100 g food	Cholesterol free
	(mg)	
Ice cream, non-dairy	7	Vegetable oil
Milk, skimmed	2	Vegetable margarine
Cottage cheese	13	Egg white
Low-fat yogurt	4	Fruit
		Vegetables
		Cereals
		Sugar

IV.33 GLUTEN CONTENT OF FOODS

Gluten-free foods	Gluten-containing foods
Cereals	**Cereals**
Corn or maize, cornmeal, grits	Wheat, rye, barley, oats
Rice and wild rice	Spelt, triticale, kamut
Arrowroot, amaranth, buckwheat, millet, quinoa, sorghum, teff	Bulgar wheat, durum wheat
Specially manufactured gluten-free wheat starch, flour and mixes*	Semolina, couscous
Sago, tapioca, cassava	Wheat and oat bran
Rice bran	Wheatgerm
Popcorn	
Flour*	**Flour**
Cornflour, polenta	Wheat, rye, barley, oat, spelt and triticale flours, graham flour
Rice flour and ground rice	
Soy flour	
Potato flour, potato starch	
Bean flours, chickpea (gram) flour, split-pea flour	
Modified starch	**Modified starch**
Modified maize starch	Commercial wheat starch
Modified starch	
Bread, cake and biscuits	**Bread, cake and biscuits**
Gluten-free (and part-baked) bread and rolls	All ordinary bread and bread products
Gluten-free biscuits, crispbread and crackers	All ordinary biscuits, crispbreads, crackers, matzos, rusks
Gluten-free cakes	All ordinary cakes and pastries
Gluten-free pastry	All ordinary pizzas, croutons, pancakes, chapatti, naan, wheat tortillas
Gluten-free pizza bases	
Rice cakes	
Pasta	**Pasta**
Gluten-free pasta	All other fresh, dried or canned pasta
Corn and rice pasta	
Rice noodles	All other noodles
Breakfast cereals	**Breakfast cereals**
Cornflakes, Rice Krispies – check additives	All other breakfast cereals
Gluten-free muesli	

*May not be allowed on a gluten-free diet as can contain small traces of gluten.

Gluten-free foods	Gluten-containing foods
Meat and poultry	**Meat and poultry**
All fresh, smoked or cured pure meat	Meat or poultry cooked in batter or breadcrumbs
Gluten-free sausages	Meat pies and puddings
	Haggis
	Ordinary sausages and sausage meat
	Burgers, faggots and rissoles (unless homemade)
	Meat paté and meat paste[†]
Fish and shellfish	**Fish and shellfish**
All fresh, smoked and kippered fish and seafood	Fish in batter or breadcrumbs
Fish canned in oil, water or brine	Fish cakes
Frozen, plain fish and shellfish	Fish fingers
	Taramasalata
	Fish in sauces; fish pastes and patés[†]
Cheese and eggs	**Cheese and eggs**
All plain cheese, cottage cheese and cream cheese	Cheese spreads and processed cheese[†]
Cheese with added fruit, nuts and herbs	
Eggs	Scotch eggs
Milk and milk products	**Milk and milk products**
Fresh, condensed and evaporated milk	Artificial cream
Yogurt – check ingredients	Oat milk
	Yogurt and fromage frais containing muesli, cereals or sweets[†]
Fats and oils	**Fats and oils**
Butter, margarine, lard, cooking oils	Shredded suet
Reduced-fat and low-fat spreads	
Fruits, vegetables and nuts	**Fruits, vegetables and nuts**
All fresh, frozen, canned and dried pure fruits and vegetables	Vegetables and potatoes in batter, breadcrumbs or dusted with flour
Plain, salted nuts	Vegetables in sauce, including baked beans[†]
	Oven, microwave and frozen chips/french fries[†]
	Potato croquettes, potato waffles
	Instant mashed potato[†]
	Fruit pie fillings, fruit sauces
	Dry roasted nuts

Gluten-free foods	Gluten-containing foods
Savory snacks	**Savory snacks**
Plain potato-crisps/potato chips	Flavored crisps/potato chips[†]
Rice Krispie squares	All other snack products made from wheat, barley, rye and oats
Preserves and spreads	**Preserves and spreads**
Jam/jelly, honey, golden syrup, treacle, marmalade	Mincemeat[†]
Nut butters – check ingredients	Lemon curd[†]
Soups, sauces and seasonings	**Soups, sauces and seasonings**
Soups, sauces or gravy made with gluten-free ingredients or thickened with gluten-free flours	Canned and packet soups[†]
Herbs and spices	Packet sauces and sauce mixes[†]
Wine and cider vinegars	Bottled sauces and ketchups[†]
	Stock and stock cubes[†]
	Gravy browning and gravy mixes[†]
Tamari soy sauce	Soy Sauce
	Mustard powder and curry powder[†]
	Mayonnaise and salad cream[†]
	Salad dressings[†]
Confectionery	**Confectionery**
Plain hard fruits Check ingredients for other sweets/candy	Liquorice
Puddings	**Puddings**
Jello/jelly	All other puddings
Homemade and milk puddings made using gluten-free ingredients	Instant desserts[†]
	Ice cream and ice lollies[†]
	Custard powders[†]
Drinks	**Drinks**
Tea, coffee, fruit juice, fruit squash	Herbal tea[†]
Cocoa	Instant coffee containing barley
	Barley fruit drinks
	Cloudy fizzy drinks
	Vending-machine chocolate drinks
	Chocolate powder and drinks[†]
	Milkshakes and milkshake mixes[†]
	Malted milk drinks
Miscellaneous	**Miscellaneous**
Gelatin	Baking powder/soda[†]
Bicarbonate of soda, cream of tartar	Cake coverings and cake decorations[†]

Gluten-free foods	Gluten-containing foods
Fresh and dried yeast	Marzipan[†]
Tofu, quorn	Meat, vegetable and yeast extracts[†]

*Ensure that flours are not cross-contaminated and are milled in 'clean' mills.

†These products need to be checked in the food lists published by the UK and the American Celiac Societies. The Food List must be updated with deletions monthly.

IV.34 PROCESSED FOODS THAT MAY CONTAIN GLUTEN

Check the food lists published by the UK and American Celiac Societies

Condiments

Ketchup, savory sauces, mustards, baking powder; stock cubes and granules; mayonnaise and salad cream

Soups

All chilled, canned and packet soups

Meat and fish

Any fish or meat in a sauce, marinated or coated in seasonings

Ready-sliced meat products

Savory spreads (e.g. meat and fish paste), savory crisps/chips and snacks

Vegetables

Any vegetable products in a sauce, marinated or coated in seasonings

Puddings/desserts

Dessert mixes, custard and blancmange/pudding mixes, dessert toppings, artificial creams and aerosol-packed creams

Drinks

'Bedtime' drinks and chocolate-type drinks

Confectionery

All confectionery and ice cream

Miscellaneous

Textured vegetable protein and hydrolyzed vegetable protein, packaged suet

IV.35 SELECTED PRODUCTS AVAILABLE FOR GLUTEN-FREE DIETS

Low-protein products are usually suitable for a gluten-free diet but the reverse is not true. Gluten-free products may have milk and/or egg included in the ingredients, thus significantly increasing the protein content.

The following table provides a selection of gluten-free products, some of which are also low in protein, but it is important to note that products are constantly changing and may be marketed by different companies or under different names in countries outside the UK. Check with your national celiac society for the most up-to-date information and for advice on availability. In the UK and other countries, some of these products are available on prescription.

Product type	Name	Manufacturer
Biscuits/Cookies	Arnott's rice cookies	Ultrapharm
	Bi-aglut gluten-free biscuits	Ultrapharm
	Glutafin gluten-free biscuits	Nutricia Dietary Care
	Glutafin gluten-free tea biscuits	Nutricia Dietary Care
	Glutafin gluten-free sweet biscuits	Nutricia Dietary Care
	Glutafin gluten-free digestive biscuits	Nutricia Dietary Care
	Glutafin gluten-free savoury biscuits	Nutricia Dietary Care
	Glutano gluten-free biscuits	Gluten-free Foods
	Juvela gluten-free digestive biscuits	SHS
	Juvela gluten-free tea biscuits	SHS
	Juvela gluten-free savoury biscuits	SHS
	Polial gluten-free biscuits	Ultrapharm
	Schar Biscuits	Dr Schar
	Schar Savoy Biscuits	Dr Schar
Bread	Barkat white rice bread (sliced)	Gluten-free Foods
	Barkat brown rice bread (sliced)	Gluten-free Foods
	Glutano gluten-free par-baked (white sliced bread)	Gluten-free Foods
	Glutano gluten-free par-baked (rolls)	Gluten-free Foods
	Glutano gluten-free par-baked (baguette)	Gluten-free Foods
	Ener-G brown rice bread (sliced)	General Dietary
	Ener-G brown rice and maize bread (sliced)	General Dietary
	Ener-G rice loaf (sliced)	General Dietary
	Ener-G white rice bread (sliced)	General Dietary
	Ener-G tapioca bread (sliced)	General Dietary
	Glutafin white loaf (sliced and unsliced)	Nutricia Dietary Care
	Glutafin fiber loaf (sliced and unsliced)	Nutricia Dietary Care
	Glutafin multigrain white loaf (sliced and unsliced)	Nutricia Dietary Care

Product type	Name	Manufacturer
	Glutafin multigrain fiber loaf (sliced and unsliced)	Nutricia Dietary Care
	Glutafin multigrain white rolls	Nutricia Dietary Care
	Glutafin multigrain fiber rolls	Nutricia Dietary Care
	Glutafin part-baked white loaf	Nutricia Dietary Care
	Glutafin part-baked fiber loaf	Nutricia Dietary Care
	Glutafin part-baked white rolls	Nutricia Dietary Care
	Glutafin part-baked fiber rolls	Nutricia Dietary Care
	Glutafin part-baked long white rolls	Nutricia Dietary Care
	Glutafin part-baked long fiber rolls	Nutricia Dietary Care
	Glutafin pizza bases	Nutricia Dietary Care
	Glutafin canned bread with added soya	Nutricia Dietary Care
	Glutano gluten-free sliced wholemeal bread	Gluten-free Foods
	Glutano gluten-free wholemeal par-baked bread	Gluten-free Foods
	Barkat white rice pizza crust	Gluten-free Foods
	Barkat brown rice pizza crust	Gluten-free Foods
	Juvela gluten-free loaf (sliced and whole)	SHS
	Juvela gluten-free fiber loaf (sliced and whole)	SHS
	Juvela gluten-free bread rolls	SHS
	Juvela gluten-free fiber bread rolls	SHS
	Juvela gluten-free part-baked rolls	SHS
	Lifestyle Healthcare brown bread (sliced and unsliced)	Lifestyle Healthcare
	Lifestyle Healthcare white bread (sliced and unsliced)	Lifestyle Healthcare
	Lifestyle Healthcare high fiber bread (unsliced only)	Lifestyle Healthcare
	Lifestyle Healthcare bread rolls	Lifestyle Healthcare
	Lifestyle Healthcare high fiber bread rolls	Lifestyle Healthcare
	Rite-Diet white bread (sliced or unsliced)	Nutricia Dietary Care
	Rite-Diet fiber bread (sliced or unsliced)	Nutricia Dietary Care
	Rite-Diet part-baked white loaf	Nutricia Dietary Care
	Rite-Diet part-baked long white rolls	Nutricia Dietary Care
	Rite-Diet white rolls	Nutricia Dietary Care
	Rite-Diet fiber rolls	Nutricia Dietary Care
	Rite-Diet part-baked fiber loaf	Nutricia Dietary Care
	Rite-Diet part-baked long fiber rolls	Nutricia Dietary Care

Product type	Name	Manufacturer
	Schar bread	Dr Schar
	Schar wholemeal bread	Dr Schar
	Schar bread rolls	Dr Schar
	Schar white bread rolls	Dr Schar
	Schar lunch rolls	Dr Schar
	Schar French bread baguette	Dr Schar
	Schar pizza bases (250 g)	Dr Schar
	Ultra gluten-free baguette	Ultrapharm
	Ultra gluten-free pizza bases	Ultrapharm
	Ultra high fiber bread	Ultrapharm
	Ultra wheat-free bread	Ultrapharm
	Ultra wheat-free bread rolls	Ultrapharm
	Valpiform country loaf (sliced)	General Dietary
	Valpiform petites baguettes	General Dietary
Crackers	Bi-Aglut crackers	Ultrapharm
	Bi-Aglut cracker toast	Ultrapharm
	Glutafin crackers	Nutricia Dietary Care
	Glutafin high fiber crackers	Nutricia Dietary Care
	Glutano gluten-free crackers	Gluten-free Foods
	Juvela gluten-free crispbread	SHS
	Schar cracker toast	Dr Schar
	Schar crispbread	Dr Schar
	Ultra crackerbread	Ultrapharm
	Ultra gluten-free crackers	Ultrapharm
Flours	Aproten flour	Ultrapharm
	Glutano G/F pasta (animal shapes)	Gluten-free Foods
	Barkat G/F bread mix	Gluten-free Foods
	Clara's kitchen gluten-free flour	Gluten-free Foods
	Clara's kitchen gluten-free high fiber flour	Gluten-free Foods
	Dietary specialties brown bread mix	Nutrition Point
	Dietary specialties white bread mix	Nutrition Point
	Dietary specialties corn bread mix	Nutrition Point
	Dietary specialties white cake mix	Nutrition Point
	Glutafin white mix	Nutricia Dietary Care
	Glutafin fiber mix	Nutricia Dietary Care

Product type	Name	Manufacturer
	Glutafin multigrain white mix	Nutricia Dietary Care
	Glutafin multigrain fiber mix	Nutricia Dietary Care
	Glutano gluten-free flour mix	Gluten-free Foods
	Juvela gluten-free mix	SHS
	Juvela gluten-free fiber mix	SHS
	Juvela gluten-free harvest mix	SHS
	Schar flour mix	Dr Schar
	Schar wholemeal flour mix	Dr Schar
	Schar bread mix	Dr Schar
	Schar cake mix	Dr Schar
	Tritamyl gluten-free flour	Gluten-free Foods
	Tritamyl gluten-free brown bread mix	Gluten-free Foods
	Tritamyl gluten-free white bread mix	Gluten-free Foods
	Trufree No 1 Bread flour	Larkhall Natural Health
	Trufree No 2 Flour with rice bran	Larkhall Natural Health
	Trufree No 4 White bread flour	Larkhall Natural Health
	Trufree No 5 Brown bread flour	Larkhall Natural Health
	Trufree No 6 Plain flour	Larkhall Natural Health
	Trufree No 7 Self raising flour	Larkhall Natural Health
	Trufree No 8 White bread flour	Larkhall Natural Health
Flour mixes	Valpiform bread mix	General Dietary
	Valpiform pastry mix	General Dietary
Pasta	Bi-Aglut – spaghetti, fusilli, penne, macaroni, lasagne	Ultrapharm
	Ener-G – cannelloni, lasagne, macaroni, shells, small shells, spaghetti, tagliatelle, vermicelli	General Dietary
	Ener-G Brown Rice Pasta – lasagne, macaroni, spaghetti	General Dietary
	Glutafin – long spaghetti, macaroni, penne, spirals, lasagne, tagliatelle, shells	Nutricia Dietary Care
	Glutano G/F pasta (animal shapes)	Gluten-free Foods
	Glutano Pasta – macaroni, spaghetti, spirals, tagliatelle	Gluten-free Foods
	Schar – bavette, fusilli, penne, rigati, spaghetti, lasagne, macaroni, alphabet, rings, shells and strands	Dr Schar
	Tinkyada Brown Rice Pasta – spaghetti, spirals, penne, shells, elbows, fusilli, fettuccini	General Dietary

IV.36 SOY CONTENT OF FOODS

Foods that may include soy as an ingredient include:

Protein foods – sausages, burgers, canned and frozen meat dishes in a sauce, shaped and minced (ground) meat products, vegetable burgers, vegetarian dishes.

Cereal products – bread (information should be sought from individual bakeries), biscuits/cookies/crackers, cakes and pastries, baking mixes, pancake mixes.

Dairy products – malted milk-type beverages, yogurts.

Miscellaneous – meat and vegetable extracts/stock, savory canned/dried and bottled sauces, canned and dehydrated soups, soy sauce, miso, salad dressing.

IV.37 FIBER CONTENT OF FOODS

Good fiber sources	Lesser fiber sources
Cereals	
Bran (wheat)	
Bread – wholemeal/wholewheat, brown	Bread – white Cornbread/tortilla
Chapatti – wholemeal	Chapatti – chapatti flour
Rice, boiled – wholegrain	Rice, boiled – white
Biscuits/cookies/crackers – wholegrain (e.g. 'Digestive', graham crackers)	Biscuits/cookies – white flour
Crispbread – rye	Crackers
Breakfast cereals – bran based, wholewheat, corn based, muesli type	Breakfast cereals – rice based
Fruits	
Berry fruits	Strawberries
Banana	Apple – raw
Dates – fresh	Grapes
Damsons – raw	Orange
Prunes – stewed	Mango
Raisins, sultanas	Melon
Nuts	
Peanuts	
Peanut butter	
Coconut – fresh	
Other nuts	
Vegetables	
Potatoes, boiled – old, new	Cucumber
Potato-crisps/chips	Lettuce
Root vegetables	Tomato
Leafy vegetables	
Spinach	
Beans – green, dried, boiled/refried, baked	
Peas, boiled	
Lentils, boiled – dhal	

IV.38 MINIMAL-RESIDUE AND LOW-RESIDUE FOODS

Foods free of fiber	Low fiber foods
Egg	Cornstarch or cornflour
Fish and shellfish	White polished rice (boiled)
Meat*, poultry*	Tapioca
Milk*	Spaghetti (white)
Cheese*	Sponge cake (plain)
Butter and margarine*	Asparagus
Cooking fats and oils*	Cucumber
Ice cream*	Pumpkin
Plain yogurts*	Tomato flesh (no skin or pips)
Meringues	Grapes (no skin or pips)
Jelly/Jello	Melon
Sugar	Fresh/canned fruit juice
Honey	
Jam/Jelly (no pips)	
Clear sweets/candies	
Clear soups and broths	
Fruit-flavored juice drink	
Fizzy drinks/sodas	
Tea and coffee	

*Although animal foods such as meat, milk and milk products contain no dietary fiber, they are incompletely digested in the small intestine. Food residue passes into the large intestine, providing a substrate for bacterial action and increasing the bulk of intestinal contents; therefore, these foods cannot be regarded as being residue free. Milk and milk products result in appreciable quantities of stool bulk and may need to be restricted if a very-low-residue diet is required.

In malabsorption syndromes, all foods are likely to result in food residue passing into the large bowel and thus increasing stool bulk.

IV.39 ELIMINATION REGIMEN

Stage I

Until symptoms have been absent for 1 week, use foods of low reported allergenicity:
- Lamb – cooked without the addition of meat or yeast extracts or manufactured 'gravy mixes'
- Green vegetables – such as cabbage or green beans, boiled in water
- Potatoes – boiled in water
- Rice – boiled in water, or ground rice cooked with water and sweetened with glucose as a cereal substitute
- Table salt may be added to taste
- Fluids should consist only of water sweetened with glucose
- Fresh pears – may be poached in water and sweetened with glucose

No other foods or drinks should be taken. An elemental diet may be used to supplement this regimen and to supply minerals, vitamins and trace elements.

The ten stages of the elimination diet need not be introduced in the order given. Only one item of food should be introduced in any one day and a record should be kept of any symptoms that arise.

Stage II

Other foods of low allergenicity.

Sugar, root vegetables (e.g. carrot, turnip, swede), olive oil (for frying), other green vegetables (e.g. lettuce, Brussels sprouts, cauliflower, broccoli).

Stage III

Citrus fruits and foods containing salicylate.

Apples, apricots, bananas, cucumber, grapes, oranges, peaches, rhubarb, tomato.

Stage IV

Yeast.

Yeast extract (e.g. Marmite) used as gravy.

Stage V

Cereals.

Homemade wheat bread, flour, wholewheat pasta, plain wheat pasta (no additives), cornflour, cornmeal, corn oil, oats, wholemeal pasta.

Stage VI

Protein foods.

Chicken, egg, pork, ham, bacon (not sausages).

Stage VII

Dairy products.

Butter (not margarine), cheese, evaporated milk, whole milk, beef, veal.

Stage VIII
Pulses/legumes.

Peas (if Stage III is tolerated), broad beans, soy milk, peanuts, vegetable oil, lentils.

Stage IX
Chocolate (if Stages VII and VIII are tolerated), fish.

Stage X
Food additives.

Bread, biscuits, colorings (red, yellow and green), soft drinks, sausages (if beef, yeast and wheat are tolerated), fish fingers/fish sticks (if fish and wheat are tolerated), chicken nuggets (if chicken is tolerated).

Other items that appear on the initial diet record can then be introduced at the rate of one every 1–3 days. In this way, the true allergens in foods containing many ingredients can be pinpointed, rather than whole classes of foods being arbitrarily removed from the diet.

IV.40 SALICYLATES AND ADDITIVES IN FOODS

Foods that contain natural salicylate

Vegetables – cucumber, peas, tomato.

Fruit and nuts – almonds, apples, apricots, bananas, berry fruits (including raspberries and strawberries), blackcurrants, cherries, grapes (including sultanas, raisins and currants), oranges and similar fruits, peaches, prunes, rhubarb.

Foods that may contain additives (check the label)

Protein foods – canned, dehydrated and frozen meat or fish products, fresh products coated with breadcrumbs such as ham and fried fish or chicken, sausages, luncheon meats, burgers.

Cereal products – breakfast cereals, biscuits/cookies/crackers, bought cakes, bread, pastry, cake mixes, popcorn, pasta, noodles, tinned spaghetti in sauce.

Dairy products – ice cream, milkshakes, processed cheese; dessert mixes and puddings, flavored yogurts, margarines.

Confectionery: hard and soft sweets or candies, chocolate containing fruit or almonds, mints, cough sweets, fruit squash drinks, fruit flavoured drinks, carbonated or 'fizzy' drinks, chewing gum, jam/jelly, lemon curd.

Miscellaneous: canned and dehydrated soups, sauces, vinegar, pickles, salad dressings, potato crisps/chips and similar products, vegetables in sauce (e.g. baked beans), beer, wine, cider.

Non-food items – aspirin and similar drugs, toothpaste, mouthwashes, throat lozenges, perfumes, any pills or tablets with colored surround, colored medicines or cough mixtures.

IV.41 QUANTIFICATION OF TYRAMINE IN CHEESES

Cheese type	Quantity of tyramine (μg/g)
Cottage cheese	Not detectable
Quark (skimmed-milk soft cheese)	Not detectable
Cream cheese	Not detectable
Curd cheese	Not detectable
Edam	216
Brie	240
Wensleydale	312
Leicester	312
Lancashire	360
Melbury	456
Processed Cheddar	552
Goat cheese	576
Vegetarian Cheddar	601
Derby	648
Mild Cheddar	768
Lymeswold	787
Swiss Emmental	864
Low-calorie Cheddar	912
Mature Cheddar	1036
Italian gorgonzola	1248
Fully matured Cheddar	1440
Danish blue	3840
Blue stilton	4200

By kind permission of S Gray and CS Evans, London.

DIETS USED FOR THE MODIFICATION OF NITROGEN AND MINERAL INTAKE

V.1 PROTEIN CONTENT OF FOODS AND PROTEIN EXCHANGES

High-protein foods (quantity containing approx 6 g protein)	Moderate-protein foods (quantity containing approx 2 g protein)	Low-protein foods (usually allowed freely except on minimal protein diets)
Dairy products		
Milk (full or low fat) 180 ml Infant milks 380 ml Condensed milk 60 ml Evaporated milk 70 ml Drinking yogurt 200 ml Fruit/flavored yogurt 150 g Hard cheeses (e.g. Cheddar) 25 g Full-fat soft/cream cheese 70 g Cottage cheese 45 g Feta cheese 40 g Eggs (raw weight) 50 g	Single cream 80 g Double/heavy cream 120 g Ice cream 55 g Sorbet 200 g Coffee creamers 75 g	Low-protein milks Low-protein egg replacer Butter Margarine
Cereals		
Soya flour 15 g	Wheat flour 20 g Maize flour/cornmeal 25 g Popcorn 20 g Breads 25 g Breakfast cereals (plain unsweetened) – corn/maize cereals 25 g, rice cereals 30 g, wheat cereals 20 g Biscuits/cookies 30 g Pasta/noodles, cooked 50 g Rice, cooked 100 g	Cornstarch, wheat starch, potato starch, sago, tapioca Custard powder Low-protein products – bread, biscuits/cookies, breakfast cereal, crackers, rice, pasta
Fruits and vegetables		
Lentils, dahl 120 g Dried beans 25 g Cooked beans 90 g Baked beans 125 g Hummus, tofu 75 g Nuts – almond, cashew, pistachio 35 g Peanuts, peanut butter 25 g Coconut (fresh) 190 g	Raisins, sultanas 80 g Asparagus 60 g Avocado 100 g Broccoli, Brussels sprouts, cauliflower, spinach* 65 g Potato – boiled 140 g Potato chips/fries 65 g Peas* 30 g Mushrooms (fried) 80 g Sweetcorn* 45 g	All fruits except dried All other vegetables and pickles
Meat, fish and substitutes		
Meat (cooked) 20 g Meat substitutes, quark 40 g Sausages (cooked) 45 g Fish (cooked), prawns 30 g Fish fingers 45 g	Meat and fish paste/ spread 15 g Meat or yeast extract 5 g	

High-protein foods (quantity containing approx 6 g protein)	Moderate-protein foods (quantity containing approx 2 g protein)	Low-protein foods (usually allowed freely except on minimal protein diets)
Drinks		
Milk based drinks 180 ml		Tea, coffee, fruit juice, cordials**, fruit squash**, fizzy drinks/sodas**
Sugars		
Chocolate 40 g	Toffee 90 g Fruit gums 30 g Marshmallow 50 g Fudge 60 g Jelly/jello (made up) 160 g	Sugar, glucose polymer, jam, honey, syrup, vegetarian jelly/jello, boiled sweets (candies), low protein chocolate substitute
Fats and oils		
		Lard, solid vegetable fat, oils, fat emulsions (Liquigen, Calogen, Microlipid, etc.)
Miscellaneous		
	Potato crisps/chips 30 g	Vinegar, salt, pepper, spices, mustard powder, gravy browning, baking powder, food essences and flavors, agar, ketchup

*All vegetables are cooked weight unless otherwise stated.
**Foods containing Aspartame or Nutrasweet are contra-indicated on restricted phenylalanine diets.

V.2 ONE-GRAM PROTEIN EXCHANGES

The following weights of food contain approximately 1 g of protein

Milk	
Cow milk	30 ml
Yogurt (fruit or plain)	20 g
Ice cream	30 g
Single cream	40 ml
Double/heavy cream	60 ml

Cereals	
Wheat flour – white	10 g
Oats	10 g
Bread – white	12 g
Semi-sweet biscuit	15 g
Cornflakes	14 g
Rice Krispies	16 g
Weetabix, Wheatflakes	10 g
Pasta – boiled	30 g
Rice – boiled	45 g

Vegetables	
Baked beans	20 g
Lentils, dahl (cooked)	12 g
Broccoli leaf (cooked)	30 g
Brussels sprouts (cooked)	35 g
Cauliflower (cooked)	35 g
Peas (boiled)	20 g
Corn – kernels and baby corn	35 g

Potatoes	
Boiled	55 g
Baked (flesh only)	45 g
Roast	35 g
Chips/fries	65 g
Sweet potato	90 g

For diets with PKU where phenylalanine content of food is unknown, 1 g of protein can be considered approximately equivalent to 50 mg phenylalanine.

Food composition varies between different countries.

V.3 LOW-PROTEIN MILKS

Liquids that can be used in place of milk for drinks, cooking and adding to cereal can either be prepared in the home or can be obtained ready prepared. They are generally low in sodium, potassium and phosphorus as well as protein. They contain no micronutrients and their function is to increase the energy content of the diet and enhance palatability.

Minimal-protein milk substitute

	Protein	Fat	Carbohydrate	Energy		Sodium	Potassium	Phosphorus
	(g)	(g)	(g)	(kcal)	(kJ)	(mmol)	(mmol)	(mmol)
10 ml Calogen/ Microlipid	–	5.0	–	45	188	–	–	–
5 g sugar	–	–	5.0	20	84	–	–	–
Water to make up to 100 ml								
Total	–	5.0	5.0	65	272	–	–	–

Low-protein milk substitute

	Protein	Fat	Carbohydrate	Energy	
	(g)	(g)	(g)	(kcal)	(kJ)
30 ml double/ heavy cream	0.5	14.4	0.81	135	565
5 g sugar	–	–	5.00	20	84
Water to make up to 100 ml					
Total	0.5	14.4	5.81	155	649

	Sodium		Potassium		Phosphorus	
	(mmol)	(mg)	(mmol)	(mg)	(mmol)	(mg)
30 ml double/ heavy cream	0.48	11	0.50	18	0.48	14.88
5 g sugar	–	–	–	–	–	–
Water to make up to 100 ml						
Total	0.48	11	0.50	18	0.48	14.88

Ready-prepared low-protein milk substitutes (per 100 ml)

Product	Protein	Energy		Sodium		Potassium		Phosphorus	
	(g)	(kcal)	(kJ)	(mmol)	(mg)	(mmol)	(mg)	(mmol)	(mg)
Milupa Lpd	0.4	40	167	1.04	24	2.15	84	1.09	33.79
SHS Sno-Pro	0.2	67	281	3.26	75	1.28	50	0.96	29.76

V.4 Low salt diets: Sodium content of foods

High-sodium foods	Moderate-sodium foods	Low-sodium foods (generally allowed freely)
Salt[†]		
Canned savory pasta and rice dishes, savory 'nibbles', canned and packet soups	Ordinary breads*, breakfast cereals*, biscuits/cookies, cakes, pastries, crispbreads Eggs	Plain flours, dietetic low-salt bread, rice, pasta Fresh meat, poultry, offal/ organ meats, fish
Canned, smoked, dried and fermented meat and fish, sausages, 'cold cuts', savory spreads, meat extracts	Shellfish Cow milk and milk products*, fermented milks and yogurts (depends on local customs)	Whey-dominant infant formulas
Cheeses		
Canned in brine, dried and fermented vegetables and pulses, olives, pickles, tomato juice, potato crisps/chips, salted nuts	Dried fruit Vegetables (cooked in salted water)	Fresh and frozen vegetables, (cooked without salt) nuts, pulses; fresh, frozen and canned fruit and fruit juice, tomato juice (no salt added)
	Salted butter and margarines	Unsalted butter, double cream, lard, cooking and salad oils
Sauces, ketchup, relish, salad dressing, food additives, flavor enhancers, stock and gravy makers, yeast extract Vegemite, Marmite	Golden syrup, treacle, chocolate-filled sweets and candies, fruit cordials, instant tea and coffee, malted milk, mineral water, fizzy drinks	Sugar, jam/jelly, jelly/jello, clear sweets or candies, ice lollies or popsicles Yeast, herbs, spices, pepper, vinegar Cocoa powder, tea, coffee
Baking aids, baking powder, bicarbonate of soda, baking soda	Drinking water (depends on area)	Distilled water Salt substitutes (contain potassium or ammonium salts)

*These moderate sodium foods are generally allowed in limited quaantities on a low-salt diet. One or more foods (depending on the degree of restriction required), in a quantity that is appropriate to the age of the child, can be taken each day, e.g. one egg daily, one cup (200 ml) cow milk daily, etc.
[†]Salt may be allowed in cooking depending on the level of sodium restriction required.

V.5 POTASSIUM CONTENT OF FOODS

High-potassium foods	Moderate-potassium foods	Low-potassium foods
Wholemeal flour cereals and bread, bran, soy flour and soy products	Refined (white) flour cereals, breads and pasta	Cornflour/cornstarch, wheatstarch, tapioca, sago, low-protein breads and flours
Potatoes, tomatoes, leafy green vegetables, vegetable juices, pulses, nuts, fresh fruit and fruit juices, dried fruits	Runner and French beans, celery, cauliflower, baked beans, root vegetables (e.g. carrot), mushrooms, apple, pear, canned fruits in syrup	Boiled/steamed rice Butter, margarine, fats, oils, double/heavy cream Sugar, glucose and glucose polymer, jam/jelly, honey
Milk and milk products	Egg	
Meat and fish, meat extracts	Whey-dominant infant formulas	
Salt substitutes, stock and gravy makers, potato-crisps, low-salt canned dietetic products, yeast extract	Corn snacks	Herbs, spices, salt, pepper, vinegar
Blackcurrant cordials, malted milks, chocolate, some fruit juice drinks	Ground and instant coffee, instant tea, drinking water*	Tea, fruit cordials and fizzy drinks/sodas, distilled water

*Drinking water may contain high quantities of potassium in some areas.

The potassium content of cooked foods can be significantly reduced by prior soaking of the food in a large volume of water. This water is discarded and the food is cooked in a further large volume of water. Sauces and gravies should not be prepared from the cooking water. This process also reduces the vitamin C content of foods.

Foods in the high and moderate groups may be restricted on low potassium diets according to the level of tolerance and the child's food preferences.

V.6 PHOSPHORUS CONTENT OF FOODS

High-phosphorus foods	Moderate-phosphorus foods	Low-phosphorus foods
Wholemeal/wholewheat bread, flours and cereals, bran, soy flour and products	Refined (white) bread, flours, cereals and pasta	Cornflour, wheatstarch, tapioca, sago, rice
Organ meats/offal, game, meat extracts, sardines, fatty fish, fish roe	Meat, fish, eggs	
Cow milk, and products, yogurt, cheese, milk chocolate	Whey-dominant infant milk formulas, single cream, cream cheese	Butter, margarine, fats, oils, double/heavy cream
Peas, beans, spinach, mushrooms, baked beans, dried fruit, nuts, peanut butter	Potato, fresh, frozen and canned green and root vegetables, lentils, dates, figs	Fresh, frozen and canned fruit
Malted milks, cocoa powder	Instant coffee, mineral water, cola drinks, drinking water (dependent on area)	Tea, coffee, fruit cordials/fruit juice drinks and fizzy drinks/sodas, distilled water Sugar, glucose and glucose polymer, jam/jelly, honey, clear sweets and candies
Yeast extract, baking powder, baking aids	Stock and gravy makers	Herbs, spices, salt, pepper, vinegar

Foods in the high and moderate groups may be restricted on a low phosphorus diet according to the level of tolerance and the child's food preferences.

V.7 SELECTED LOW-PHENYLALANINE PROTEIN SUBSTITUTES

Protein substitutes for use in a phenylalanine-restricted diet must be used with a prescribed quantity of phenylalanine, usually derived from natural protein. Protein substitutes derived from hydrolysis and filtration of a whole protein (such as casein) do contain some residual phenylalanine, which needs to be considered when prescribing the phenylalanine intake. Products derived from amino acids are phenylalanine free. All products are supplemented with tyrosine, which becomes an essential amino acid in phenylketonuria.

Protein substitutes for infants are generally nutritionally complete, containing fat, carbohydrate, vitamins, minerals and trace elements. They are available as a powder, that is reconstituted with water in the same way as standard infant formulas. Products for older children are available in a variety of formats – powder, capsules, tablets and a confectionery-type bar. They contain varying amounts of fat and carbohydrates and will need supplementation with other foods as well as with a source of phenylalanine. Some products are not fortified with a full range of minerals and vitamins. The manufacturers' instructions should be followed carefully.

SHS[†]	XP Analog
	Analog LCP
	XP Maxamaid
	Anamix Flavoured and Unflavoured
	XP Maxamum
	Phlexy-10 Drink Mix
	Phlexy-10 Capsules
	Phlexy-10 Bar
	PK Aid 4
Mead Johnson	Lofenalac
	Phenyl-Free
Milupa*	PKU 2
	PKU 3
Ultra-Pharm*	Aminogran Food Supplement
	Aminogran Tablets
Ross Products/Abbott	Phenex-1
	Phenex-2

*Not available in the USA.
[†]Some products may not be available in the USA, check with company literature.

V.8 COMPOSITION OF LOW–PHENYLALANINE PROTEIN SUBSTITUTES

	Protein equivalent	L-Amino acids	Phenylalanine	Tyrosine
	(g)	(g)	(mg)	(mg)
Aminogran Food Supplement per 100 g	97.00	100.0	Nil	6.42 g
Aminogran Food Supplement Tablets per tablet	0.97	1.0	Nil	64.20
Analog LCP per 100 g	13.00	15.5	Nil	1.44
Anamix Flavoured per 29 g sachet	8.40	10.0	Nil	0.91
Anamix Unflavoured per 29 g sachet	8.40	10.0	Nil	0.91
Lofenalac per 100 g	15.00	Nil	0.08	0.78
Phlexy-10 Drink Mix per 20 g sachet	8.33	10.0	Nil	0.97
Phlexy-10 Capsules per 20 capsules	8.33	10.0	Nil	0.97
Phlexy-10 Bar per 42 g bar	8.33	10.0	Nil	0.97
PK Aid 4 per 100 g	79.00	95.0	Nil	9.23 g
PKU 2 per 100 g	66.80	80.1	Nil	4.5 g
PKU 3 per 100 g	68.00	81.6	Nil	6.0 g
XP Analog per 100 g	13.00	15.5	Nil	1.44
XP Maxamaid per 100 g	25.00	30.0	Nil	2.70
XP Maxamum	39.00	47.0	Nil	4.24
Phenex-1 per 100 g	15.00	Nil	Trace	1.5 g
Phenex-2 per 100 g	30.00	Nil	Trace	3.0 g
Phenyl-Free per 100 g	20.00	Nil	Nil	2.0 g

| | Fat | CHO | Energy | | Is product vitamin, mineral or trace element supplemented? |
	(g)	(g)	(kcal)	(kJ)	
Aminogran Food Supplement per 100 g	–	–	400	1675	No – use in conjunction with Aminogran Mineral Mixture and Ketovite tablets
Aminogran Food Supplement Tablets per tablet	<0.1	0.30	5	21	No – use in conjunction with Aminogran Mineral Mixture and Ketovite tablets
Analog LCP per 100 g	23.0	54.00	475	1989	Yes
Anamix Flavoured per 29 g sachet	13.5	9.80	108	452	Yes
Anamix Unflavoured per 29 g sachet	13.5	11.00	113	473	Yes
Lofenalac per 100 g	18.0	60.00	462	1934	Yes
Phlexy-10 Drink Mix per 20 g sachet	Nil	8.80	69	289	No
Phlexy-10 Capsules per 20 capsules	Nil	0.45	35	147	No
Phlexy-10 Bar per 42 g bar	4.5	20.50	156	653	No – use in conjunction with Phlexy Vits
PK Aid 4 per 100 g	Nil	4.50	334	1398	No
PKU 2 per 100 g	–	8.20	300	1256	Yes
PKU 3 per 100 g	–	3.90	288	1206	Yes
XP Analog per 100 g	23.0	54.00	475	1989	Yes
XP Maxamaid per 100 g	<0.5	51.00	309	1294	Yes
XP Maxamum	<0.5	34.00	297	1243	Yes
Phenex-1 per 100 g	23.9	46.30	480	2016	Yes
Phenex-2 per 100 g	15.5	30.00	410	1722	Yes
Phenyl-Free per 100 g	6.8	66.00	410	1722	Yes

CHO = carbohydrate

V.9 Low phenylalanine diet

Low-protein foods**	Fruits and vegetables** 1 average-size portion contains 15–20 mg phenylalanine
Sugar, glucose, glucose polymer, jam/jelly, honey, jelly/jello	Asparagus, beansprouts, broccoli, beans (green beans only), Brussels sprouts, cabbage, carrots, cauliflower, celery, cucumber, eggplant, kale, leeks, lettuce, okra, onion, parsley, parsnips, peppers, pumpkin, radishes, squash, tomato, turnip, spring greens, swede
Clear fruit sweets and candies, vegetarian jelly/jello*	
Ice lollies, popsicles, saccharin*	
Fruit juice, fruit-flavored squash/cordial, fizzy drinks/'pop'/soda	
Tea, coffee	Apple, apricot, avocado, banana, berries, dates, figs, grapes, guava, mango, melon, orange, peach, pear, pineapple, plum
Vegetarian margarine, pure white shortening, cooking and salad oils, protein-free fat emulsion (e.g. Calogen)	
Salt, pepper, mustard, vinegar, herbs, spices	
Flavorings and colorings, baking powder*	
Special low-protein products prepared from wheatstarch[†] e.g. low-protein flour, low-protein bread and bread mix, low-protein biscuits or cookies, low-protein pasta	

*The artificial sweetener Aspartame or NutraSweet is a dipeptide that is hydrolyzed in the small intestine to phenylalanine and so cannot be used for this diet. The level of aspartame in soft drinks may be up to 700 mg/l (400 mg phenylalanine per liter) and in sweetening tablets 18 mg (10 mg phenylalanine).

**In the UK many of these foods are allowed freely, but some may be calculated as part of the phenylalanine allowance in other countries. The degree of restriction may also depend on the level of enzyme activity.

†Gluten-free products may contain protein.

V.10 PHENYLALANINE EXCHANGES

Phenylalanine exchanges (UK)

Food	Weight (g) of food containing 1 × 50 mg Phe exchange (UK)
Cow milk	30
Potato – boiled	55
Potato – chips/fries	25
Rice – boiled	45
Peas – boiled	15
Sweetcorn – canned	35
Cornflakes	15
Rice Krispies	15
Wheat cereals	10

Exchange system for phenylalanine restricted diets (USA)

	Phenylalanine	Tyrosine	Protein	Energy
	(mg)	(mg)	(g)	(kcal)
Breads/cereals	30	20	0.6	30
Fats	5	4	0.1	60
Fruits	15	10	0.5	60
Vegetables	15	10	0.5	10
Free Foods A	5	4	0.1	65
Free Foods B	–	–	–	55

Detailed food lists can be found in Acosta PB, Yanicelli S. Nutrition Support Protocols, 3rd ed. Columbus, OH: Ross Products Division, Abbott Laboratories; 1997.

V.11 PROTEIN SUBSTITUTES FOR INBORN ERRORS OF METABOLISM

Protein substitutes are essential in conditions where intakes of natural protein are restricted, in order for the normal requirements for nitrogen and essential amino acids to be met. Errors of metabolism involving essential amino acids (e.g. maple syrup urine disease) are treated by a product that is low in one or more essential amino acid, which must be provided in a prescribed quantity from natural protein foods. Inborn errors of organic acids metabolism, urea cycle disorders and non-essential amino acids require a protein substitute that contains adequate quantities of essential amino acids and appropriate quantities of suitable non-essential amino acids. Products are usually available in powder form and are reconstituted to form a milk substitute for infants or a drink or paste for older children. Manufacturers' instructions on mineral and micronutrient supplementation should be followed carefully.

Condition	Product	Manufacturer
Maple syrup urine disease	MSUD Analog	SHS
	MSUD Maxamaid	SHS
	MSUD Maxamum	SHS
	MSUD Aid	SHS
	MSUD Diet Powder	Mead Johnson
	Ketonex-1	Ross
	Ketonex-2	Ross
Hereditary tyrosinemia	XPT Analog	SHS
	XPT Maxamaid	SHS
	XPT Maxamum	SHS
	XPT Tyrosidon	SHS
	XPTM Analog	SHS
	XPTM Maxamaid	SHS
	XPTM Tyrosidon	SHS
	Tyrex-1	Ross
	Tyrex-2	Ross
Methylmalonic acidemia and proprionic acidemia	XMTVI Analog	SHS
	XMTVI Maxamaid	SHS
	XMTVI Maxamum	SHS
	XMTVI Amino Acid Mix	SHS
	Propimex-1	Ross
	Propimex-2	Ross
	OS 1	Mead Johnson
	OS 2	Mead Johnson
Urea cycle disorders	Dialamine	SHS
	Essential Amino Acid Mix	SHS
	Cyclinex-1	Ross
	Cyclinex-2	Ross
Fatty acid oxidation disorders – LCAD	Monogen	SHS
Histidinemia	Histidon	SHS

Homocystinuria and hypermethioninemia	XMet Analog	SHS
	XMet Maxamaid	SHS
	XMet Maxamum	SHS
	XMet Amino Acid Mix	SHS
	Hominex-1	Ross
	Hominex-2	Ross
Glutaric aciduria Type 1	XLys LowTry Analog	SHS
	XLys LowTry Maxamaid	SHS
	XLys LowTry Maxamum	SHS
	XLys Xtry Amino Acid Mix	SHS
	Glutarex-1	Ross
	Glutarex-2	Ross
Sulfite oxidase deficiency	XMet XCys Analog	SHS
	XMet XCys Maxamaid	SHS
Isovaleric acidemia and disorders of leucine metabolism	XLeu Analog	SHS
	XLeu Maxamaid	SHS
	XLeu Maxamum	SHS
	XLeu Amino Acid Mix	SHS
	I-Valex 1	Ross
	I-Valex 2	Ross
Hyperlysinemia	XLys Analog	SHS
	XLys Maxamaid	SHS
	XLys Amino Acid Mix	SHS

LCAD = long-chain 3-hydroxyacyl CoA dehydrogenase

V.12 MINIMAL-PROTEIN REGIMEN FOR INFANTS TO GIVE 1.5 G PROTEIN PER KG BODY WEIGHT

12 g whey-dominant baby-milk powder per kg body weight
15 g glucose polymer per kg
120 ml fluid per kg

For example, for a 3 kg infant:

	Protein	Energy	
	(g)	(kcal)	(kJ)
36 g whey-dominant powder	4.5	213	891
45 g glucose polymer powder	–	180	752
Water to make up to total volume of 360 ml			
Total:	**4.5**	**393**	**1643**
Total per kg:	**1.5**	**131**	**548**

In addition, a full vitamin supplement and a mineral/trace element supplement containing electrolytes, iron and calcium Appendix II.14 should be given.

V.13 EMERGENCY PROTEIN-FREE REGIMEN FOR INBORN ERRORS OF PROTEIN METABOLISM (PRE-DIAGNOSIS OR DURING INFECTION)

Day 1	10% dextrose saline		
	100 ml/kg actual body weight = 40 kcal/kg (167 kJ/kg)		

Day 2	15% carbohydrate with electrolytes		
			Carbohydrate (g)
	1 sachet Infalyte (p. 364) or 920 ml Pedialyte RTF*		23
	130 g glucose polymer		130
	Water to make total volume of 1000 ml		
		Total:	153
	100 ml/kg = 60 kcal/kg (251 kJ/kg)		
	170 ml/kg = 102 kcal/kg (427 kJ/kg)		

Day 3	20% carbohydrate with electrolytes		
			Carbohydrate (g)
	1 sachet Infalyte or 920 ml Pedialyte RTF*		23
	180 g glucose polymer		180
	Water to make total volume of 1000 ml		
		Total:	203
	Plus 3 Ketovite tablets and 5 ml Ketovite Liquid* or alternative multivitamin supplement (p. 368)		
	100 ml/kg = 80 kcal/kg (335 kJ/kg)		
	130 ml/kg = 104 kcal/kg (435 kJ/kg)		

*If alternative ready-to-feed (RTF) oral rehydration solution is used or alternative powdered preparation, check amount required to provide similar carbohydrate level.

V.14 FORMULAS USED IN RENAL DISEASE

Casilan, Protifar, Vitapro and Maxipro are high in protein and low in sodium and are suitable for inclusion in a high-protein, high-energy, salt-restricted diet. Details of the composition of these powders can be found in the section on protein modules.

Nepro   Abbott/Ross

Nutritionally complete, casein-dominant feed. The carbohydrate source is predominantly corn syrup and the fat source is safflower and canola oils.

Use with caution in children aged 1–5 years. Not suitable for children under 1 year of age. Recommended for tube or oral feeding.

Composition of Nepro (per 100 ml of feed)

Energy		Protein	Carbohydrate	Fat	Sodium	
(kcal)	(kJ)	(g)	(g)	(g)	(mmol)	(mg)
200	837	6.99	21.5	9.6	3.48	83

Potassium		Phosphorus		Osmolality
(mmol)	(mg)	(mmol)	(mg)	mOsm/kg
2.69	106	2.32	72	635

V.15 HIGH-PROTEIN, MODERATE-SODIUM MILK FOR SALT-RESTRICTED DIETS

Recipe for 1000 ml	Protein	Fat	Carbohydrate
	(g)	(g)	(g)
130 g powder, whey-dominant baby milk	15.0	38.0	70.0
30 g Casilan powder*	27.0	Trace	Trace
30 g sugar/glucose	–	–	30.0
40 ml fat emulsion or 20 ml oil	–	20.0	–
Water to make up to 1000 ml			
Total:	42.0	58.0	100.0

Recipe for 1000 ml	Energy		Sodium		Phosphorus	
	(kcal)	(kJ)	(mmol)	(mg)	(mmol)	(mg)
130 g powder, whey-dominant baby milk	650	2721	7.8	179.0	9.0	279.0
30 g Casilan powder*	113	473	Trace	Trace	Trace	Trace
30 g sugar/glucose	120	502	Trace	Trace	Trace	Trace
40 ml fat emulsion or 20 ml oil	180	754	–	–	Trace	Trace
Water to make up to 1000 ml						
Total:	1063	4450	7.8	179.0	9.0	279.0

* US alternatives include:

35 g Promod (Abbott) provides 26 g protein, 164 kcal, 25 mg (1.1 mmol) sodium, and 136 mg (4.39 mmol) phosphorus.

30 g Casec (Mead Johnson) provides 27 g protein, 111 kcal, 36 mg (1.6 mmol) sodium, and 240 mg (7.74 mmol) phosphorus.

The protein in the milk can be increased to a total of 60 g/l, provided that enough extra non-protein energy is supplied in the form of, for example, high-energy drinks.

appendix VI

DIETS USED FOR MODIFICATION OF ENERGY OR CARBOHYDRATE INTAKE

VI.1 ADVICE FOR REDUCING DIETS

Choose meals from these foods:

Lean meat
Poultry
Fish
Eggs
Cheese

Vegetables: all varieties of green and root vegetables and salads

Fruit: all varieties of fresh fruit or fruit canned in natural juice

Drinks:
Low-calorie squash/cordial and cola
Unsweetened fruit juice
Tea and coffee, without sugar
Unthickened soups

Cereals: include one portion from exchange list at each meal

Seasonings, herbs, spices and artificial sweeteners if desired

Allowances:
0.5–1 pint (284–568 ml) low-fat milk daily
240 g butter or margarine weekly

Useful isocaloric exchanges (70 kcal or 293 kJ):
1 slice bread (preferably wholemeal)
or 1 tablespoon boiled rice
or 3 tablespoons unsweetened breakfast cereal
or 1 potato (not fried)
or 2 crispbreads
or 4 tablespoons cooked porridge

Foods to avoid:

Sugar	Fizzy drinks e.g. cola
Sweets/candy	Cakes, pastries
Chocolate	Pies
Glucose	Sweet biscuits, cookies
Honey	Cream
Syrup	Fried foods
Treacle	Potato-crisps
Jam/jelly	Proprietary slimming foods except sugar
Marmalade	free low energy drinks
Sorbitol	
Fruit squash, cordials	

VI.2 LOW-CARBOHYDRATE, LOW-ENERGY FOODS – DIABETES UK

Vegetables

Group A – negligible energy or carbohydrate, 1–3 g fiber per small portion.
Allowed freely:

Asparagus

Brussels sprouts

Cauliflower

Celery

Cucumber

French, runner or snap beans

Green leafy vegetables and salads

Mushrooms

Peppers

Radish

Tomato

Group B – contain approx. 5 g carbohydrate, 45 kcal (188 kJ), 3–5 g fiber per small portion.
May be allowed freely:

Beetroot

Carrots

Onions

Peas

Squash – winter and summer

Turnip

Fruits – contain approx. 5 g carbohydrate, 45 kcal (188 kJ), 2–6 g fiber per small portion.
May be allowed freely:

Berry fruits

Blackcurrants

Cranberries

Grapefruit

Lemon

Rhubarb

Watermelon

Other foods – negligible content.
Allowed freely:

Artificial sweeteners: Saccharin, Aspartame (NutraSweet)

Coffee, tea

Gelatin

Herbs, spices, seasonings

Sugar-free, low-energy drinks

Stock or bouillon cubes

Vinegar

VI.3 LOW-CARBOHYDRATE FOODS CONTAINING ENERGY – DIABETES UK

Animal foods

Allowed in moderation by Diabetes UK, not measured as exchanges.

Measured as meat exchanges by the American Diabetic Association. One meat exchange contains 75 kcal (314 kJ), 7 g protein, 5 g fat.

Fatty foods

Allowed in small quantities by Diabetes UK, not measured as exchanges.

Measured as fat exchanges by the American Diabetic Association. One fat exchange contains 45 kcal (188 kJ), 5 g fat, no protein.

VI.4 CARBOHYDRATE EXCHANGES – DIABETES UK

CHO Exc = 10 g CHO, ~ 50 kcal (210 kJ) and 1.5 g protein

Food	Quantity	Approx. weight of food containing 10 g CHO (g)
Bread		
White	½ large thin slice	20
Wholemeal	1 small medium cut slice	25
Chapatti	1 small	20
Biscuits		
Plain or semi-sweet	2	15
Digestive	1	15
Crackers (plain)	2	15
Crispbread	2	15
Breakfast Cereals		
All-bran	5 tbsp	20
Branflakes	5 tbsp	20
Cornflakes	5 tbsp	10
Muesli	2 tbsp	15
Puffed Wheat	15 tbsp	15
Rice Krispies	6 tbsp	10
Shredded Wheat	⅔ of 1	10
Special K	8 tbsp	15
Weetabix	1	15
Porridge	4 tbsp	120
Flour and Grains		
Flour – white	1 tbsp	10
Flour – wholemeal	1½ tbsp	15
Rice – cooked	1 heaped	30
Pasta – cooked	2 tbsp	30

Food	Quantity	Approx. weight of food containing 10 g CHO (g)
Beans		
Baked beans and cooked beans	3 tbsp	70
Lentils – dhal	2 tbsp	60
Vegetables		
Parsnip – cooked	1 small/1 ½ tbsp	70
Potato:		
cooked	1 small	50
chips	4 large	25
crisps	1 small packet	25
mashed	1 small scoop	50
roast	½ medium	40
Sweetcorn	5 tbsp	60

Diabetes UK no longer publishes lists of carbohydrate exchanges and they are rarely used in the UK.

Milk

CHO Exc = 10 g CHO, ~ 170 kcal (710 kJ)

	1 exchange (g)	Measurement
Milk, liquid, whole	200	7 fl oz
Dried whole milk powder	25	1 heaped tablespoon
Dried skimmed milk powder*	20	1 rounded tablespoon
Evaporated milk	80	4 tablespoons
Ice cream	90	2 tablespoons or scoops
Plain yogurt, unsweetened	150	1 (5oz) tub
Fruit flavored yogurt, sweetened	60	1/2 (5oz) tub
'Diet' yogurts	150	1 (5oz) tub

*Low in fat: less than 1 g fat/10 g carbohydrate exchange.

Fruits

One exchange = 40 kcal (167 kJ), 10 g CHO

	Approx. weight of food containing 10 g CHO (g)	Measurement
Apple	110	1 medium
Apricot: Fresh	160	3 medium
Dried	25	4 small
Banana (no skin)	50	1/2 medium
Blackberries	150	10
Cherries	100	12
Dates, fresh	50	3 medium
Figs, fresh	100	1
Grapes	75	10 large
Mango	100	1/2 medium
Melon	300	1 slice
Nectarine	90	1
Orange	150	1 large
Papaya	70	1/3 medium
Peach	125	1 large
Pear	130	1 large
Plum	110	2 large
Pineapple	90	1 thick slice
Raisins, sultanas, etc.	15	2 tablespoons
Raspberries	175	12 tablespoons
Strawberries	160	15 medium
Tangerine	175	2 large
Unsweetened fruit juice	100	3 1/2 oz

VI.5 EXCHANGE LISTS FOR MEAL PLANNING – US

Nutrient content of exchanges

Groups/Lists	Carbohydrate (g)	Protein (g)	Fat (g)	Calories
Carbohydrate Group				
Starch	15	3	1 or less	80
Fruit	15	–	–	60
Skimmed milk	12	8	0–3	90
Low-fat milk	12	8	5	120
Whole milk	12	8	8	150
Other carbohydrates	15	varies	varies	varies
Vegetables	5	2	–	25
Meat and Meat Substitute Group				
Very lean	–	7	0–1	35
Lean	–	7	3	55
Medium-fat	–	7	5	75
High-fat	–	7	8	100
Fat Group	–	–	5	45

Reprinted with permission from Exchange Lists for Meal Planning. Chicago Il1: American Diabetes Association and The American Dietetic Association; 1995.

Starch List	
Bread (white or whole wheat)	1 slice (1 oz)
Hot dog or hamburger bun	½ (1 oz)
Rice	⅓ cup
Pasta	½ cup
Cereals (cooked, bran, sugar-frosted)	½ cup
Starchy vegetables (corn, peas)	½ cup
Saltines	6
Popcorn (popped, no fat added)	3 cups
Animal crackers	8
Fruit List	
Apple or banana (small)	1 (4 oz)
Juice (apple, orange)	½ cup
Canned fruit (peaches, pears)	½ cup
Grapes	17 (3 oz)
Raisins	2 tbsp
Milk List	
Nonfat, low-fat, reduced-fat, whole	1 cup (8 oz)
Nonfat or low-fat fruit-flavored yogurt sweetened with a nonnutritive sweetener	1 cup (8 oz)
Vegetable List	
Broccoli	½ cup
Green beans	cooked or
Carrots	1 cup raw
Spinach	
Free Foods List	
Cream cheese (fat-free)	1 tbsp
Mayonnaise (fat-free)	1 tbsp
Syrup (sugar-free)	1 tbsp
Condiments	1 tbsp
Sugar substitutes	
Seasonings	
Diet soft drinks	
Gelatin dessert (sugar-free)	
Salsa	¼ cup

Meat and Meat Substitutes List

Very lean:		Lean:	
Poultry (white meat, no skin)	1 oz	Beef (round, sirloin, chuck)	1 oz
Fish (cod, flounder, tuna in water)	1 oz	Pork (ham, Canadian bacon)	1 oz
Cheese (1 g fat or less)	1 oz	Poultry (dark meat, no skin)	1 oz
Egg whites	2	Cheese (3 g fat or less)	1 oz
Hot dog (1 g fat or less)	1 oz	Lunch meat (3 g fat or less)	1 oz
Medium:		**High-fat:**	
Beef (ground beef, Prime)	1 oz	Cheese (American, cheddar)	1 oz
Poultry (with the skin)	1 oz	Bacon	3 strips
Fish (fried)	1 oz	Lunch meat (8 g fat)	1 oz
Cheese (5 g fat or less)	1 oz	Peanut butter	2 tbsp
Egg	1		

Fat List

Monounsaturated:			
Oil (canola, olive, peanut)	1 tsp		
Peanut butter	2 tsp		
Polyunsaturated:			
Margarine	1 tsp	low-fat	1 tbsp
Mayonnaise (regular)	1 tsp	reduced-fat	1 tbsp
Oil (corn, safflower)	1 tsp		
Salad dressing (regular)	1 tbsp	reduced-fat	2 tbsp
Saturated:			
Sour cream (regular)	2 tbsp	reduced-fat	3 tbsp
Bacon	1 slice		
Butter	1 tsp		
Cream cheese (regular)	1 tbsp	reduced-fat	2 tbsp

Other Carbohydrates List

1 carbohydrate:		1 carbohydrate, 1 fat:	
Gingersnaps	3	Brownie, small, unfrosted	2 in square
Gelatin, regular	1/2 cup	Sandwich cookie with creme filling	2 small
Fruit juice bars, frozen, 100 % juice	1 bar (3 oz)	Granola bar	1 bar
Cookie, fat free	2 small	Ice cream, light	1/2 cup
Ice cream, fat free, no sugar added	1/2 cup	Vanilla wafers	5
Pudding, sugar free, reduced-fat milk	1/2 cup		

*Partial listing; shows amounts to equal one exchange.
Reprinted with permission from Exchange Lists for Meal Planning, I11: American Diabetes Association and The American Dietetic Association; 1995.

VI.6 THE FOOD GUIDE PYRAMID

The food guide pyramid provides the basis for healthy eating guidelines as recommended for the population of the United States of America. It can be used as a guide for healthy food choices for weight management, with the emphasis being to encourage children and adolescents to eat more fruits, vegetables and cereal foods, and reduce intake of high-fat foods. The food guide pyramid for young children also emphasizes the importance of exercise. Further information can be obtained from the website USDA (United States Department for Agriculture) (http://www.nal.usda.gov/fnic/Fpyr/pyramid.html).

appendix VII

NAMES AND ADDRESSES OF SELECTED MANUFACTURERS AND AVAILABILITY OF THEIR PRODUCTS

Not every product manufactured by a company is available in all areas indicated below. There are likely to be formulation differences between products of the same name marketed in different countries; in addition, the size of scoops supplied with some milk substitutes may differ from country to country. It is important to read the manufacturer's instructions for each product prior to use.

Address of Manufacturer	Availability of product
Abbott International 625 Cleveland Avenue Columbus OH 43215-1724 USA	Africa, Asia, Australia, Canada, Caribbean, Europe, Far East, Middle East, New Zealand, S. Africa, S. America, USA
Abbott Laboratories Ltd Norden Road Maidenhead Berkshire SL6 4XE UK	UK
Allen & Hanbury Ltd Stockley Park West Uxbridge Middlesex UB11 1BT UK	UK
Alliance Pharmaceuticals Ltd Avonbridge House Bath Road Chippenham Wiltshire SN15 2BB UK	UK

AstraZeneca Kings Court Water Lane Wilmslow Cheshire SK9 5AZ UK	Australia, Canada, Europe, UK
Beecham Products See SmithKline Beecham	
Bencard See SmithKline Beecham	
Biosearch Medical Products Inc 35A Industrial Parkway Somerville NJ 08876 USA	Canada, USA
The Boots Company plc 1 Thane Road Nottingham NG2 3AA UK	UK
Bristol-Myers Squibb Pharmaceuticals See Mead Johnson	
Carnation Co Nutritional Products Division 5045 Wilshire Blvd Los Angeles CA 90036 USA	USA
Ciba See Novartis Pharmaceuticals	
Cow & Gate Nutricia Ltd White Horse Business Park Trowbridge Wiltshire BA14 0XQ UK	Australia, Europe, Middle East, UK

Dr Schar
PO Box 126
Worcester
WR5 2ZN
UK

Canada, Europe, USA, UK

Evans
See Medeva Pharmaceuticals Ltd

Farley
See Heinz

Fisons plc
Pharmaceutical Division
Coleorton Hall
Ashby Road
Coleorton
Coalville
Leicestershire
LE67 8GP
UK

Australia, Canada, Europe, S. Africa,
USA, UK

Fresenius Kabi Ltd
Hampton Court
Manor Park
Runcorn
Cheshire
WA7 1UF
UK

Australia, Europe, Middle East, S. Africa,
UK

Friesland Nutrition
PO Box 226
8901 MA
Leeuwarden
Pieter Stuyvesantweg 1
The Netherlands

Africa, Asia, Europe, Far East, Middle East

Geistlich Sons Ltd
Newton Bank
Long Lane
Chester
CH2 3QZ
UK

UK

General Dietary Ltd
PO Box 38
Kingston upon Thames
Surrey
KT2 7YP
UK

Canada, UK, USA

Gerber Products Co
445 State Street
Freemont
MI 49412
USA

Europe, USA

Gluten Free Foods Ltd
Unit 10 Honeypot Business Park
Parr Road
Stanmore
Middlesex
HA7 1NL
UK

Canada, UK, USA

Goldshield Pharmaceuticals Ltd
NLA Tower
12–16 Addiscombe Road
Croydon
Surrey
CR9 6BP
UK

UK

Heinz H J Co Ltd
Hayes Park
Hayes
Middlesex
UB4 8AL
UK

UK

HK Pharma
PO Box 105
Hitchin
Herts
SG5 2GG
UK

UK

Larkhall Natural Health   UK
PO Box 99
Trowbridge
Wiltshire
BA4 0YN
UK

Lifestyle Healthcare Ltd   UK, USA
Centenary Business Park
Henley-on-Thames
Oxon
RG9 1DS
UK

Link Pharmaceuticals Ltd   UK
7/8 Sterling Buildings
Carfax
Horsham
Surrey
West Sussex
RH12 1DR
UK

Mead Johnson International   Africa, Asia, Australia, Far East, Middle
Evansville   East, New Zealand, S. America, S. Africa,
IN 47708   USA
USA

Mead Johnson Nutritionals   UK
Division of Bristol-Myers Squibb
Pharmaceuticals Ltd
141–149 Staines Road
Hounslow
Middlesex
TW3 3JA
UK

Medeva Pharma Ltd   UK
Medeva House
Regent Park
Kingston Road
Leatherhead
Surrey
KT22 7PQ
UK

Merck Pharmaceuticals Harrier House High Street Yiewsley West Drayton Middlesex UB7 7QG UK	Asia, Europe, Far East, UK
Milupa Ltd White Horse Business Park Trowbridge Wilts BA14 0XQ UK	UK
Milupa GmbH & Co 61379 Friedrichsdorf West Germany	Australia, Canada, Europe, Middle East
Napp Pharmaceuticals Cambridge Science Park Milton Road Cambridge CB4 4GW UK	Australia, UK
Nestlé UK Ltd St. George's House Croydon Surrey CR9 1NR UK	Australia, Europe, UK
Novartis Pharmaceuticals UK Ltd Frimley Business Park Frimley Camberley Surrey GU16 5SG UK	UK

Nutricia Healthcare PO Box 1 2700 MA Zoetermeer The Netherlands	UK, Ireland, Europe, Middle East, South Africa, Brazil, Australia, New Zealand
Nutrition Point Ltd Murlain House Union Street Chester Cheshire CH1 1QP UK	UK
Paines & Byrne See Yamanouchi	
Parke-Davis Research Laboratories Lambert Court Chestnut Avenue Eastleigh Hants SO5 3ZQ UK	UK
Reckitt & Colman Products Ltd Dansom Lane Hull N. Humberside HU8 7DS UK	UK
Ross See Abbott Laboratories Ltd	
Sandoz Nutrition 5320 West 23rd Street Minneapolis Minnesota 55416 USA	USA
Scientific Hospital Supplies International Ltd 100 Wavertree Boulevard Liverpool L7 9PT UK	Australia, Europe, New Zealand, USA, UK

Searle
Lane End Road
High Wycombe
Bucks
HP12 4HL
UK

Africa, Asia, Caribbean, Middle East,
S. Africa, S. America, UK

SMA Nutrition
Huntercombe Lane South
Taplow
Maidenhead
Berks
SL6 0PH
UK

UK

SmithKline Beecham Pharmaceuticals
Mundells
Welwyn Garden City
Herts
AL7 1EY
UK

Africa, Asia, Australia, Far East, Middle
East, New Zealand, S. America, S. Africa,
USA, UK

Sutherland Health Ltd
Unit 5 Rivermead
Pipers Way
Thatcham
Berkshire
RG13 4TP
UK

UK

UCB (Pharma) Ltd
Star House
69 Clarendon Road
Watford
Herts
WD1 1DJ
UK

UK

Ultrapharm Ltd
Centenary Business Park
Henley-on-Thames
Oxon
RG9 1DS
UK

UK

Vitaflo Ltd 11 Summers Road Century Building Brunswick Business Park Liverpool L3 4BL UK	UK
Wallace Manufacturing Chemists Ltd Randles Road Knowsley Industrial Park Merseyside L34 9HX UK	UK
Wyeth Laboratories Huntercombe Lane South Maidenhead Berks SL6 0PH UK	Australia, Canada, Far East, Middle East, S. Africa, S. America, USA
Wyeth Pharmaceuticals (SMA) 50 Arcola Road Collegeville PA 19426 USA	USA
Yamanouchi Pharma Ltd Yamanouchi House Pyford Road West Byfleet Surrey KT14 6RA UK	UK

index